A MANUAL OF
NEONATAL INTENSIVE CARE

A MANUAL OF
NEONATAL INTENSIVE CARE

FOURTH EDITION

Janet M Rennie MA MD FRCP FRCPCH DCH
Consultant and Senior Lecturer in Neonatal Medicine,
King's College Hospital, London, UK

and

NRC Roberton MA MB FRCP FRCPCH
Formerly Consultant Paediatrician and Neonatologist,
Rosie Maternity Hospital, Cambridge and Fellow,
Fitzwilliam College, Cambridge, UK

A member of the Hodder Headline Group
LONDON NEW YORK NEW DELHI

First published in Great Britain in 2002 by
Arnold, a member of the Hodder Headline Group,
338 Euston Road, London NW1 3BH

http://www.arnoldpublishers.com

Distributed in the USA by
Oxford University Press Inc.
198 Madison Avenue, New York, NY10016
Oxford is a registered trademark of Oxford University Press

British Library Cataloguing in Publication Data
A catalogue record for this book is available from the British Library

Library of Congress Cataloging-in-Publication Data
A catalog record for this book is available from the Library of Congress

ISBN 0 340 72010 7
ISBN 0 340 76343 4 (International Students' Edition)

1 2 3 4 5 6 7 8 9 10

Typeset in 9/11pt New Baskerville by
Cambrian Typesetters, Frimley, Surrey
Printed and bound in Italy by Giunti

What do you think about this book? Or any other Arnold title?
Please send your comments to feedback.arnold@hodder.co.uk

CONTENTS

CONTRIBUTOR

___

Vanessa Wright MB BS LRCP FRCS
Consultant Paediatric Surgeon,
Queen Elizabeth Hospital for Children,
London UK

PREFACE

Our aim in this manual is to provide a guide for the management of the acute medical and surgical problems a resident is likely to encounter on a modern neonatal intensive care unit. This will of course include certain aspects of neonatal care which apply to both asymptomatic and ill low birth weight infants, but the emphasis will always be on those aspects which are particularly germane to the care of sick infants. It is not the purpose of this book to describe the basic principles of the medical and nursing care of healthy premature or mature newborn infants. These are dealt with in detail in the companion volume (Roberton, N.R.C. (1996) *Manual of Normal Neonatal Care* 2nd Edition, Arnold, London). All the chapters have been revised, and much new material added, to reflect changes in neonatal practice since the third edition was written in 1993. We have maintained the emphasis on practical common sense advice with background reasoning and physiology. We have referred to the baby throughout as "he" for simplicity.

JMR
NRCR
London and Skye,
2001

ACKNOWLEDGEMENTS

Dr Ian Huggen
Fetal and Paediatric Cardiologist,
King's College Hospital,
London UK

ABBREVIATIONS

A

A-aDO$_2$	Alveolar–arterial oxygen difference (of PaO$_2$)
AAP	American Academy of Pediatrics
ACE	Angiotensin converting enzyme
AD	Autosomal dominant
ADH	Antidiuretic hormone
ANP	Atrial natriuretic peptide
APTT	Activated partial thromboplastin time
AR	Autosomal recessive
ARF	Acute renal failure
ASD	Atrial septal defect
ATN	Acute tubular necrosis
AV	Atrioventricular

B

BAPM	British Association of Perinatal Medicine formerly BAPP – British Association of Perinatal Paediatrics
BCG	Bacille Calmette-Guérin
BP	Blood pressure
BPD	Bronchopulmonary dysplasia Biparietal diameter
BW	Birth weight

C

CAH	Congenital adrenal hyperplasia
CBF	Cerebral blood flow
CCAM	Congenital cystic adenomatoid malformation
CDH	Congenital diaphragmatic hernia
CHD	Congenital heart disease
C$_L$	Lung compliance
CLD	Chronic lung disease

CMV	Cytomegalovirus
CNS	Central nervous system
CONS	Coagulase negative staphylococci
CPAP	Continuous positive airways pressure
CPD – A	Citrate phosphate dextrose – adenine
CPIP	Chronic pulmonary insufficiency of prematurity
CRIB	Clinical risk index for babies
CRP	C-reactive protein
CSF	Cerebrospinal fluid
CT	Computerized tomography
CTG	Cardiotocogram (cardiotocography)
CVP	Central venous pressure
CXR	Chest X-ray

D

DA	Ductus arteriosus
DBM	Drip/donor breast milk
DC	Direct current
DCT	Direct Coombs' test
DDH	Developmental dysplasia of the hip
DDI	didanosine
DHT	Dihydrotestosterone
DIC	Disseminated intravascular coagulation
DL_{CO}	Diffusion capacity for carbon monoxide
DMSA	Dimercaptosuccinic acid
DNA	Deoxyribonucleic acid
2,3 DPG	2,3 Diphosphoglycerate
DPL	Dipalmitoyl lecithin
DPPC	Dipalmitoyl phosphatidyl choline
DQ	Development quotient
DTPA	Diethylenetriaminepentacetic acid

E

EBM	Expressed breast milk
ECF	Extracellular fluid
ECG	Electrocardiogram
ECM	External cardiac massage
ECMO	Extracorporeal membrane oxygenation
EEG	Electroencephalogram
ELBW	Extremely low birth weight (<1.0 kg birth weight)

EMLA	Eutectic mixture of local anaesthetic
EPO	Erythropoietin
ET	Exchange transfusion
ETA	Estimated time of arrival
ETT	Endotracheal tube

F

FBC	Full blood count
FDP	Fibrin degradation products
FFP	Fresh frozen plasma
FG	French gauge
F_ICO_2	Fractional inspired CO_2 concentration
F_IO_2	Fractional inspired oxygen concentration
FISH	Fluorescent *in situ* hybridization
FRC	Functional residual capacity

G

GA	Gestational age
GABA	Gamma-aminobutyric acid
GBS	Group B beta haemolytic streptococcus
GFR	Glomerular filtration rate
GIT	Gastrointestinal tract
GMH-IVH	Germinal matrix-intraventricular haemorrhage
GOR	Gastro-oesophageal reflux
GP	General Practitioner
G6PD	Glucose-6-phosphate dehydrogenase

H

HCG	Human chorionic gonadotrophin
HDN	Haemolytic disease of the newborn
	Haemorrhagic disease of the newborn (better termed VKDB)
HFO(V)	High frequency oscillatory (ventilation)
HIE	Hypoxic ischaemic encephalopathy
HIV	Human immunodeficiency virus
HMD	Hyaline membrane disease
HPA	Human platelet antigen
HTLV	Human T-cell lymphotropic virus
HVS	High vaginal swab
Hz	Hertz (cycles/second)

I

ICF	Intracellular fluid

ICP	Intracranial pressure
IDM	Infant of diabetic mother
I:E	Inspiratory:expiratory ratio
IEM	Inborn error of metabolism
IgA, D, G, and M	Immunoglobulins A, D, G and M
IM	Intramuscular
IMV	Intermittent mandatory ventilation
INAH	Isonicotinic acid hydrazide (Isoniazid)
INR	International normalized ratio
IPL	Intraparenchymal lesion
IPPV	Intermittent positive pressure ventilation
IQ	Intelligence quotient
ITP	Idiopathic thrombocytopenic purpura
IUCD	Intra-uterine contraceptive device
IUGR	Intra-uterine growth retardation/restriction
IV	Intravenous
IVC	Inferior vena cava
IVH	Intraventricular haemorrhage
IVIG	Intravenous immunoglobulin
IVU	Intravenous urogram

K

kPa	kiloPascal (= 7.6 mmHg)

L

LBW	Low birth weight (<2.50 kg)
LCPUFA	Long chain polyunsaturated fatty acids
LP	Lumbar puncture
L:S	Lecithin:sphingomyelin (ratio)
LV	Left ventricle

M

MAG 3	Mercaptoacetyl triglycine
MAP	Mean airway pressure
MAPCA	Major aorto – pulmonary communicating arteries
MAS	Meconium aspiration syndrome
MCAD	Medium chain acyl-CoA dehydrogenase
MCH	Mean corpuscular haemoglobin
MCHC	Mean corpuscular haemoglobin concentration
MCT	Medium chain triglycerides

MCU	Micturating cysto-urethrogram
MCV	Mean corpuscular volume
MMC	Meningomyelocele
mm Hg	Millimetres of mercury
MMR	Mumps, measles and rubella (vaccine)
MRC	Medical Research Council
MR(I)	Magnetic resonance (imaging)
MRSA	Methicillin resistant *Staphylococcus aureus*
ms	millisecond
mV	milliVolt

N

NAITP	Neonatal alloimmune thrombocytopenic purpura
NEC	Necrotising enterocolitis
NG	Nasogastric
NICU	Neonatal intensive care unit
NMDA	N-methyl-d-aspartate
NND	Neonatal death
NNM	Neonatal mortality
NNU	Neonatal unit
NO	Nitric oxide
NO_2	Nitrogen dioxide

O

OFC	Occipitofrontal circumference
17-OHP	17-hydroxyprogesterone
OI	Oxygenation index

P

P_{50}	Partial pressure at which the haemoglobin molecule is 50% oxygen saturated
PA	Pulmonary artery
$PaCO_2$	Partial pressure of CO in arterial blood
$PACO_2$	Partial pressure of CO_2 in alveolar gas
PaO_2	Partial pressure of oxygen in arterial blood
PAO_2	Partial pressure of oxygen in alveolar gas
PCKD	Polycystic kidney disease
PCR	Polymerase chain reaction
PCV	Packed cell volume
PD	Peritoneal dialysis
PDA	Patent ductus arteriosus

PEEP	Positive end expiratory pressure
PET	Pre-eclamptic toxaemia
PG	Phosphatidylglycerol
pH	Hydrogen ion concentration
PHLS	Public Health Laboratory Service
PHVD	Post haemorrhagic ventricular dilatation
PIE	Pulmonary interstitial emphysema
PIP	Peak inflating pressure
PKU	Phenylketonuria
PPD	Purified protein derivative (for Mantoux test)
PPHN	Persistent pulmonary hypertension of the newborn
PPROM	Preterm premature rupture of the membranes
PROM	Prolonged rupture of the membranes
PSV	Patient support ventilation
PT	Prothrombin time
PTT	Partial thromboplastin time
PTV	Patient triggered ventilation
PUJ	Pelvi-ureteric junction
PVH	Periventricular haemorrhage
PVL	Periventricular leukomalacia

Q

Q_c	Pulmonary capillary blood flow

R

R_{AW}	Airways resistance
RA	Right atrium
RBC	Red blood cell
RCOpth	Royal College of Ophthalmologists
RCT	Randomized controlled trial
RDS	Respiratory distress syndrome
RIP	Respiratory inductive plethysmography
R_L	Total pulmonary resistance
RNA	Ribonucleic acid
ROP	Retinopathy of prematurity
RSV	Respiratory syncytial virus
RTA	Renal tubular acidosis
RV	Right ventricle

S

SAG-M	Sodium chloride, adenine, glucose-mannitol (blood preservative)
SAH	Subarachnoid haemorrhage
SaO_2	true oxygen saturation (measured with a co-oximeter on arterial blood)
SFD	Small-for-dates
SG_{AW}	Specific airways conductance
SGA	Small for gestational age
SHO	Senior House Officer
SIADH	Syndrome of inappropriate ADH secretion
SIMV	Synchronous intermittent mandatory ventilation
SLE	Systemic lupus erythematosus
SpO_2	transcutaneous oxygen saturation (measured with pulse oximeter)
SVC	Superior vena cava
SVT	Supraventricular tachycardia

T

T_3, T_4	Tri-iodothyronine, Thyroxine
TAPVD	Total anomalous pulmonary venous drainage
TAR	Thrombocytopenia and absent radius syndrome
TCT	Thrombin clotting time
$TcPCO_2$	Transcutaneous PCO_2
$TcPO_2$	Transcutaneous PO_2
T_E	Expiratory time
TGV	Thoracic gas volume
THAM	Tris-hydroxymethyl-aminomethane
Ti	Inspiratory time
TOF	Tracheo-oesophageal fistula
TORCH	Toxoplasma, rubella, cytomegalovirus, herpes
tPA	Tissue plasminogen activator
TPN	Total parenteral nutrition
TPR	Temperature, pulse and respiration rate
TRH	Thyrotrophin releasing hormone
TT	Thrombin time
TTN	Transient tachypnoea of the newborn

U

UAC	Umbilical artery catheter

UK	United Kingdom
URTI	Upper respiratory tract infection
UTI	Urinary tract infection
UV	Umbilical vein
UVC	Umbilical venous catheter

V

$\dot{V}_A$	Alveolar capacity
V_C	Vital capacity
V_D	Dead space
$\dot{V}_E$	Minute volume
V_T	Tidal volume
v.i.	*Vide infra* (see below in text)
VKDB	Vitamin K deficiency bleeding
VLBW(I)	Very low birth weight (infants) (<1.5 kg)
VMA	Vanillyl mandelic acid
VP	Ventriculoperitoneal (shunt)
V/Q	Ventilation/perfusion ratio
v.s.	*Vide supra* (see above in text)
VSD	Ventricular septal defect
VT	Ventricular tachycardia
VUJ	Vesico-ureteric junction
VUR	Vesico-ureteric reflux
VWF	von Willebrand factor

W

| WBC | White blood cell (count) |
| WPW | Wolff-Parkinson-White (syndrome) |

Z

| ZIG | Zoster immune globulin |

1

ORGANIZATION OF NEONATAL CARE

- *Do not admit babies to neonatal units without a good reason; unnecessary admissions include babies of diabetic mothers, babies delivered by instrumental means.*
- *Postnatal transfer of a sick baby is preferable to leaving him in a unit which is not staffed or equipped to manage him.*
- *Allow parents, grandparents and siblings free access to their baby at all times, and keep them informed of progress.*

ORGANIZATION OF NEONATAL CARE; DEFINITION OF LEVELS OF CARE

More than half a million babies are born every year in the UK; less than 1% of these babies will die. At least half the deaths occur in very premature babies with a birth weight less than 1.5 kg. About 10% of all babies are admitted to UK neonatal units, with a wide range between hospitals from 4 to 35% (Audit Commission 1992). Most of these admissions are for "special care"; for example jaundice requiring phototherapy or blood glucose monitoring. Maternity units, which provide "transitional care", usually on postnatal wards staffed with midwives with experience and expertise in the care of the well small baby, have reduced admissions to their special care nurseries to 5%. About 2% of babies need full intensive care, mainly because they are born very prematurely and need artificial ventilation for respiratory distress syndrome. The definitions of levels of care are given in Table 1.1.

For intensive care the BAPM and the Neonatal Nurses Association recommend a nurse:cot ratio of at least 5:1 to cover each 24 hour period, and for high dependency care a ratio of 3:1. For babies requiring less continuous therapy or observation in special care baby units, a nurse:cot ratio of 1.25:1 to cover each 24 hour period is required.

Table 1.1 Categories of babies requiring neonatal care (BAPM 1992)

Level 1 Intensive Care (Maximal Intensive Care)

Care given in an intensive care nursery which provides continuous skilled supervision by qualified and specially trained nursing and medical staff.

Level 1 intensive care includes babies:

(1) receiving assisted ventilation (including CPAP) and in the first 24 hours following withdrawal.

(2) <27 weeks gestation for the first 48 hours post delivery.

(3) <1000 gms for the first 48 hours post delivery.

(4) requiring major surgery, for the preoperative period and post operatively for 48 hours.

(5) on the day of death.

(6) during transport by a team including medical and nursing staff.

(7) receiving peritoneal dialysis.

(8) requiring exchange transfusion complicated by other disease process.

(9) with severe respiratory disease in the first 48 hours of life requiring F_IO_2 >0.6.

(10) who have recurrent apnoea needing frequent intervention, e.g. over five stimulations in 8 hours or resuscitation with IPPV two or more times in 24 hours.

(11) who have a significant requirement for circulatory support, e.g. inotropes, 3 or more transfusions of colloid in 24 hours, infusions of prostaglandins.

Level 2 Intensive Care (High Dependency Intensive Care)

Care given in an intensive care nursery which provides continuous skilled supervision by qualified and specially trained nursing staff who may care for more babies than in Level 1 care. Medical supervision is not so immediate as in Level 1 care.

Level 2 intensive care includes babies:

(1) requiring parenteral nutrition.

(2) who are having convulsions.

(3) being transported by a trained skilled neonatal nurse alone.

(4) with arterial line or chest drain.

(5) with respiratory disease in the first 48 hours of life requiring F_IO_2 0.4–0.6.

(6) with recurrent apnoea requiring stimulation up to 5 times in an 8 hour period or any resuscitation with IPPV.

(7) who require an exchange transfusion alone.

(8) more than 48 hours post-operation and require complex nursing procedures.

(9) with tracheostomy for the first two weeks.

Special Care

Care given in a special care nursery, transitional care ward, or postnatal ward which provides care and treatment exceeding normal routine care. Some aspects of special care may be undertaken by a mother supervised by qualified nursing staff.

Special care should be provided for these babies:

(1) those requiring continuous monitoring of respiration of heart rate or by transcutaneous transducers.

(2) receiving additional oxygen.

(3) with tracheostomy after the first 2 weeks.
(4) being given intravenous glucose and electrolyte solutions.
(5) who are being tube fed.
(6) who have had minor surgery in the previous 24 hours.
(7) who require terminal care but not on the day of death.
(8) being barrier nursed.
(9) undergoing phototherapy.
(10) receiving special monitoring (for example frequent glucose or bilirubin estimations).
(11) needing constant supervision (for example babies whose mothers are drug addicts).
(12) being treated with antibiotics.

Normal Care
Care given by the mother or mother substitute with medical or nursing advice if needed

For the purpose of this book we will refer to all units as neonatal units rather than intensive care or special care units, and readers will no doubt have a clear – if not altogether unbiased – opinion of what level of care their own units provide.

PROVISION OF INTENSIVE CARE FACILITIES

UK neonatal units have evolved into a three-tier structure, similar to the structure in the USA and Australia:

- Level 1: Hospitals providing only special care and emergency resuscitation. Babies requiring any intensive care support are transferred out;
- Level 2: Hospitals capable of providing short-term intensive care, for example ventilation for RDS in a baby of 30 weeks likely to require ventilation for a few days. More complex cases, very tiny babies, surgical and cardiac cases transferred out;
- Level 3: Hospitals providing the full range of intensive care techniques. The London review group have classified hospitals providing neonatal surgical services in addition as level 3S.

The BAPM (1996) recommend 1–1.5 intensive care cots per 1000 births, and suggest that prolonged intensive care (level 3 care) should only be undertaken by those units providing more than 500 days of intensive care per year.

Although a three-tier system has much to commend it, and similar systems have evolved in other specialties which are "high-cost low-volume" it does require an organized transport structure, which does not exist at present in the UK. There are disadvantages in

Table 1.2 Conditions for which *in utero* transfer to a level 3 neonatal unit should be considered

Gestation	Less than 28 weeks
Estimated fetal weight	Less than 1.25 kg
Multiple pregnancy	Less than 32 weeks
Fetal disease	e.g. rhesus isoimmunization, hydrops
Congenital malformation likely to require treatment	e.g. congenital heart disease, diaphragmatic hernia, duodenal atresia

transferring small, sick babies long distances after delivery although careful management during transfer (see Appendix E) can reduce the risks. Peaks in demand and lack of resource mean that postnatal transport will never be entirely avoided. The alternative is *in utero* transport, which has its own drawbacks. One is that the mother may need to remain undelivered in the accepting institution for several weeks. Indications for *in utero* transfer are given in Table 1.2. *In utero* transfer should always be discussed with a consultant; contra-indications include mothers with advanced pre-eclampsia, mothers with antepartum haemorrhage, and mothers in advanced labour. Embarking on a long ambulance journey in these situations risks the health of both the mother and her child.

CRITERIA FOR ADMISSION TO AND DISCHARGE FROM NNUS

Too many babies are admitted to NNUs when their mothers could look after them just as well, if not better, on the postnatal ward. Early separation of mother and baby is damaging for both and should be avoided unless it is absolutely necessary. For this reason the basic criteria for admission to a NNU should be:

- illness in the baby;
- birth weight less than 1.8 kg.

Asymptomatic babies over 1.8 kg, more or less irrespective of gestation, may be nursed with their mothers on the postnatal wards. Instrumental or surgical delivery does not require NNU admission. Furthermore, many minor problems in the neonatal period can be managed while keeping the baby with his mother on the postnatal ward (Table 1.3).

Once a baby who weighs more than 1.8–2.0 kg has recovered from the conditions that precipitated his admission to the NNU, he

Table 1.3 Unjustifiable causes for admission to NNU for babies weighing >1.8 kg. These babies can be managed on a suitably staffed postnatal ward

Forceps delivery	
Caesarean section	
Breech delivery	Providing the baby is in good condition
Ventouse extraction	
Other malpresentations	
Multiple pregnancy	
Mild birth depression	IPPV for resuscitation but baby vigorous by 10 minutes of age. Consider NNU admission if: cord pH <7.0, or CTG with late decelerations and/or reduced base line variability plus thick meconium in liquor
Birth weight 1.8–2.5 kg including SFD babies	Baby in good condition >33 weeks gestation
Meconium stained liquor	Baby in good condition with no respiratory symptoms
Traumatic cyanosis	
Previous obstetric complications in maternal history e.g. stillbirth, early NND	Baby in good condition, check no history of group B streptococcal disease (p. 240)
Maternal illness or therapy e.g. epilepsy, asthma, thyroid disease	Baby in good condition. See p. 281–2 for advice on maternal thyroid disease
Babies of diabetic mothers >1.8 kg	Require glucose monitoring on the postnatal ward (p. 287)
Jittery	Does not need investigation unless severe (p. 286, 311)
Jaundice	Treat with phototherapy on postnatal ward; admit to NNU when nearing exchange levels (p. 426–430)
Feeding problems	
Mucousy	But be careful as this can be an early symptom of oesophageal atresia
Vomiting	Only if no persisting weight loss or signs of intestinal obstruction. Bile stained vomiting is a sign of intestinal obstruction.
Infections	Those not causing systemic upset; skin, eye, UTI
Malformations	Those not requiring surgical intervention or special nursing supervision
Social problems	

can go home. If his mother is still in hospital, he can be reunited with her on the postnatal ward, since this makes it much more likely that breast feeding will be established.

Well babies who weigh 1.8–2.0 kg and who are feeding satisfactorily – albeit three-hourly – may be discharged from hospital. Most homes are safe for the baby who has reached this weight, particularly if the mother can be relied on to keep her baby well swaddled in a room at 70–75°F, (21–24°C approx). It is, of course, important to inform the mother's general practitioner, midwife and health visitor prior to discharge.

PARENTAL ACCESS

One of the major advances in neonatology over the last 20 years has been the recognition of the psychological problems which can be caused by even short separation of a well neonate from his mother (Davis *et al.* 1983, Richards and Hawthorne 1999). The emotionally more arduous and much more protracted separation of a sick, very low birth weight baby from his mother may have more severe effects, including an increased risk of non-accidental injury and "failure to thrive" after discharge from the NNU.

It is therefore essential that all the family should have free access to their baby in the NNU. They should be encouraged to hold their baby's hand and soothe him no matter how ill he is and how much complicated monitoring paraphernalia he is connected to. Their baby's illness and his progress must be continuously explained to them by senior members of both the nursing and medical staff. Siblings and grandparents should always be allowed into the units. As the baby's condition improves, parents should be encouraged to take him out of the incubator for a cuddle, and to help with bathing and tube feeds.

REFERENCES

Audit Commission (1992) *Children First: a study of hospital services.* Audit Commission Services report No. 7. London: HMSO.

BAPM (1992) Categories of babies requiring neonatal care. *Archives of Disease in Childhood* **67**: 868–869.

BAPM (1996) *Standards for Hospitals Providing Neonatal Care.* London: BAPM; www.bapm-London.org

Davis, J.A., Richards, M.P.M. and Roberton, N.R.C. (1983) *Parent–Baby Attachment in Premature Infants.* Croom Helm, Beckenham, Kent.

Richards, M.P.M. and Hawthorne, J.T. (1999) Psychological aspects of neonatal care. In: *Textbook of Neonatology,* 3rd edn, Rennie, J.M. and Roberton, N.R.C. (eds). Churchill Livingstone, Edinburgh, pp. 61–72.

2

TEMPERATURE CONTROL

▬

- *Cold can kill.*
- *Babies should be kept in the thermoneutral range, with a core body temperature as close to 37°C as possible.*
- *Body temperature below 36°C or above 37.5°C, or a core-peripheral difference of more than 3°C which does not respond to environmental manipulation is a marker of serious illness until proved otherwise.*
- *Body temperature above or below this range increases mortality and morbidity.*
- *Adequate humidity, reduction of draughts and covering (dressing) babies after drying them makes control of their thermal environment easier.*

In this era of sophisticated incubators and complex infant care centres with overhead radiant heaters, it should not be assumed that the control of a premature infant's thermal environment is either unimportant or easy. Indeed there is evidence that overhead radiant heaters have made the infant's thermal environment more dangerous and difficult to control.

PHYSIOLOGY

HEAT LOSS

Physical

The neonate has a large surface area (0.1 m^2 at 28 weeks and 0.2 m^2 at term) for a small body mass, and loses heat rapidly. The smaller the baby the greater this loss will be, particularly if he is naked. Heat is lost in four ways: conduction, convection, evaporation and radiation.

1. Conductive losses are small, unless the baby is laid on a cold uninsulated surface!

2. Evaporative heat loss is due to the latent heat of evaporation of water on the baby's skin and is dependent on three things:
   (a) How wet is the baby from sweating or being covered with liquor at delivery?
   (b) How immature and water permeable is his skin?
   (c) How much is he exposed to drying factors such as air movement or radiant heaters?
3. Convective heat loss is due to the cooling effect of air currents around the baby, and is normally small, unless the baby is in a cool draught.
4. The baby loses heat by radiation on to nearby objects. When this is the incubator wall, the effective temperature is a function of the temperature inside and outside the incubator. To obtain the "operative" temperature, 1°C needs to be deducted from the incubator temperature for every 7°C the room temperature falls below the incubator temperature. This form of heat loss is much greater when the baby, particularly if naked, is outside an incubator and is radiating heat on to the walls and windows of a labour ward or a NNU.

Physiological

Babies who are too warm can lose heat by sweating (only possible >36 weeks gestation), by vasodilatation and by lying in an extended posture.

HEAT CONSERVATION

The simplest way in which babies can conserve heat is to lie curled up in as tightly flexed a position as possible. This is the natural position for a mature baby, and it can be imposed on a prone premature baby. The sick neonate tends to lie supine in the "frog" position with all his surfaces showing, thereby maximizing heat loss.

Skin vasoconstriction in response to cold in neonates and adults is similar, but even in the chubby full-term baby the insulation provided by the subcutaneous tissues is less than half that of the adult, and in low birth weight babies it is even less.

HEAT PRODUCTION

When a neonate is exposed to cold he becomes restless, but only shivers when the environmental temperature falls to 15°C or lower.

During the first weeks of life non-shivering thermogenesis is the main mechanism for generating heat. This is achieved by the hydrolysis of triglycerides in brown fat to free fatty acids and glycerol, and their subsequent resynthesis. These pathways are exothermic and by liberating approximately 2.5 cal/g of brown fat/min, warm the blood passing through these tissues.

During brown fat metabolism oxygen is consumed, and if the baby is hypoxic his response to cold will be jeopardized (Fig. 2.1). Hypoxic babies therefore drop their body temperatures rapidly if transiently exposed to a cool environment. Drugs, intracranial haemorrhage, hypoglycaemia and central nervous system malformations also inhibit thermogenesis in brown fat.

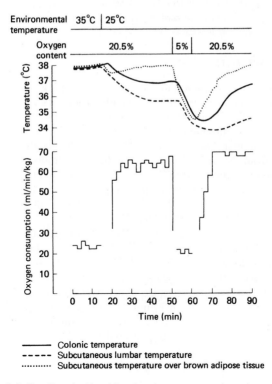

——— Colonic temperature
- - - - - Subcutaneous lumbar temperature
·········· Subcutaneous temperature over brown adipose tissue

Figure 2.1 The effect of cold and hypoxia on oxygen consumption and temperature in the neonatal rabbit. (From Dawkins and Hull, 1964.)

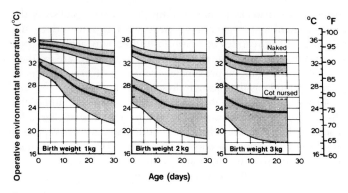

Figure 2.2 Temperature at which newborn babies should be nursed in a draught-free environment at 50% relative humidity. The dark line indicates the optimum temperature and the shaded areas denote the range of temperatures within which the baby can maintain a normal body temperature. (From Hey, 1971.)

THERMONEUTRALITY

Since oxygen is consumed in the process of keeping a baby warm, or when he is too hot and restless, the ideal thermal environment is one where the baby's oxygen consumption is minimal. This is known as the neutral temperature range.

The minimal oxygen consumption rises during the neonatal period from 4.6 ml/kg/min in the first few hours, to 7.0–7.5 ml/kg/min at one month. The lower end of the neutral temperature range varies with body weight and postnatal age, being higher in babies of lower birth weight and steadily falling in all birth weight groups with increasing postnatal age.

By noting the environmental temperature at which oxygen consumption is minimal, the ideal temperature in which to nurse naked and clothed newborn babies of different birth weights and postnatal ages has been determined (Fig. 2.2).

It is important to emphasize that babies can keep their core temperature normal at environmental temperatures outside the thermoneutral range, but only at the cost of consuming oxygen to generate heat or sustain cooling mechanisms.

MEASURING TEMPERATURE

Rectal temperature measured using a thermocouple/thermistor inserted to a distance of 3 cm is the gold standard, and all babies should have a rectal temperature of 36.5–37.5°C (Rutter, 1999). Axillary temperatures are also accurate and reproducible, but may be up to 0.5–1.0°C lower than simultaneously measured rectal values.

CORE-PERIPHERAL DIFFERENCES

Comparing core temperature with a peripheral site (e.g. big toe) is a useful marker of peripheral perfusion. A difference of more than 3°C is often an early marker of serious illness, especially infection (p. 106, 230).

CLINICAL EFFECTS OF COLD

The deleterious effects of cold on the premature baby are listed in Table 2.1. Even if the neonate's temperature does not fall, cooling can cause problems. Once the baby's physiological responses to cold are overcome and his body temperature falls, the effects of a cold environment become much more serious.

The most dramatic effect of allowing babies to get cold is the increase in morbidity and mortality. Blackfan and Yaglou (1933) showed that keeping babies warmer significantly reduced mortality, and this observation has been reconfirmed (Silverman and Blanc 1957, Stanley and Alberman 1978) (Table 2.1).

CLINICAL EFFECTS OF OVERHEATING

There are also dangers from overheating (Yashiro *et al.* 1973). Although the exact mechanisms are not clear, the various associations which have been reported are listed in Table 2.2.

Table 2.1 Neonatal mortality and temperature on admission to NNU (From Stanley and Alberman 1978)

Temperature on admission	NNM/1000 live births	
	BW <1.5 kg	BW 1.5 to 2.0 kg
<32.9°C	864	836
33–39.4°C	415	153
>35°C	373	38

Table 2.2 Deleterious effects of thermal stress on low birth weight babies

(a) COLD	(b) HEAT
↓ Surfactant synthesis	↑ Fluid loss (evaporative, sweating)
↓ Surfactant efficacy	↑ Postnatal weight loss
↓ pH	Hypernatraemia (hyperosmolarity)
↓ PaO_2	↑ jaundice
hypoglycaemia	Recurrent apnoea
↑ O_2 consumption	↑ NEONATAL MORTALITY
Diversion of cardiac output to brown fat	
↑ Utilization of calorie reserves	
↑ Postnatal weight loss	
↓ Later weight gain	
Neonatal cold injury (? sclerema)	
↓ Blood coagulability	
↑ NEONATAL MORTALITY	

MANAGEMENT OF TEMPERATURE CONTROL

NORMAL OR ILL BABIES

Control of the thermal environment

Since babies who get cold or who are overheated have a much higher morbidity and mortality, it is essential to make every effort to keep their core temperature as close to 37°C as possible. The following practices should be routine in all maternity hospitals and all NNUs:

1. Keep labour wards as warm and as draught-free as possible, and make special efforts when a premature baby is being delivered. Ideally the room should be warmed to 23–24°C. The resuscitation area must be draught-free, away from windows and air conditioning, and the resuscitation carried out under an overhead radiant heater.
2. Dry all babies after delivery with a warm towel, and thereafter keep them either wrapped up, or under the radiant heat source.
3. Avoid bathing babies on the labour ward.
4. Keep nurseries and NNUs hot enough (26–28°C) to minimize radiant heat loss.
5. Nurse babies in incubators set at the temperatures given in Fig. 2.2.
6. Minimize radiant heat loss in incubators by:

(a) using double-glazed incubators;

(b) covering the baby with a radiant heat shield;

(c) covering the baby with an insulating fabric (silver swaddlers, bubble-wrap, clingfilm);

(d) using hats and bootees/leggings even in neonates requiring intensive care;

(e) dressing babies once they no longer require intensive care and meticulous observation.

7. Minimize evaporative heat loss by:

(a) avoiding very dry environments. Put water in the incubator humidifier for babies of less than 30 weeks gestation who are having any problem maintaining their temperature;

(b) covering the baby with clingfilm or an insulating fabric (see above) to create a humid microenvironment. Clothing has a similar effect;

(c) avoiding overhead radiant heaters for thin skinned ELBW babies in the first week.

8. Avoid convective heat loss by:

(a) wrapping the babies in clingfilm or dressing them (*v.s.*);

(b) blocking off one end of a radiant heat shield with clingfilm to prevent a wind tunnel effect.

9. Warm and humidify all medical gases administered to babies.

10. Warm up operating theatres and anaesthetic rooms before the baby arrives.

Incubators or overhead radiant heaters

Overhead radiant heaters on "infant nursing units" are now extensively used. They have the enormous advantage of superb access to the patient. However, compared with incubators they increase considerably the evaporative and convective heat losses from the babies. Although the smallest ELBW neonate can be kept warm under radiant heaters they have higher oxygen consumption in this situation and their fluid balance is much more difficult to control. For this reason we prefer to use incubators, often humidified, for most babies <1.0 kg BW and 28 weeks GA (Hull and Chellappah 1983, Rutter 1999).

Servo control

Modern incubators can be controlled accurately to a preset temperature by a proportional controller on the heater unit, or run in a "servo" controlled mode from a probe attached to the baby. We have found no benefit from servo control. The units are more expensive and more likely to break down, and if the patient probe malfunctions or falls off the baby may cook or freeze.

Practical environmental temperature control

We find that by setting incubator temperatures according to Fig. 2.2, using the humidifier if necessary, wrapping babies up in cling-film or clothes and checking the baby's temperature every 3–6 hours, we experience very few problems with temperature control even in sick small babies, and we retain the benefit of pyrexia and hypothermia as useful clinical signs. For the occasional 500–600 g baby who remains cold, an external radiant heat source or a "sauna" (*v.i.*) may be necessary in the short term before replacing the wrapped warm baby in a warm humidified incubator in a warm room.

COLD BABIES

Hypothermia (temperature below 35°C) is most commonly seen when the baby is admitted to the NNU following thermal stress in the labour ward (*v.s.*). If it occurs later it suggests either that the control of the baby's thermal environment has been sloppy, or that he is suffering from some serious problem such as sepsis, brain damage, hypoxia or hypoglycaemia which must be excluded and treated. In addition to specific therapy the baby should be nursed in an incubator with its temperature set according to Hey's chart (Fig. 2.2) and should be covered with a radiant heat shield. He should be dressed in as much clothing as is compatible with his monitoring and treatment.

If his temperature is not rising within an hour, the following steps should be taken:

1. Increase the incubator temperature further.
2. Increase the room temperature – i.e. increase the environmental temperature.
3. Close off the end of the heat shield (*v.s.*).
4. Put water in the incubator humidifier to prevent evaporative loss: in the short term this can be hot water which, by giving the baby a 'sauna', will raise his temperature more quickly.
5. Add an overhead radiant heat source.

Profound hypothermia, <30°C is rarely seen in the UK. However when it does occur there is no contraindication to rewarming the baby rapidly at 1–2°C/h using radiant heaters and/or a heated water mattress (Rutter 1999).

PYREXIAL BABIES

A temperature of 37.5°C, or sometimes even higher, in a baby in an NNU or on a postnatal ward is usually due to:

1. Incubator/room temperature too high.
2. Lying in direct sunlight or phototherapy – effectively a radiant heat source.
3. Over-swaddling the baby – causing heat stroke!
4. Some combination of all three (common).

These errors should be remedied, and if the temperature falls within an hour no further action is usually required. However, if none of the common precipitating factors are present and the baby looks unwell, or if he is still febrile 60 minutes later, the following should be considered:

1. Infection (p. 232–234). A full infectious disease work-up should be carried out. The normal core-peripheral temperature difference is less than 2°C, and a higher difference suggests sepsis.
2. Dehydration fever (usually a term baby who has fed poorly and lost more than 10% of his birth weight). His serum osmolarity will exceed 300 mosm/kg water, and rehydration with milk or intravenous or oral glucose electrolyte solution rapidly restores the temperature to normal.
3. Brain damage with injury to hypothalamic centres.

REFERENCES

Blackfan, K.D. and Yaglou, C.P. (1933) The premature infant: a study of the effects of atmospheric conditions on growth and on development. *American Journal of Diseases of Children* **46**: 1175–1236.

Dawkins, M.J.R. and Hull, D. (1964) Brown adipose tissue in the response of newborn animals to cold. *Journal of Physiology* **172**: 216–238.

Hey, E.N. (1971) The care of babies in incubators. In: *Recent Advances in Paediatrics*, Gairdner, D.T.M., Hull, J. and Churchill, A. (eds). London, pp. 171–216.

Hull, D. and Chellappah, G. (1983) On keeping babies warm. In: *Recent*

Advances in Perinatal Medicine, Vol. 1, Chiswick, M.L. (ed). Churchill Livingstone, Edinburgh, pp. 153–168.

Rutter, N. (1999) Temperature Control and its Disorders. In: *Textbook of Neonatology*, 3rd edn, Rennie, J.M. and Roberton, N.R.C. (eds). Churchill Livingstone, Edinburgh, pp. 289–303.

Silverman, W.A. and Blanc, W.A. (1957) The effect of humidity on survival of newly born premature infants. *Pediatrics* **20**: 477–487.

Stanley, F.J. and Alberman, E.D. (1978) Infants of very low birth weight: I – Perinatal factors affecting survival. *Developmental Medicine and Child Neurology* **20**: 300–312.

Yashiro, K., Adams, F.H., Emmanouilides, G.C. and Mickey, M.R. (1973) Preliminary studies on the thermal environment of low birth weight infants. *Journal of Pediatrics* **82**: 991–994.

3

FLUID AND ELECTROLYTE BALANCE

- *Newborn babies, particularly VLBWI, can only regulate their fluid and electrolyte balance within narrow limits.*
- *VLBWI easily become dehydrated due to large transepidermal fluid losses and an inability to concentrate urine.*
- *A postnatal diuresis and natriuresis is normal, and sodium should not be added to the intravenous fluids until this has occurred.*
- *Weight and serum sodium are the keys to correct management of fluid balance in the newborn.*

Renal function in the neonate is limited. In essence, the neonate, especially the preterm neonate, can only regulate fluid and electrolyte homeostasis within narrow limits. The basic principles of management are standard, and consist of providing maintenance fluid and electrolyte requirements and providing for ongoing losses. In neonatal medicine, the rapid changes which are seen, make this a challenging aspect of intensive care requiring meticulous attention to detail.

NEONATAL RENAL FUNCTION AND PHYSIOLOGY

Human glomerulogenesis and nephrogenesis are complete by 34–35 weeks gestation, although at term the glomeruli are still much smaller than in the adult. The tubules are not fully grown even at term, and only those of the juxtamedullary glomeruli extend deep into the medulla. These factors contribute to the low GFR of the neonate, and his inability to concentrate urine. Expressing GFR per unit of surface area is inappropriate in the neonate, and GFR should be expressed per kilogram. When this is done the preterm neonate has a GFR of 0.5 ml/kg/min and the term neonate a GFR of 1.5 ml/kg/min compared to an adult value of 2 ml/kg/min. In clinical practice the serum creatinine concentration is the best guide to GFR.

The renal blood supply arises from the aorta between T12 and L2 and umbilical artery catheters must be positioned to end above or below this region (p. 99). Renal blood flow is around 100 ml/min/1.73 m^2 at term, and is lower in preterm babies or when a baby is ill.

Although healthy babies excrete the majority of a water load adequately, being able to reduce urine osmolality to <100 mosmol/kg H$_2$O, when they are ill they are less able to do this, in part due to the lower GFR. Babies can only concentrate urine to a maximum osmolality of 600–800 mosmol/kg H$_2$O until they establish an adequate medullary osmotic gradient. This occurs much later in the neonatal period; by adult life a urine concentration of 1500 mosmol/kg H$_2$O can be achieved. Urinary sodium losses are high in the early neonatal period with up to 5% of the filtered sodium being excreted in the urine in the first few days, yet the natriuretic response to salt overload is also defective.

Plasma levels of mineralocorticoids and ADH in neonates are within, or just above, the normal adult range, though the distal tubule, particularly in VLBW babies, responds poorly to the mineralocorticoids. ANP levels are high in the early neonatal period and although the kidney may be relatively insensitive, high ANP may contribute to the high rate of sodium excretion.

WATER

At term, 75% of the baby's body weight is water, and this percentage is higher in preterm babies. Part of the normal adaptation to extrauterine life is a marked reduction in body water, especially from the ECF. A reduction in ECF accounts for the early fall in body weight, and there is a change in the ratio of ECF to ICF from the 2:1 seen in fetal life to the 1:1 ratio which is normal for the neonate. After an initial period of 12–24 hours without diuresis the baby enters a diuretic phase (which is also a natriuresis) and then, after postnatal homeostasis is achieved, has normal sodium and water balance (Lorenz et al. 1995, Fig. 3.1). In ill preterm babies, characteristically those with RDS, the onset of the diuretic and natriuretic phase is delayed.

The key to the management of fluid balance in the ill baby lies in recognizing and adapting to these phases of water and sodium balance, and in such babies fluid overload and dehydration readily occur.

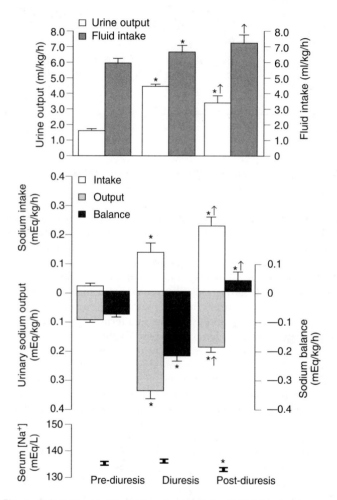

Figure 3.1 Fluid and sodium intake and output during the first few days in preterm neonates with and without RDS. Prediuresis lasted on average 25 hours and diuresis completed on average by 96 hours. Reproduced from Lorenz *et al.* 1995, with permission. Significant differences (P <0.05) are marked thus*.

Table 3.1 Transepidermal water loss (g/kg/24 h) at an ambient humidity of 50% (From Hammarlund *et al.* 1983)

Gestational age (weeks)	Postnatal age (days)			
	0–1	3	7	14
25–27	129 ± 39	71 ± 9	43 ± 9	32 ± 10
28–30	42 ± 13	32 ± 9	24 ± 7	18 ± 6
31–36	12 ± 5	12 ± 4	12 ± 4	9 ± 3
37–41	7 ± 2	6 ± 1	6 ± 1	6 ± 1

INSENSIBLE WATER LOSS: TRANSEPIDERMAL AND RESPIRATORY TRACT LOSS

The main route of insensible water loss is transepidermal water loss, and this is particularly high in preterm infants (Table 3.1). Insensible water loss also occurs via the respiratory tract. Respiratory tract water loss ranges from 4 mg/kg/min when a term baby is asleep to 10 mg/kg/min when he is crying furiously (Riesenfeld *et al.* 1987). This corresponds to a loss of about 6–9 ml/kg/24 h, which means that respiratory tract loss accounts for about half of the daily insensible loss in a term infant (Table 3.1). Respiratory losses are eliminated when a baby is artificially ventilated with humidified gas. Overhead heaters, draughts and phototherapy lamps, increase transepidermal water loss and can be significantly reduced by high ambient humidity and covering the baby. Evaporation of water from the skin causes the baby to lose heat, and reducing transepidermal water loss is an important component of thermoregulation (Chapter 2). When calculating water replacement, an estimate of the insensible water loss needs to be added to the urine volume and any other losses (remember gut losses in babies who have undergone surgery).

OBLIGATORY URINE WATER LOSS

This is the volume of water needed to excrete the urea and other waste products generated from the baby's diet. Obligatory urine water depends on the renal solute load of the diet, which in turn varies according to the type of milk or other feed the baby is receiving. The renal solute load of breast milk is much lower than that of formula milks. The obligatory urine water is approximately 2–4 ml/kg/h.

STOOL WATER

In babies the water lost in stool is approximately 7 ml/kg/day (Patrick and Pittard 1988) although clearly the water loss varies with the number of stools, and the fat content of the stool.

FLUID OVERLOAD, FLUID RETENTION AND OEDEMA

In the first week of life, particularly in ill VLBW neonates, the first indication of fluid overload or retention is a weight loss of less than 1% per day, or weight gain. After the first week fluid retention results in a weight gain of more than 20 g/kg/24 h. The signs of fluid overload include oedema, which is often hidden around the back and flank of a baby who is nursed supine.

Fluid overload occurs with:

1. excessive maintenance intravenous fluid including sodium, particularly when the normal postnatal diuresis and natriuresis has not yet occurred (see above);
2. large boluses of bicarbonate, dextrose, plasma or blood being given to sick babies without making allowances in the maintenance fluid intake;
3. excessive infusion through arterial catheters (umbilical or peripheral);
4. human error or mechanical failure in the pumps controlling the IV fluid.

Fluid retention – and, if severe, oedema – occurs with:

1. renal failure e.g. caused by asphyxia, hypotension, acidaemia (p. 373–375);
2. congestive cardiac failure e.g. with a patent ductus;
3. CNS damage (e.g. asphyxia, meningitis) causing inappropriate ADH secretion (p. 22, 318);
4. leaky capillaries owing to severe RDS, asphyxia, endotoxaemia, sepsis;
5. a rise in central venous pressure due to CPAP or IPPV;
6. a combination of (4) and (5) – commonly seen in babies with RDS who, in addition, have been paralysed. Paralysis eliminates the action of muscle activity on venous and lymphatic drainage;

7. extravasation of fluid into the extracellular space owing to hypoalbuminaemia;
8. Indomethacin used to treat PDA (p. 355–356).

Effects of excess fluid (overload or retention)

These include the following:

1. heart failure, including massive pulmonary haemorrhage (p. 188);
2. pulmonary oedema – in lung disease this exacerbates the hypoxaemia;
3. in babies recovering from RDS, an increased incidence of PDA (p. 172), and perhaps CLD (p. 202–203);
4. hyponatraemia, hypokalaemia;
5. oedema of kidneys, liver and gut, making these organs (respectively) less effective at excreting urine, conjugating drugs and bilirubin, and more prone to NEC (p. 386);
6. cerebral oedema, especially if there is coexisting asphyxial brain damage;
7. sclerema (p. 231).

TREATMENT

There are seven clinical situations commonly encountered:

1. **In a seriously ill neonate oedema is often accompanied by hypoalbuminaemia and leaky capillaries.** This is very common in the early stages of RDS, and recovery from the underlying disease is heralded by a spontaneous diuresis and clearing of the subcutaneous oedema (Fig. 3.1). However, while the baby is oedematous with weight gain, or no weight loss, he must have his fluid intake restricted to the minimum consistent with maintaining blood pressure and replacing transepidermal loss and urine water. For an average baby this corresponds to about 40–60 ml/kg/24 h.
2. **The baby with heart disease who develops heart failure** (treatment pp. 355).
3. **Oedema due to fluid overload**. Restrict fluids to 30–40 ml/kg/24 h. This may be all that is necessary; but if symptoms are present, give frusemide 2 mg/kg IV.
4. **Oedema due to inappropriate ADH secretion.** The presence of an abnormally low serum osmolality combined with a urinary osmolality above 300 mosmol/kg H_2O establishes the diagnosis.

The treatment is that of the underlying condition, together with fluid restriction to 30–40 ml/kg/24h IV of an electrolyte solution containing the daily electrolyte requirements.

5. **Oedema following indomethacin treatment.** This can be anticipated and fluid input reduced by one third for the duration of treatment. If it does develop the fluid retention will usually clear spontaneously.
6. **Hydrops fetalis** (p. 456–460).
7. **After surgery.** Perhaps due to a combination of replacement fluids leaking out, paralysis and some pre-renal renal impairment, fluid retention is commonly seen in the post-operative neonate who should have his fluids restricted as in 3) above.

If, in any of these situations, on clinical or radiological grounds oedema appears to be significantly adding to the baby's lung problem, exacerbating hypoxaemia, frusemide 2 mg/kg IV should be tried. Repeated doses can be given as necessary. If oedema is severe or progressive with a poor urinary output and/or a rising serum creatinine, dialysis or haemofiltration can be considered (p. 376).

DEHYDRATION

In the first week in neonates this is a weight loss of ≥3% per 24 h. Thereafter the standard criteria for dehydration apply. A weight loss of more than 2.5% is clinically significant, more than 5% moderate, and more than 10% severe.

Signs of dehydration

Dehydration in the neonate is easy to recognize. In addition to weight loss the baby develops decreased skin turgor, sunken eyes, a depressed fontanelle, and a reduced urinary output. The value of these clinical signs is much greater than any biochemical abnormality.

Dehydration readily develops in neonates and is likely to occur with:

1. a high insensible transepidermal water loss (*v.s.* and Chapter 2);
2. an osmotic diuresis due to glycosuria in VLBW babies;
3. gut fluid loss in diarrhoea and vomiting;
4. inadequate intake – tissued infusion, fluid deliberately withheld to avoid overload, and very occasionally due to inadequate breast milk supply (p. 15);

5. over vigorous use of diuretics;
6. pyrexia.

The effects of the fluid loss are:

1. progressive reduction of the plasma volume leading to hypoxia and acidaemia, gut under-perfusion predisposing to NEC, pre-renal uraemia, and ultimately to shock;
2. jaundice (p. 420);
3. electrolyte problems, in particular hypernatraemia (*v.i.*).

Treatment

In a baby who is clinically dehydrated his fluid intake should:

1. consist of a maintenance of 120–150 ml/kg/24 h;
2. replace fluid losses (if the dehydration is of sudden onset the weight loss can be assumed to be just water and can be replaced as extra intravenous fluid over the next 12–24 h);
3. allow for insensible loss from overhead radiant heaters (an extra 50–75 ml/kg/24 h);
4. keep up with ongoing losses in diarrhoea, NG aspirate, CSF leak, etc;
5. allow for pyrexia (an increased intake of 10 ml H_2O/kg/24 h for each degree C above 37°C).

Overall, this may mean an intake of 250–300 ml/kg/24 h. Such babies require meticulous reassessment of their fluid requirements every 8–12 hours.

SODIUM

The normal serum sodium concentration is 130–145 mmol/l. Values between 125 and 150 mmol/l are well tolerated but outside this range urgent treatment is required. The requirement for sodium in the neonate is 2–3 mmol/kg/24 h, and it is usually possible to calculate an electrolyte input, which keeps healthy neonates in balance. However, in sick babies many factors are present which severely disrupt sodium homeostasis.

Hyponatraemic babies (serum sodium <125 mmol/l) become listless, develop an ileus and may become hypotensive and convulse. With hypernatraemia (>150 mmol/l) the major hazard is CNS damage from the changes in intracerebral fluid distribution which occur during both the acute illness and recovery.

HYPONATRAEMIA

Hyponatraemia is relatively rare in the first 48–72 hours. It is vitally important to understand that low serum sodium can reflect either a low body sodium or can result from dilution, because the management of the two situations is quite different. Hyponatraemia is found in the following situations:

Water excess (dilutional hyponatraemia)

1. in babies born to hyponatraemic mothers, usually due to excess intravenous infusion of salt free fluids during labour. This is the only common cause of first day hyponatraemia;
2. with CNS injury causing inappropriate ADH production (p. 22, 318);
3. in renal failure or with reduced urine output secondary to indomethacin therapy.

Sodium depletion

1. in very small premature babies with poor renal conservation of sodium;
2. in preterm babies on a low sodium intake (e.g. just breast milk, or plain 10% dextrose IV);
3. following frusemide, both acutely and in babies with CLD on "maintenance" diuretics;
4. with diarrhoea or vomiting owing to excessive sodium losses. Similar losses may occur through an ileostomy;
5. "sequestered" sodium loss into the gut or into damaged cells (e.g. NEC – a low serum sodium is common in early NEC – or associated with sepsis);
6. following external drainage of CSF for the treatment of hydrocephalus;
7. salt losing forms of congenital adrenal hyperplasia (p. 277–279).

Treatment of hyponatraemia

Treatment depends on the cause; leaving aside the baby with GIT loss, CSF loss and CAH there are three common clinical situations;

1. **Hyponatraemia in the ill neonate.** This requires careful assessment. Examination of the intravenous fluid charts, urine output records and the baby's weight trend should help. The baby with

total body sodium depletion needs more sodium whereas one who is retaining fluid does not need more sodium, merely fluid restriction. Alternatively the hyponatraemia may be a marker of intravascular volume depletion, to which there has been an appropriate release of ADH resulting in water retention and a dilutional hyponatraemia. This requires volume replacement with a sodium-containing fluid.

2. **Hyponatraemia, usually after the first week in an otherwise healthy baby who may be growing poorly.** All this baby requires is an increased sodium intake, sometimes to as much as 10 mmol/kg/day or more, plus regular monitoring of his serum sodium.

3. **True inappropriate ADH secretion (SIADH).** Usually as a result of brain (hypothalamic) injury excess ADH is produced despite normovolaemia, normal blood pressure and normal renal function. There is hyponatraemia and a low plasma osmolarity with an inappropriately high urinary sodium and osmolarity. As well as treating the primary CNS disorder, the treatment is fluid restriction (40–50 ml/kg/day) with judicious sodium supplementation (at least the normal daily requirement).

HYPERNATRAEMIA

Hypernatraemia develops if water losses exceed sodium losses or if too much sodium is given. It is primarily seen in ill ELBW neonates in the first 24–72 hours of life. Causes include:

1. an inadequate fluid intake for any reason;
2. small ill premature babies with a marked transepidermal water loss (more marked in those nursed under overhead radiant heaters, p. 13). This is the most common cause of early hypernatraemia;
3. phototherapy, which has a similar effect to radiant heaters and also causes diarrhoea (p. 429);
4. hyperglycaemia in premature babies receiving excessive dextrose causing an osmotic water loss;
5. diarrhoea;
6. too much sodium as bicarbonate or from other sources such as drugs.

Treatment of hypernatraemia

Ideally hypernatraemia should be avoided by careful control of the baby's microenvironment, avoiding excess sodium intake (bicarbonate, blood and blood products, drugs and saline catheter flushes) and by maintaining appropriate fluid balance. However if the serum sodium is above 150 mmol/l the following action should be taken:

1. minimize transepidermal water loss (humidify incubator, wrap baby in clothes or plastic);
2. exclude osmotic diuresis;
3. stop added sodium;
4. if the weight loss has been more than 3% per day, the baby is likely to be volume depleted. Increase fluid intake (sodium-free) accordingly. If the weight loss has been 1–3 % be careful to avoid fluid overload with its attendant hazards.

POTASSIUM

The normal serum potassium concentration is 3.5–5.5 mmol/l. Neonates tolerate levels of 3.0–6.5 mmol/l extremely well, but outside this range treatment is required. The normal neonate needs 1–3 mmol/kg/24h of potassium, and disorders of potassium homeostasis are rare. Hypokalaemia is usually the result of careless control of intravenous fluid prescriptions and is readily treated by increasing the potassium intake. Hyperkalaemia is seen in ill VLBW babies who have been hypotensive and are in renal failure. The emergency treatment of hyperkalaemia and the management of renal failure is discussed on page 375.

HYDROGEN IONS AND BICARBONATE

(See Table 11.4, p. 123, for normal values.)

There are five important reasons for a neonate having a metabolic acidaemia – that is, a base deficit greater than 8–10 mmol/l. They are:

1. accumulation of lactic or other acids with asphyxia (p. 80–81), hypotension (p. 86, 138), sepsis (p. 233), hypoxia (p. 86, 138), or various inborn errors of metabolism (p. 297);
2. the hydrogen ion load resulting from growth and the metabolism of high protein milks (p. 48);
3. defective urinary acidification due to the low GFR, reduced urinary phosphate production, and reduced capacity of the neonatal kidney to make ammonia;

4. tubular bicarbonate leak. The bicarbonate threshold in a preterm baby may be as low as 12 mmol/l;
5. total parenteral nutrition with hyperchloraemic metabolic acidosis (p. 56).

Nothing can or should be done for factors (3) and (4), although occasionally a full-blown Fanconi tubular defect (p. 381) is seen after severe neonatal illness and needs bicarbonate replacement. Factor (2) rarely needs treatment. The treatment of the causes of acidaemia listed under (1) and (5) are dealt with elsewhere.

CALCIUM AND PHOSPHATE

The normal serum calcium concentration is in the range 2.2 to 2.6 mmol/l (1.0–1.4 mmol/l ionized calcium). Serum phosphate levels vary from between 2.0–2.6 mmol/l at birth to 1.5–2.9 mmol/l after the first week. Calcium and phosphate levels are higher in cord blood than in maternal plasma. Calcium is actively transported from the mother into the fetus, and the fetal phosphate level rises due to hypoparathyroidism induced by the high calcium concentration.

Postnatally, neonatal plasma phosphate may rise further owing to the low GFR and the relatively high phosphate intake in bottle-fed babies. Parathormone levels rise slowly in small sick babies, and will therefore have little phosphaturic effect on the neonatal renal tubule. Neonatal vitamin D metabolism is probably normal.

HYPOCALCAEMIA

Hypocalcaemia is common in the neonatal period, but allowance must be made for coexistent hypoalbuminaemia. On average, the serum calcium falls by 0.1 mmol/l for each 4 g by which the serum albumin falls below the mean for the baby's gestation.

Serum calcium levels above 1.75 mmol/l rarely cause any problem, but symptoms (see below) may develop if the serum calcium falls below 1.5 mmol/l. This happens in the following situations:

1. during the first 24–48 hours in severely ill babies. This accounts for 95% of neonatal hypocalcaemia. The babies have a subnormal parathormone response to the low calcium level, but have high circulating levels of hormones such as glucocorticoids and calcitonin which depress plasma calcium;
2. in babies of diabetic mothers;

3. during an exchange transfusion with citrated blood. The citrate chelates the calcium, causing a rapid drop in the plasma level.

Other rare causes of neonatal hypocalcaemia, which should be sought if the problems listed above are not present, include the following:

1. maternal and fetal hypovitaminosis D. This may be particularly common in babies from ethnic groups that are at risk of rickets;
2. babies fed on high phosphate milks (e.g. unadulterated cow's milk). This used to be common, but is now fortunately very rare;
3. renal failure;
4. primary hypoparathyroidism, including Di George syndrome;
5. maternal hypercalcaemia including that due to hyperparathyroidism, causing prolonged neonatal parathyroid depression.

The symptoms of hypocalcaemia depend on the age at presentation. In babies less than 72 hours old convulsions are rare; but these babies may be jittery, particularly if they are on IPPV. Hypocalcaemia that develops during an exchange transfusion may cause convulsions, cardiac arrhythmias or tetany with a positive Chvostek sign. At the end of the first week in an otherwise well baby hypocalcaemia causes clonic fits (p. 313). Hypocalcaemia may cause heart failure and apnoea at any time in the neonatal period.

Hypocalcaemia should be avoided by adequate treatment of the illnesses which predispose to it. Convulsions should be controlled pharmacologically (p. 314–5) while investigating the cause of the hypocalcaemia, and the plasma calcium increased with oral or intravenous calcium supplements.

To prevent early hypocalcaemia in ill neonates, appropriate intravenous supplements of 10% calcium gluconate should be given. In general, 5–10 ml of 10% calcium gluconate (1.125–2.25 mmol of calcium) IV each 24 hours is all that is usually necessary.

Depending on the cause, specific therapy may be required with phosphate restriction, calcium supplements, or treatment with vitamin D. In general, if vitamin D is required, we use the standard vitamin D preparations rather than the newer much more potent vitamin D metabolites such as 1–α-vitamin D or 1:25 vitamin D.

The dose of calcium for tetany or hypocalcaemic arrhythmias during an exchange transfusion is 1 ml of 10% calcium gluconate (equivalent to 0.225 mmol calcium) infused over 2 minutes under ECG control.

HYPERCALCAEMIA

Neonatal hypercalcaemia is rare and usually iatrogenic. Occasionally, hypercalcaemia of 3.0–3.5 mmol/l may develop in the ELBW baby who has become profoundly hypophosphataemic (<0.5 mmol/l). Treatment is with phosphate supplements, giving 2–3 mmol/kg/24 h of neutral phosphate (p. 38). Rare cases of neonatal hyperparathyroidism have been described.

HYPOPHOSPHATAEMIA

Hypophosphataemia is now being seen with increasing frequency in VLBW babies on TPN (p. 56) or in those receiving low phosphate milks. In enterally fed babies this can be prevented by adding phosphate to breast milk (p. 38). When severe it causes hypercalcaemia (*v.s.*).

MAGNESIUM

Abnormalities of magnesium homeostasis are now rare with the withdrawal of the high phosphate milks. Magnesium sulphate is used for treating maternal pre-eclampsia and can give rise to high levels of magnesium in the neonate. The baby is usually asymptomatic but hypermagnesaemia can cause floppiness. Hypomagnesaemia may occasionally occur during parenteral nutrition. Giving 0.2 ml/kg of a 50% solution of $MgSO_4$ intramuscularly can treat it.

PRACTICAL FLUID AND ELECTROLYTE MANAGEMENT

The single most useful measurement for assessing a baby's fluid requirement is his weight. In the first week of life the very premature baby should lose about 1–3% of his body weight per day. If he is not doing this he is being overhydrated; if he is losing more than this he needs more fluid. It is, therefore, essential that sick VLBW neonates are weighed at least daily, and in some cases twice daily, as part of their intensive care.

The information required for assessing fluid requirements other than weight, includes urinary output, PCV, BP, serum sodium and creatinine estimations and a clinical assessment of the baby's state of hydration and perfusion. Weighing the nappies is the easiest way of measuring urine output and should be standard practice whilst babies are requiring intensive care. Controlling the fluid intake by aiming to achieve some set biochemical goal such as a normal urinary osmolality or a specific urinary output without taking note of the clinical state and weight of the baby is ill-advised, and frequently results in serious over hydration. Nevertheless since the changes in the electrolyte concentrations in ill neonates are to some extent unpredictable all such babies should have measurement of their plasma electrolytes, urea and creatinine at least daily whilst they are in intensive care. Table 3.2 summarizes our approach to the

Table 3.2 Outline of fluid therapy in the newborn

Indicator	Frequency of estimation during intensive care	Response
Weight	Daily or twice daily	Aim for a weight loss of 1–2% per day for 5 days. Adjust volume of maintenance fluid accordingly.
Urine output	Continuous, using nappy weights, or urine collection system. Review results 8 hourly.	Aim for a urine output of at least 0.5 ml/kg/24 h on the first day, and 2–7 ml/kg/h thereafter. Adjust maintenance fluid, blood pressure support to achieve this. Urine output below 1 ml/kg/24 h for more than 8 hours requires renal failure management (p. 374–376).
Sodium	Daily or twice daily	**Omit** added sodium a) until urine output is established and b) if plasma sodium >145 mmol/l **Increase** input if low sodium (<125 mmol/l considered to be due to sodium depletion) — otherwise restrict fluid (p. 25–26).
Glucose	At least 6 hourly during intensive care	Maintain level between 2.6 and 10 mmol/l by adjusting glucose concentration of fluid. Usual requirement 8–12 mmol/kg/min.
Potassium	Daily or twice daily	**Omit** a) on day 1 b) if potassium >5.5 mmol/l c) renal failure developing **Increase** a) if potassium <2.5 mmol/l.
Calcium	Daily	Give 5 ml 10% calcium gluconate/kg/24 h if serum calcium <1.75 mmol/l Give 10 ml/kg/24 h if calcium <1.5 mmol/l.

interpretation of results. We start with a maintenance fluid of 10% dextrose, and vary the concentration to keep the blood glucose between 2.5 and 10 mmol/l (p. 284, 294). An alternative approach is to use a Y connection to mix 5% and 50% glucose (Modi 1999).

REFERENCES

Hammarlund, K., Sedin, G. and Stromberg, B. (1983) Transepidermal water loss in the newborn VIII. Relation to gestational age and postnatal age in appropriate and small for gestational age infants. *Acta Paediatrica Scandinavica* **72**: 721–728.

Lorenz, J.M., Kleinman, L.I., Ahmed, G. and Markarian, K. (1995) Phases of fluid and electrolyte homeostasis in the extremely low birth weight baby. *Pediatrics* **96**: 484–489.

Modi, N. (1999) Renal function, fluid and electrolyte balance and neonatal renal disease. In: *Textbook of Neonatology*, 3rd edn. Rennie, J.M. and Roberton, N.R.C. (eds), Churchill Livingstone, Edinburgh, pp. 1009–1037.

Patrick, C.H. and Pittard, W.B. (1988) Stool water loss in very low birth weight neonates. *Clinical Pediatrics* **27**: 144–6.

Riesenfeld, K., Hammarlund, K. and Sedin, G. (1987) Respiratory water loss in relation to activity in fullterm infants on their first day after birth. *Acta Paediatrica Scandinavica* **76**: 889–893.

FURTHER READING

Modi, N (1999) Renal function, fluid and electrolyte balance and neonatal renal disease. In: *Textbook of Neonatology*, 3rd edn. Rennie, J.M. and Roberton, N.R.C. (eds), Churchill Livingstone, Edinburgh, pp. 1009–1037.

Sedin, G. (1996) Fluid management in the extremely preterm infant. In: *Current Topics in Neonatology* vol 1, T.N. Hansen and N. McIntosh (eds), pp 50–66

4

NEONATAL ENTERAL NUTRITION

- *Breast milk is the ideal food for babies of all weights and all gestations.*
- *When starting enteral nutrition in VLBWI breast milk is better tolerated than formula.*
- *Once enteral nutrition is established, breast milk alone is not suitable as sole diet in VLBWI.*
- *Minimal enteral feeding should be started early and only stopped if there is clear evidence of gastrointestinal disease.*

In order to grow and develop normally babies must have enough energy and the correct balance of carbohydrate, fat and protein with vitamins and minerals. Enteral feeding is the best way in which to deliver nutrition, and we are depressed by the current tendency to stop even minimal enteral feeding (*v.i.*) at the least excuse. For guidance on when to stop see p. 46. The aim of all nutritional support is to achieve a growth rate of about 15 g/kg/day whilst maintaining a normal body composition. Provision of nutrition by the enteral route is safer and easier than parenteral nutrition (Chapter 5). For a full discussion of this vast subject the reader is referred to Hay (1991), Tsang *et al.* (1993) and Fewtrell and Lucas (1999).

INFANT NUTRIENT REQUIREMENTS

ENERGY

A well preterm baby who is in a thermoneutral environment (p. 10) needs about 50 kcal/kg just to maintain essential body functions. If he is to grow he requires another 5 calories for every gram of weight gain. Sick babies need more, and although some babies grow well on 90–120 kcal/kg/day, particularly if the fat in their diet is well absorbed, many need 140–160 kcal/kg/day. The clear differences in caloric value of different milks can be seen in Tables 4.1, 4.2 and 4.3. Enough calories need to be provided to ensure that the baby

Table 4.1 Composition of commonly used formula feeds compared to mature breast milk (manufacturer's data)

	Mature breast milk	SMA Gold (Wyeth)	Cow & Gate Premium	Farley's First Milk	Milupa Aptamil
Carbohydrate (g/100 ml)	7.0	7.2	7.5	7.0	7.2
Fat (g/100 ml)	4.2	3.6	3.5	3.82	3.6
Protein (g/100 ml)	1.34	1.5	1.4	1.45	1.5
Casein:lactalbumin ratio	2:3	2:3	2:3	2:3	2:3
Kilocaloriess /100 ml	70	67	67	68	67
Sodium mmol/l	6.5	7.0	8.2	7.4	10.0
Potassium mmol/l	15	16.7	16.7	14.6	19.2
Calcium mg%	35	46	54	39	66
Phosphate mg%	15	33	27	27	42
Iron mg%	0.08	0.8	0.51	0.69	0.7
Vitamin A μg/100 ml	60	75	84	100	60
Vitamin D μg/100 ml	0.01	1.1	1.4	1.0	1.0
Folic acid μg/100 ml	5.2	8.0	10	3.4	10

Table 4.2 Composition of different types of human breast milk compared to cow's milk

	Cow	Mature breast milk*	Term (mother's own) day 7[+]	Preterm milk day 7[+]	Drip breast milk[~]
Carbohydrate (g/100 ml)	4.6	7.0	6.4	6.4	7.1
Fat (g/100 ml)	3.9	4.2	2.9	3.1	2.2
Protein (g/100 ml)	3.4	1.34	2.6	2.7	1.35
Casein:lactalbumin ratio	4:1	2:3	2:3	2:3	2:3
Kilocalories /100 ml	67	70	73	74	54
Sodium mmol/l	23	6.5	9.5	17	4.8
Potassium mmol/l	40	15	17	17	16
Calcium mg%	124	35	29	29	28
Phosphate mg%	98	15	17	13	14
Iron mg%	0.05	0.08	0.08	0.15	
Vitamin A μg/100 ml	40	60			
Vitamin D μg/100 ml	0.02	0.01			
Folic acid μg/100 ml	5	5.2	2.1		

* data of working party on the medical aspects of food policy: composition of mature human milk (Fewtrell and Lucas 1999).

[+] data from Lemons et al. (1982). Note that the protein content of term breast milk on day 7 is about 2.5 g/100 ml — considerably higher than that found in mature breast milk, column 2.

[~] data of Lucas, Gibbs and Baum (1978) from milk 30–90 days postpartum.

Table 4.3 Composition of preterm formulas (manufacturer's data)

	SMA low birth weight	Cow & Gate Nutriprem	Farley's Osterprem	Milupa Prematil
Carbohydrate (g/100 ml)	8.6	8.0	7.65	7.7
Lactose (g/100 ml)	4.3	4.0	6.0	4.9
Maltodextrin (g/100 ml)	4.3	4.0	1.65	2.8
Fat (g/100 ml)	4.4	4.4	4.61	3.5
Protein (g/100 ml)	2.0	2.2	2.0	2.0
Casein:lactalbumin ratio	2:3	2:3	2:3	2:3
Kilocalories /100 ml	82	80	80	70
Sodium (mmol/l)	14	14	18	12
Potassium (mmol/l)	19	18	18	19
Calcium (mg%)	77	108	110	70
Phosphate (mg%)	33	54	63	42
Iron (mg%)	0.67	0.90	0.40	1.0
Vitamin A (μg/100 ml)	74	100	100	53
Vitamin D (μg/100 ml)	1.2	2.4	2.4	2.0
Folic acid (μg/100 ml)	49	48	50	43

uses all the protein in his diet for cell building and does not break protein down for energy. This is the reason why the protein: non protein calorie ratio is important (*v.i.*).

FAT

Fat is the main energy source for babies, and dietary fat should constitute at least 30% of the total caloric intake per day, giving 5–9 g/kg/24 h. In addition to supplying energy, fats are required to build new cell membranes, particularly in the brain, and to carry essential fat soluble vitamins (p. 39). Fat can be stored in large quantities, in contrast to carbohydrate and protein for which the storage capacity of the body is limited. For the newborn, using fat for energy marks a major change from fetal life, during which the main energy source was glucose. The fat component of various milks is listed in Tables 4.1, 4.2 and 4.3.

There are four major lipid types; glycerides, phospholipids, sterols and fatty acids. The fat globules in human milk consist mainly of triglyceride, with some cholesterol, phospholipid and fatty acids. Formula milks contain only traces of cholesterol, and have few long-chain fatty acids. The amount of fat in breast milk changes with gestation and the phase of feeding. The fat content of formula milk is constant, and is derived from cow's milk and/or vegetable oils such as corn oil. These fats are less well digested and absorbed than fat from breast milk. Artificially fed premature babies may lose up to 50% of ingested long chain fat in their stools. Despite this, formula fed babies become fatter than their breast fed counterparts, although a link between formula feeding and later obesity or arteriosclerosis is not proven.

Recently, formula manufacturers have added long chain polyunsaturated fatty acids (e.g. eicosapentanoic acid, docosahexanoic acid) and essential fatty acids like linoleic and linolenic, together with other factors required in fat metabolism such as carnitine and choline. There is some evidence that retinal function depends on the provision of LCPUFAs in the diet at a critical stage of development. Whether these effects are permanent, and whether the current composition of these more humanized milks is optimal has not yet been established.

PROTEIN

The growing preterm baby requires a higher protein intake than the term baby, an intake that is higher than it is possible to achieve using breast milk (Table 4.2). It is generally recommended that preterm babies should have a protein intake of 2.9–4.0 g/kg/24 h given in a whey predominant formula (Table 4.3) containing a total of 2.0–2.2 g protein/100 ml (Table 4.3). This protein intake can also be achieved by adding fortifiers to breast milk (Table 4.4). Term babies require about 2.2 g/kg/day of protein. No more than 7–12% of the daily calorie intake should be derived from protein. In addition to the amino acids which are essential for adults, histidine, cysteine and tyrosine may be essential for newborn babies. The protein:non protein calorie ratio is equally important in enteral as parenteral nutrition.

Protein intakes of more than 4 g/kg/24 h should be avoided particularly if casein predominant formulas are used, as these may cause problems such as hyperaminoacidaemia, metabolic acidaemia and poor growth (Raiha *et al.* 1976).

CARBOHYDRATE

The main carbohydrate in human milk and term formulas is lactose (Table 4.1 and 4.2), whereas in preterm formulas it is a mixture of

Table 4.4 Major nutrient composition in one sachet/scoop of breast milk fortifiers available in the UK (this is the amount added to 100 ml of human milk): manufacturer's data

	Cow and Gate Nutriprem	Milupa Eoprotein	Mead Johnson Enfamil	SMA Breast Milk Fortifier
Energy (kJ)	44	47	58	64
Energy (kcal)	10	11	14	15
Protein (g)	0.7	0.6	0.7	1.0
Carbohydrate (g)	2.0	2.1	2.73	2.4
Fat (g)	Nil	0.02	0.05	0.16
Sodium (mg)	6.0	20	7.0	18
Potassium (mg)	4.0	2.4	45	27
Calcium (mg)	60	38	90	90
Phosphorus (mg)	40	26	45	45
Magnesium (mg)	6.0	2.1	1.0	3.0
Vitamin A (μg)	130	30	234	270
Vitamin D (μg)	5.0	Nil	6.5	7.6
Vitamin K (μg)	6.3	0.2	9.1	11.0

lactose and glucose polymers. Lactose is split up into the monosaccharides glucose and galactose by β-galactosidase (lactase), a brush border enzyme.

MINERALS

Sodium

On formulas with a very low sodium content or breast milk, babies smaller than 1.5 kg may become hyponatraemic (sodium <125 mmol/l) since they lose much more salt in their urine than full-term babies. Hyponatraemia is much less likely with preterm formulas or if fortifier is added to breast milk (Table 4.4).

Calcium and phosphorus

Calcium is the most abundant mineral in the body, 99% of it being found in bone. Babies born prematurely suffer an interruption of supply at a time of rapid accretion (about 2.5 mmol/kg/day or 120 mg/kg/day for calcium, and 2.2 mmol/kg/day or 70 mg/kg/day for phosphorus). Consequently preterm babies require much more calcium and phosphorus than can be provided by breast milk. Metabolic bone disease of prematurity (p. 309–310) is mainly due to this dietary deficiency. Hypocalcaemia is discussed on p. 28–29.

Preterm babies require 60–100 mg of calcium and 40–70 mg of phosphorus/100 ml milk – values which are only achieved using preterm formulas. Babies weighing less than 1.2 kg who are fed on breast milk without fortifier should receive an extra 0.5 mmol of phosphate per 100 ml feed (Bishop 1999) given as a neutral phosphate solution (a mixture of Na_2HPO_4 + NaH_2PO_4). If their serum phosphate is still <1.25 mmol/l, an extra 0.5 mmol phosphate and 1 mmol calcium/100 ml should be put in their feeds, the phosphate being added first in order to avoid precipitation.

Iron

Commercial formulas have iron added to them (Table 4.1, 4.3), whereas all forms of breast milk are very low in iron (Table 4.2), although the iron is in a form which is more readily absorbed than the iron in formulas (Saarinen and Siimes 1979).

Babies of 32–34 weeks gestation or less are born before their body iron stores are laid down by transplacental transfer. Preterm babies need iron supplements after they are 6 weeks old. Iron supplementation is not then required if they are fed on an iron supplemented preterm formula (Table 4.3). However, preterm babies who are fed on breast milk should receive 2.5 mg/kg/day of iron up to a maximum of 15 mg/day, and should stay on this treatment until they are taking an adequate mixed diet. Iron supplementation in this way does not prevent the physiological anaemia of prematurity (p. 437) but it does prevent later iron deficiency. There is also some research linking iron deficiency in infancy with a lower IQ later in childhood.

Trace minerals

Humans require zinc, copper, selenium, chromium, molybdenum, manganese and iodine in addition to iron. Copper and zinc deficiency do occur rarely in ELBW neonates at 2–4 months of age, usually only in those who have been given prolonged TPN with inadequate trace mineral supplementation (Fewtrell and Lucas 1999). Manganese toxicity has been reported with long-term TPN (Fell *et al.* 1996). Aluminium is not an essential trace mineral, but can also accumulate during TPN (Bishop *et al.* 1997).

VITAMINS

Vitamins A, D, K and E are fat-soluble; the B vitamins, folic acid and vitamin C are water-soluble. Unsupplemented breast milk is lacking in some vitamins, and we routinely supplement all premature babies with Abidec (containing vitamins A B_1 B_2 B_6 C and D) 0.3 ml daily until discharge and then 0.6 ml daily till the age of 6 months. Whilst still in the neonatal unit VLBW babies who are not being fed on supplemented breast milk or a preterm formula receive an additional 400 units of vitamin D per day. If this is done, together with an adequate provision of calcium and phosphate (*v.s.*), osteopenia of prematurity will be very rare (Bishop 1999).

Vitamin K deficiency bleeding (p. 447–449) is much more common in breast fed babies. To prevent it, all babies should receive 0.5–1.0 mg of vitamin K intramuscularly at birth (p. 74, 446).

Folic acid deficiency may reduce growth, and may rarely cause a megaloblastic anaemia both in babies weighing less than 2.0 kg at birth and in survivors of haemolytic disease. We give these babies 1 mg of folic acid weekly until discharge.

WHICH MILK TO GIVE?

For the healthy term baby all paediatricians will recommend breast feeding, though it has to be admitted that in Western society there is little evidence that harm comes to babies who are fed on the newer formulas (Table 4.1).

For preterm babies there are five milk preparations available:

1. standard infant formulas (Table 4.1);
2. special "preterm" formulas (Table 4.3);
3. "mother's own" expressed breast milk (Table 4.2);
4. banked breast milk (Table 4.2);
5. Supplemented breast milk (Table 4.4).

STANDARD INFANT FORMULA

These milks have been extensively modified from that originally produced by the cow, and the various brands have similar compositions (Table 4.1). In general the mineral content of the milks has been reduced so that it is more similar to that of breast milk. In addition, the protein has been modified to produce a casein: lactalbumin ratio and an amino acid pattern which approximate to those of breast milk. Finally, the fat has been modified to include more unsaturated and polyunsaturated fatty acids – again to be more like breast milk.

PRETERM FORMULA

For a newborn preterm baby to grow and accumulate sufficient nutrients and minerals to parallel intrauterine growth, he requires a higher protein and mineral intake than would be provided by a standard infant formula or human breast milk. Special preterm formulas have therefore been produced with higher protein and mineral contents (Table 4.3).

"MOTHER'S OWN" EXPRESSED BREAST MILK

The expressed breast milk from mothers who produce preterm babies has a higher protein and mineral content than term expressed breast milk (Table 4.2). The reason for this singularly sensible adaptation by the female breast remains obscure, but it may be nothing more than "concentrated" breast milk which is all that can be expressed from the breast after a preterm delivery when the breast has not been fully primed for lactation by a full 40 weeks of pregnancy.

BANKED BREAST MILK

EBM from women who have delivered at term, and who have been lactating for several weeks or months, contains less protein and minerals than preterm EBM (Table 4.2). The milk in breast milk banks is derived largely from this source, plus drip milk collected from the contra-lateral breast during suckling, and this is even more dilute (Table 4.2).

SUPPLEMENTED BREAST MILK

Various supplements have been designed which can be added to breast milk, to increase the protein and mineral content to provide an adequate intake for VLBW neonates (Table 4.4).

Which of these five options should be given to preterm babies, particularly those recovering from severe neonatal illnesses, is currently subject to widespread research and debate. However, the following factors should be considered when selecting the most appropriate milk for a specific baby.

ANTI-INFECTION AGENTS

There are many anti-infection agents in breast milk; these include lysozymes, lactoferrin, immunoglobulins and complement. Boiling destroys most of these anti-infection factors, and their concentration is reduced even by gentle pasteurization (Evans *et al.* 1978). If there are any benefits to the baby on the NNU from these anti-infection factors, they will only be available if he receives fresh EBM from his own mother.

Recently Lucas and Cole (1990) have shown that feeding breast milk, whether pasteurized or not, protects against NEC (p. 387). Whether this is an anti-infectious property or due to some other factor in EBM or formula is unclear.

INFECTION

Various viruses such as CMV, herpes, hepatitis B, HTLV I and HIV can be transmitted in breast milk, of which the most important are HIV and HTLV I (Oxtoby 1988, Lawrence and Howard 1999). It is for this reason that breast milk banks should only use milk which has been pasteurized and obtained from women who have been tested and are known to be HIV and Hepatitis B and C negative.

DRUGS

These may get into breast milk if they are not protein bound. However, it is very unusual for drugs taken by the mother to have any serious implications for the breast fed baby. Table 4.5 lists those which do, and which should therefore be avoided.

Table 4.5 Drugs which are contraindicated in breast feeding mothers (See also American Academy of Pediatrics 1994, Lawrence and Howard 1999)

Amiodarone
Ergot alkaloids
Etretinate (vitamin A derivative)
Gold salts
Immunosupressive drugs, cytotoxic drugs e.g. cyclosporin, cyclophosphamide, methotrexate
Lithium
Morphine, methadone heroin and other drugs of addiction when used by addicts — postoperative use OK
Oral contraceptives
Phenindione
Radiopharmaceuticals
Tetracycline

TOLERANCE

There is a wealth of clinical experience which shows that when starting to feed enterally low birth weight babies who have been ill or who have had bowel problems, breast milk is better tolerated than formula. This is supported by scientific research which shows that breast milk passes through the stomach faster, releases gut hormones into the circulation, and increases gut motility. Time to achieve full feeds is significantly shorter when breast milk is used.

SPECIAL MILKS

Goat's milk is a totally unsuitable food for any baby, term or preterm. Soy milk is not suitable for preterm babies, and should only be used at term for babies with galactosaemia, primary or secondary lactose intolerance or definite cow's milk protein allergy. A wide variety of other formulas have been designed for situations such as allergy, malabsorption and inborn errors of metabolism. None of these were designed with the preterm baby in mind, and when they are used (for example Neocate for short gut after NEC) extra vigilance is required. Many of these milks have a very high renal solute load, which can cause problems if the total fluid intake has to be restricted.

CONCLUSIONS

The ideal starting diet for a term or preterm baby is fresh, unpasteurized breast milk from his own mother, and for a term baby this diet will suffice for many months. If "mother's own" is unavailable the next best starting diet for a preterm baby is pasteurized donor breast milk thawed from a breast milk bank. Once a preterm baby is established on enteral feeds, we would prefer to continue with "mother's own" EBM, unpasteurized, and we are prepared to keep it in the fridge for up to 48 hours to avoid freezing. We do not wait for bacteriological culture results before starting to give a mother's own milk to her baby. Freeze-thawing the mother's own breast milk is sometimes necessary to bridge gaps in supply. Once full feeds are established in preterm babies weighing less than 1850 g, we supplement a diet which consists solely of breast milk with fortifier. For mothers who do not wish fortifier to be added, as a minimum we add phosphate to try to avoid metabolic bone disease of prematurity. If "mother's own" milk is not available, since there are obvious financial, social and intellectual advantages if a LBW baby gains weight rapidly and is discharged home as soon as possible, we would not continue with donor breast milk after using it to establish feeds, but would feed the baby on one of the preterm formulas (Lucas *et al.* 1984, 1990).

WHEN TO START ENTERAL FEEDS

Babies less than 34 weeks cannot usually sustain co-ordinated sucking and swallowing and require tube feeding. Healthy LBW babies should have an orogastric or nasogastric tube passed within 1–2 hours of delivery, and feeding with full strength milk can be started at once. Ideally some form of breast milk (see above) should be used to minimize the risk of NEC (p. 387) and because it is better tolerated. There is no point in starting with a clear fluid feed. For VLBW babies it is safer to give 10% glucose intravenously for the first 6–12 hours before starting to feed them. VLBWI are unlikely to tolerate sufficient enteral feed quickly enough to prevent hypoglycaemia even if they are well.

Sick babies of any birth weight often have a concomitant ileus. For this reason enteral feeds should only be started in sick babies – even those more than 2.5 kg – if:

- the baby's condition is improving – even though they are still on IPPV;
- they do not have abdominal distention;
- they have passed meconium;
- they have normal bowel sounds.

Ill babies weighing more than 2.0–2.5 kg often reach this stage within 2–3 days, but the smaller and sicker the baby the longer it may take.

Great care should be taken when starting feeds to aspirate the stomach 4–6 hourly in order to prevent pooling of milk and secretions in the stomach.

VOLUME AND FREQUENCY OF FEEDS

MINIMAL ENTERAL FEEDING (TROPHIC FEEDING)

Giving small, nutritionally insignificant volumes of milk encourages the secretion of gut hormones, improves gut motility, helps in the earlier achievement of full enteral feeds and reduces the hazards of TPN (Dunn *et al.* 1988). The presence of a UAC or a putative risk of NEC are *not* contraindications to trying enteral feeds so long as the precautions outlined below are observed. The one situation when we would definitely wait as long as a week before starting enteral feeds is in the IUGR baby who had reversed end-diastolic blood flow in his umbilical artery before birth. This is known to be a very high-risk situation for NEC (Hackett *et al.* 1987).

HEALTHY LBW BABIES

The volumes listed in Table 4.6(a) should be given. It is particularly important to feed these volumes to babies who are small for dates and at risk from hypoglycaemia (p. 287–289).

If the baby is unable to suck, then appropriate volumes of milk should be given hourly through an indwelling orogastric or naso-gastric tube. Low birth weight asymptomatic babies can be fed 2 hourly when they weigh about 1.3 kg and 3 hourly when they reach 1.5 kg. Well babies weighing more than 2.0 kg at birth usually toler-ate 2–3 hourly feeds during the first 24 hours of life. Whenever nasogastric feeding is started, the position of the nasogastric tube should be checked radiologically, by injecting air while listening over the stomach, or by aspirating acid stomach contents.

Table 4.6 Volumes of milk

(a) Volumes of milk given to healthy premature or SFD babies	
Day 1 (of life)	60 ml/kg
Day 2	90 ml/kg
Day 3	120 ml/kg
Day 4	150 ml/kg
Day 10	180 ml/kg
Day 14 (if required)	200 ml/kg

(b) Volumes of milk to give to LBW babies recovering from severe neonatal illness	
Day 1 (of life or from start of feeding)	20 ml/kg
Day 2	40 ml/kg
Day 3	60 ml/kg
Day 4	80 ml/kg
Day 5	100 ml/kg
Day 6	120 ml/kg
Day 7	150 ml/kg

Then as above.

Sustained nipple feeding (breast or bottle) is rarely possible in babies of less than 34 weeks; but putting a much less mature baby to the breast, even briefly, will boost the mother's morale enormously. Non-nutritive sucking from a dummy helps weight gain in all preterm babies and should be offered during tube feeds when the baby is awake and well enough.

SICK LBW BABIES

Certain important generalizations govern the feeding of these babies:

1. The baby less than 32 weeks gestation has caloric reserves for only 4–5 days' extrauterine existence, and enough glycogen for only a few hours.
2. An adequate caloric intake is necessary to prevent hypoglycaemia and jaundice, and may be one of the factors that affects neurological handicap in survivors.
3. The sooner a baby puts on weight, the sooner he recovers from serious neonatal illness, e.g. severe RDS.
4. If oral feeds are not tolerated or are contraindicated, intravenous feeding should be started within 3–4 days, especially in sick babies weighing less than 1.5 kg.
5. Although milk is good for premature babies it can also do harm (Table 4.7). Sick babies, especially in the first phase of their illness, have an ileus and to feed such babies is not only dangerous but also a waste of milk.

Table 4.7 Dangers of milk feeding in premature babies

Danger	Complication
Pooling in stomach	Regurgitation and aspiration
Compromised respiratory function (partly due to gastric distension and partly due to nasal obstruction)	Recurrent apnoea $\downarrow$ PaO_2 $\downarrow$ FRC
Introduction of infection (?due to indwelling tube)	Gastroenteritis Necrotising enterocolitis
Electrolyte imbalance	Hyponatraemia Acidaemia Hypophosphataemia
Milk bolus obstruction	Gut perforation

6. If enteral feeding is given to symptomatic LBW babies in the absence of an ileus, it can usually be given hourly through an indwelling nasogastric tube. In these babies the smaller volumes indicated in Table 4.6(b) should be used, and the volumes may need to be built up even more slowly at, for instance, no more than 0.5–1.0 ml per day.

7. The stomach contents must be aspirated every 4–6 hours once feeding has commenced.

8. Even when enteral feeding is established electrolyte disturbances such as hyponatraemia and hypophosphataemia may still occur and make the baby hypotonic and, for example, difficult to wean off IPPV. Serum chemistry should be checked at least weekly and, if necessary, appropriate supplements given.

9. Enteral feeds should be stopped:
   (a) When the gastric aspirate every 3–4 hours is consistently larger than the volume of milk given (except with minimal enteral feeding) or the aspirate is "dirty" – e.g. blood or bile stained.
   (b) If there are signs of intestinal obstruction (p. 396–397).
   (c) If feeding triggers apnoeic attacks.
   (d) For 12 hours post-extubation.
   (e) In babies who are having repeated convulsions.
   (f) In babies suspected of inborn errors of metabolism (Chapter 18).
   (g) During exchange transfusion.

If nasogastric tube feeding is not being tolerated, the following can be tried:

Posture

Babies' stomachs empty better if they lie on their right side or are lying prone.

Continuous infusion of milk through a nasogastric tube

Although a recent RCT (Schanler *et al.* 1999) showed no benefit from continuous NG feeds, a large body of clinical experience suggests that this method is often better tolerated when trying to establish feeds in VLBW neonates. The most satisfactory technique is to use a syringe pump to infuse the milk down the NG tube. A new supply of milk should be started every 6–8 hours. Some of the fat in the milk may adhere to the side of the tubes, thereby reducing the caloric intake.

Nasojejunal tube feeding

There is no point in using nasojejunal feeding routinely since not only is it more difficult to set up, but it aggravates the steatorrhoea of prematurity (*v.s.*) and may also increase the risk of gut infection and NEC (p. 386). It should therefore only be used if NG tube feeding results in persistent regurgitation and/or apnoea. Silastic tubes should be used. To pass them through the stomach into the duodenum, either use an introducer, or wait until the tube is carried through the pylorus by peristalsis. The position of the tube should be confirmed radiologically, and the milk given as a continuous infusion using a syringe pump. A nasogastric tube should be left *in situ* to detect regurgitation of milk back through the pylorus.

Intravenous glucose electrolyte solutions (Chapter 3)

In the short term (the first 2–4 days) this is the usual method of hydrating a baby and giving him some calories during the acute phase of any neonatal illness.

Intravenous feeding

This technique can be life saving for the baby in whom enteral feeding is going to be impossible for a period longer than 2–3 days. It is described in detail in Chapter 5.

FEEDING PROBLEMS

FAILURE TO THRIVE

Otherwise healthy premature babies may fail to gain weight at the ideal rate of 15 g/kg/24 h. The various causes for this are:

1. An inadequate protein or caloric intake (see above). This is particularly likely to occur when using banked milk derived from drip breast milk. There are four courses of action:
   (a) use a high protein "preterm" formula;
   (b) add a breast milk fortifier;
   (c) increase the intake of bank milk to 250 ml/kg/24 h;
   (d) accept the lower weight gain in exchange for the putative biological benefits of breast milk.

2. Metabolic acidaemia. Some babies develop a metabolic acidaemia (8–10 mmol/l or greater) due to their inability to excrete the hydrogen ions produced by growth and bone formation, the breakdown of nitrogen and sulphur from the amino acids in ingested protein, and the incomplete oxygenation of organic acids. All babies with poor weight gain should have their blood gases measured, and if acidaemia is confirmed, it should be treated with oral sodium bicarbonate (2–4 mmol/kg/24 h).
3. Occult urinary infection – check the urine (p.251).
4. Anaemia of prematurity (p. 437).
5. Cold stress (p. 121) – babies nursed in temperatures below thermoneutrality burn calories to sustain their body temperature.
6. CLD (p. 208).
7. The baby is "biologically" small – often very SFD at delivery.
8. All the causes of failure to thrive in older babies:
    (a) brain damage;
    (b) congenital heart disease with heart failure;
    (c) steatorrhoea, e.g. cystic fibrosis;
    (d) endocrinopathy, e.g. hypothydroidism.

Appropriate investigations for these conditions can be carried out if the more common causes of failure to thrive have been excluded and weight gain remains poor.

Following the publication of the results of Lucas *et al.* (1984), which showed that preterm formulas with their high caloric and protein content resulted in babies gaining weight faster and going home sooner, there has been a tendency to go on adding more and more caloric supplements to the feeds if convalescing babies are not gaining weight fast enough. This temptation should be resisted, unless there is clear evidence for malabsorption. It may also occasionally be justified in babies with CLD (p. 208).

EXCESS WEIGHT GAIN

Weight gain of more than 15 g/kg/day may be due to fluid retention in heart failure and renal disease, and is seen as part of the cor pulmonale that accompanies CLD (p. 203). Much more often however, such weight gain is merely catch-up growth in babies who have been ill for a long time, and are at last getting an adequate caloric intake. Such babies may also appear puffy with periorbital oedema and pitting oedema of their legs, since much of the weight gained may be water (Yeh *et al.* 1989). In the absence of other signs of heart failure this is a *normal* finding, and there is no need to reduce the feeds, or (worse still) give diuretics.

REFERENCES

American Academy of Pediatrics (1994) The transfer of drugs and other chemicals into breast milk. *Pediatrics* **93**: 137–150.

Bishop, N. (1999) Metabolic bone disease. In: *Textbook of Neonatology* 3rd edn. Rennie, J.M. and Roberton, N.R.C. (eds). Churchill Livingstone, Edinburgh, pp. 1002–1008.

Bishop, N., Morley, R., Day, J.P. and Lucas, A. (1997) Aluminium neurotoxicity in preterm infants receiving intravenous feeding solutions. *New England Journal of Medicine* **336**: 1557–1561.

Dunn, L.D., Halman, S., Weiner, J. and Kliegman, R. (1988) Beneficial effects of early hypocaloric enteral feeding on neonatal gastrointestinal tract function. Preliminary report of a randomized trial. *Journal of Pediatrics* **112**: 622–629.

Evans, T.J., Ryley, H.C., Neale, L.M., Dodge, J.A. and Lewarne, V. M. (1978) Effect of storage and heat on antimicrobial proteins in human milk. *Archives of Disease in Childhood* **53**: 239–241.

Fell, J.M.E., Reynolds, A.P., Meadows, N., Khan, K., Long, S.G., Quaghebur, G., Taylor, W.J. and Milla, P.J. (1996) Manganese toxicity in children receiving long term parenteral nutrition. *Lancet* **347**: 1218–1221.

Fewtrell, M. and Lucas, A (1999) Infant feeding. In: *Textbook of Neonatology,* 3rd edn. Rennie, J.M. and Roberton, N.R.C. (eds). Churchill Livingstone, Edinburgh, pp 305–348.

Hackett, G., Campbell, S. and Gamsu, H. (1987) Doppler studies in the growth retarded fetus and prediction of necrotising enterocolitis. *British Medical Journal* **294**: 13–17.

Hay, W.W. Jr (1991) Neonatal nutrition and metabolism. Mosby Year Book, St Louis, Missouri.

Howard, C.R. and Lawrence, R.A. (1999) Drugs and breastfeeding. *Clinics in Perinatology* **26**: 447–478.

Lawrence, R.A. and Howard, C.R. (1999) Given the benefits of breastfeeding, are there any contraindications? *Clinics in Perinatology* **26**: 479–490.

Lemons, J. A., Moyle, L., Hall, D. and Simmons, M. (1982) Differences in the composition of preterm and term human milk during early lactation. *Pediatric Research* **16**: 113–118.

Lucas, A. and Cole, T.J. (1990) Breast milk and neonatal necrotizing enterocolitis. *Lancet* **336**: 1519–1523.

Lucas, A., Gibbs, J.A.H. and Baum, J.D. (1978) Biology of human drip breast milk. *Early Human Development* **2**: 351–361.

Lucas, A., Gore, S.M., Cole, T.J. *et al.* (1984) Multicentre trial on feeding low birth weight infants: effect of diet on early growth. *Archives of Disease in Childhood* **59**: 722–730.

Lucas, A., Morley, R., Cole, T.J. *et al.* (1990) Early diet in premature babies and developmental status at 18 months. *Lancet* **335**: 1477–1481.

Oxtoby, M.J. (1988) Human immunodeficiency virus and other viruses in human milk, placing the viruses in broader perspective. *Pediatric Infectious Disease Journal* **7**: 825–835.

Raiha, N.C., Heinonen, K., Rassin, K. and Gaull, G.E. (1976) Milk protein quantity and quality in low birth weight infants; I – metabolic responses and effect on growth. *Pediatrics* **57**: 659–674.

Saarinen, U.M. and Siimes, M.A. (1979) Iron absorption from breast milk, cow's milk and iron supplemented formula. *Pediatric Research* **13**: 143–147.

Schanler, R.J., Shulman, R.J., Lau, C., Smith, E. O'B. and Heitkemper, M.M. (1999) Feeding strategies for premature infants: randomized trial of gastrointestinal priming and tube feeding method. *Pediatrics* **103**: 434–439.

Tsang, R.C., Lucas, A., Uauy, R. and Zlotkin, S. (1993) *Nutritional Needs of the Preterm Infant.* Williams and Wilkins, Baltimore.

Yeh, T.F., McClenan, D.A., Njayi, O.A. and Pildes, R.S. (1989) Metabolic rate and energy balance in infants with bronchopulmonary dysplasia. *Journal of Pediatrics* **114**: 448–451.

5

PARENTERAL NUTRITION

- *Total parenteral nutrition can be lifesaving, but is associated with complications and is always second best to enteral nutrition.*
- *TPN should be considered in VLBWI by 2–3 days if enteral nutrition is not being tolerated.*
- *TPN should be used with caution in critically ill babies, particularly VLBWI during the first days.*
- *TPN should only be administered with full pharmacy support, sterile manufacture, and biochemical monitoring.*

The caloric reserves of the neonate weighing 1.0 kg will sustain him for only 4–5 days in the absence of feeding. Giving 10% dextrose (40 kcal/100 ml) will prolong survival to some extent, but neonates who, for any reason, are still unable to tolerate enteral feeds by 3–4 days of age require some source of nitrogen and additional calories.

Full TPN – that is providing all the fat, protein, carbohydrate, vitamins, minerals and calories to support normal growth – has proved invaluable in babies who have major gastrointestinal disease which preclude enteral feeding for weeks or months (Chapters 24 and 25).

Supplementary parenteral nutrition, that is supplying, in particular protein, but also additional calories in the form of carbohydrate and fat, is now widely used in many VLBW babies such as those with severe ventilator dependent RDS whilst milk feeds are slowly introduced. No prospective study has shown short- or long-term benefits from the practice other than earlier weight gain.

Undertaking any form of intravenous nutrition demands the support of skilled personnel in pharmacy, dietetics and biochemistry, as well as the appropriate technical experience and equipment on the neonatal unit to maintain long lines (*v.i.*) and infuse small quantities accurately over prolonged periods of time.

INDICATIONS FOR IV FEEDING

Yu (1999) gives this as "the neonate whose feeding via the enteral route is impossible, inadequate or hazardous because of malformation, disease or immaturity, and in whom this state is likely to be prolonged and pose a serious threat to life and health".

CONTRAINDICATIONS TO IV FEEDING

Total parenteral nutrition should not be given during the acute phase of any illness. This includes the first 2–3 days of life in babies ventilated for RDS, or the first few days after diagnosis in babies with sepsis or NEC. Thrombocytopenia ($<50 \times 10^9$/l) and jaundice (>200 μmol/l) are often regarded as contraindications to intravenous fat because of its rare effect in reducing platelet numbers, or its potential to displace bilirubin from albumin. These anxieties are probably overstated. If the urea or creatinine is raised, as in renal failure of any cause, it is prudent to restrict the protein intake.

COMPOSITION OF PARENTERAL NUTRITION SOLUTIONS

Although this topic can be made extremely complicated, it can be broken down to a few very simple basic rules.

CARBOHYDRATE

Most neonates need at least 4–6 mg glucose/kg/min ($\cong$ 58–86 ml of 10% dextrose/kg/24 h), but larger volumes or more concentrated solutions can be used if they are tolerated (i.e. blood glucose <6–7 mmol/l; no glycosuria) to increase the caloric intake. Many babies will tolerate 12 mg/kg/min ($\cong$ 130 ml of 12.5% dextrose/kg/24 h) or more if the infusion rate is built up slowly over a period of days.

PROTEIN

The protein solutions now used are mixtures of pure l-isomers of amino acids (Table 5.1). Various solutions are available, and the newer "designer" solutions Vaminolact (formerly Infant Vamin) and Primene are probably the best choice. These solutions are certainly well tolerated although the ideal amino acid solution for preterm

Table 5.1 Composition of amino acid solutions available for use in the newborn. Composition per litre of fluid

Content per litre	Vamin 9 glucose (Pharmacia)	Primene 10% (Baxter Healthcare)	Vaminolact (Pharmacia)
Nitrogen (g)	9.4 (= 57.5 g first class protein)	15	9.3
energy (kcal/Mj)	650/2.7	250/1.05	240
sodium (mmol)	50	0	0
potassium (mmol)	20	0	0
magnesium (mmol)	1.5	0	0
calcium (mmol)	2.5	0	0
acetate(mmol)	0	25	0
chloride (mmol)	50	15.6	0
glucose (g)	100	0	0
osmolarity	1350	780	510
isoleucine	3.9 g	6.7 g	3.1 g
leucine	5.3 g	10.0 g	7.0 g
alanine	3.0 g	8.0 g	6.3 g
arginine	3.3 g	8.4 g	4.1 g
aspartic acid	4.1 g	6.0 g	4.1 g
glutamic acid	9.0 g	10.0 g	7.1 g
glycine	2.1 g	4.0 g	2.1 g
lysine	3.9 g	11.0 g	5.6 g
phenylalanine	5.5 g	4.2 g	2.7 g
proline	8.1 g	3.0 g	5.6 g
serine	7.5 g	4.0 g	3.8 g
methionine	1.9 g	2.4 g	1.3 g
threonine	3.0 g	3.7 g	3.6 g
tyrosine	0.5 g	0.45 g	0.5 g
histidine	2.4 g	3.8 g	2.1 g
tryptophan	1.0 g	2.0 g	1.4 g
valine	4.3 g	7.6 g	3.6 g
cysteine	1.4 g	1.89 g	1.0 g
taurine		0.6 g	0.3 g

babies has yet to be found. Trophamine, which is available in the USA and on the Continent, also has an acceptable composition. Vaminolact and Primene are electrolyte-free which makes it easier to tailor the electrolyte requirements to the individual baby.

It is not usually advisable to give more than 3.0–3.5 g protein/kg/24 h because of the risks of hyperammonaemia, acidaemia and hyperaminoacidaemia. It is usual to start by giving

1.0–1.5 g/kg/24 h, building up to 3.0 g/kg/24 h over several days. This corresponds to 30 ml/kg/24 h of Vaminolact or Primene. In sick preterm babies it may take up to 7 days before the full dose of protein is tolerated. To convert grams of nitrogen to grams of protein multiply by 6.25.

FAT

The provision of fat is essential if an adequate caloric intake is to be achieved in total parenteral nutrition. Although much clinical experience suggests that intravenous fat is well tolerated by ill VLBW neonates, anxieties remain that it may increase the risk of lung damage (Sosenko *et al.* 1993) and CONS sepsis (Freeman *et al.* 1990). For these reasons in the ill VLBWI, intralipid should be given initially at no more than 0.5–1.0 g/kg/24 h (2.5–5.0 ml/kg/24 h of 20% intralipid) and should probably not exceed 2 g/kg/24 h (10 ml/kg/24 h of 20% intralipid) in babies on IPPV for severe lung disease.

Even term babies receiving TPN for surgical problems rarely tolerate (or need) more than 3 g/kg/24 h (15 ml/kg/24 h of 20% intralipid) and in VLBW babies infusing more lipid may increase the incidence of CLD (Cooke 1991).

Intralipid is made from soybean oil and does not have the optimum linoleic:linolenic acid ratio for the newborn brain but it is the only product that is readily available at present. 20% intralipid is better tolerated than the 10% preparation. Using the above regimen intralipid is well tolerated; monitoring is best done with serum triglyceride levels, as plasma turbidity is a poor indicator of triglycerides (Yu 1999). The infusion rate should be reduced if the plasma triglyceride concentration exceeds 1.8 mmol/l, and certainly if it is higher than 3 mmol/l.

PROTEIN CALORIE: NON-PROTEIN CALORIE RATIO

This should be kept in the range of 1:8–1:10. Values less than 1:6 are likely to result in hyperaminoacidaemia and aminoaciduria.

VITAMINS AND TRACE ELEMENTS

If some enteral feeding is tolerated, i.e. supplemental parenteral nutrition is being given, the neonate will receive adequate trace minerals orally and can be given a standard oral vitamin supplement

Table 5.2 Contents of one 10 ml vial of Peditrace

Mineral	Amount in micrograms	Amount in micromol
Zinc	2500	38.2
Copper	200	3.15
Manganese	10	182
Selenium	20	253
Iodine	570	30

(e.g. Abidec). If TPN is to continue for more than 2 weeks then some trace elements will be required. These are zinc, selenium, copper and manganese. Iron supplementation is not required as preterm neonates receive frequent top-up transfusions. Copper and manganese should be witheld if biliary stasis is present. We use Peditrace (Table 5.2): the older Pedel contained too much manganese for preterm babies.

Solivito and Vitlipid are used to provide water and fat-soluble vitamins respectively (see Tables 5.3 and 5.4 for composition). The dose of Solivito is 0.5 ml/kg/day to a maximum of 5 ml in 24 hours, and

Table 5.3 Composition of 1 ml of Solivito (water soluble vitamins)

Vitamin	Amount
Vitamin B_1	3 mg
Vitamin B_2	3.6 mg
Nicotinamide	40 mg
Pantothenic acid	15 mg
Vitamin B_6	4 mg
Vitamin C	100 mg
Biotin	60 µg
Folic acid	0.4 mg
Vitamin B_{12}	5 µg

Table 5.4 Composition of 1 ml of Vitlipid

Vitamin	Amount
Vitamin A	230 i.u.
Vitamin D_2	1 µg
Vitamin E	0.64 mg
Vitamin K + emulsifying agents	20 µg

Vitlipid 1 ml/kg/day to a maximum of 10 ml in 24 hours. Large amounts of vitamin D and E are lost by adherence to the plastic of the tubing. These vitamins should be added as soon as TPN is begun.

ELECTROLYTES

These are prescribed on a daily basis according to the guidelines outlined in Chapter 3. Sodium and potassium are added as chlorides; this results in a hyperchloraemia when large amounts of sodium are given to replace losses in very preterm babies. A hyperchloraemic metabolic acidosis ensues, and the base deficit of babies given a proportion of their sodium requirement as sodium acetate was significantly reduced in one randomized controlled trial (Peters *et al.* 1997). These authors recommend that the daily dose of acetate should be kept to 6 mmol/kg/day when it is used in this way.

Calcium and phosphate pose major problems since their solubility product is readily exceeded and they precipitate out. Their solubility depends on the acidity of the solution, and thus mainly on the concentration of the protein solution; the higher the concentration of Vamin/Vaminolact/Primene, the larger the amount of calcium and phosphate that can be given. 1.5–2.2 mmol/kg/24 h of both calcium and phosphorus should be given in IV feeding solutions, starting with the lower dose and building up by 10% per day (Koo and Tsang 1992). The calcium should be given as calcium chloride to avoid the potentially neurotoxic concentrations of aluminium found as a contaminant in calcium gluconate preparations (Bishop *et al.* 1997).

Hypophosphataemia often develops in VLBW babies receiving TPN. If the phosphate remains below 0.8 mmol/l, the only practical solution is to give an infusion of IV phosphate using one of the formulations below (dissolved in 10% dextrose) and to stop the TPN for a few hours.

Recommendations regarding infusion:

maximum rate of potassium phosphate 0.5 mmol potassium/kg/h.
Aim to give about 0.5–1.0 mmol PO_4/kg in 12 hours.

Formulas currently available are:

Potassium phosphate 17.42%; 1 ml contains 2 mmol K and 1 mmol PO_4.
Sodium phosphate 2.5 mmol in 5 ml of monohydrogen phosphate.

Potassium acid phosphate 13.6%; 1 ml contains 1 mmol PO_4 and 1 mmol K.

Sodium glycerophosphate 1 ml contains 1 mmol PO_4 and 2 mmol Na (Costello *et al.* 1995).

INTRAVENOUS FEEDING SOLUTIONS

We use 10% Primene, and give fat as 20% Intralipid. The Primene is added to a glucose electrolyte solution by our pharmacy. The amount of Primene and the concentration of glucose and electrolytes are decided daily on the basis of the age of the baby, his tolerance of IV glucose, and in particular the desired caloric intake for the next 24 hours. Intralipid is included after the first day or so of TPN, bearing in mind the caveats outlined above. Water and fat-soluble vitamins, and trace elements, are added as discussed above. In common with most neonatal units, we no longer heparinize TPN following reports of the flocculation and destabilization of intralipid by heparin (Raupp *et al.* 1988), and because small babies can become anticoagulated if heparin is added to both TPN fluid and arterial lines. The former concern may be more theoretical than practical (Silvers *et al.* 1998), but in the past there were many reports of flocculation and creaming in neonatal TPN. If heparin is added to TPN in order to prolong the life of intravenous lines, then it must be stopped if the platelet count falls or the baby develops any bleeding problem.

ROUTE OF INFUSION

All the fluids used in intravenous feeding can be given through a peripheral vein. However, the fluids are very irritant and frequently thrombose the vessels. If extravasation occurs, permanent scarring may result. Thus, this route has limited application and should only be used for intravenous feeding lasting less than a week and for fluids with an osmolality less than 900 mosm/l (AAP 1982). Intravenous amino acids can be given safely through an umbilical artery catheter.

For long-term feeding, we prefer to use a long line sited in a major central vessel (p. 482–3). Because of the risk of introducing infection through an intravenous feeding line, it should never be used for anything other than the intravenous feeding solution. If we are merely aiming to supplement an ill, ventilated VLBW neonate with RDS, we would give the Primene/glucose solution outlined above from day 2–3. The concentration of Primene and glucose would be gradually increased over the next four days to the maximum, and we would add fat from the third or fourth day, so long as none of the contraindications were present.

Eventually in such a baby full TPN would be achieved if he had severe lung disease and was not tolerating any enteral milk. These babies, and those requiring full TPN for NEC or post-operative gut malformations, would then be receiving 30 ml/kg/day of Primene with 12.5% dextrose to provide about 12 mg/kg/min of glucose, plus Intralipid 3 g/kg/day giving approximately 100 kcal/kg/day. On this regimen the babies would receive adequate vitamin supplementation, as outlined above, and the electrolyte intake can be adjusted as required on a daily basis (Chapter 3). Trace elements are required when a baby receives prolonged TPN.

An additional peripheral infusion should be set up for intravenous antibiotics, blood transfusions, and other intravenous medications. Problems with flocculation do not occur with double lumen central catheters of the Broviac–Hickman type.

The nursing staff should change the giving sets on whatever intravenous device is used once daily. If connected to a central line this change should be carried out as a sterile procedure.

MONITORING OF IV FEEDING

The following should be monitored daily or twice daily

- Weight;
- Urinary glucose, blood glucose;
- Electrolytes;
- Haematocrit.

The following should be monitored at least weekly

- Magnesium;
- Calcium and phosphorus (daily in the first week);
- Bilirubin;
- Protein, albumin (daily in the first week);
- Liver enzymes; transaminases, alkaline phosphatase;
- Triglycerides;
- Blood gases;
- Haemoglobin, white count and platelets, CRP.

COMPLICATIONS OF TPN
(Yu and MacMahon 1992, Yu 1999)

CATHETER RELATED

Central lines are a potent cause of thrombosis in newborns, in whom venous obstruction is otherwise rare. If extravasated subcutaneously from a peripheral line, irritant TPN solutions can cause unsightly scarring. Extravasation from central lines into all sorts of spaces has been described (p. 473).

METABOLIC

Hyperglycaemia is common; although tolerance to the high glucose infusion rates required to give an adequate calorie input can be achieved if the concentration is built up slowly. Sometimes insulin has to be used. Hyperammonaemia also occurs, and urea should be monitored and kept below 6 mmol/l. Hyperchloraemic metabolic acidosis has already been discussed (p. 56). High phenylalanine levels have been detected in babies receiving amino acid solutions, but so far no adverse effect on outcome has been demonstrated.

CHOLESTATIC JAUNDICE

About a third of preterm babies who receive TPN for more than 2 weeks develop jaundice (p. 426), and this figure rises to 80% after 2 months of TPN. Biliary sludging and calculi may develop. In most cases the jaundice resolves once enteral feeding is established, but in some it progresses to cirrhosis and liver failure. Factors that increase the incidence of this complication are prematurity, duration of TPN, sepsis and surgery (Teitelbaum 1997).

INFECTION

This is the major complication of TPN, and can lead to the removal of precious central lines. The risk of infection can be minimized by a meticulously aseptic insertion technique, and rigorous adherence to the rule about not using the line for anything other than TPN.

Infection may be suspected on the basis of the routine weekly blood tests, or it may present with an insidious deterioration in the baby's condition, often accompanied by a low-grade pyrexia, changes in the WBC, a falling platelet count and a rise in CRP (p.

233). Occasionally the baby develops a full-blown septicaemic illness.

The usual pathogen isolated when there is a gradual deterioration is CONS (Freeman *et al.* 1990). If use of the long line is not essential, the safest course of action is to remove it, and to treat the baby with flucloxacillin, vancomycin or teicoplanin. If the line is crucial, and CONS is grown, it is well worth trying the effect of parenteral antibiotics given through the line, and in extreme difficulty adding Urokinase to the infusate for 24 hours (Fishbein *et al.* 1990). For more pathogenic bacteria, or for fungal infections arising from the line, there is probably no alternative but to remove it, in addition to vigorous treatment of the infection.

REFERENCES

American Academy of Pediatrics (1982) Commentary on parenteral nutrition. *Pediatrics* **71**: 547–552.

Bishop, N.J., Morley, R., Day, J.P. and Lucas, A. (1997) Aluminium neurotoxicity in preterm infants receiving intravenous feeding solutions. *New England Journal of Medicine* **336**: 1557–1561.

Cooke, R.W.I. (1991) Factors associated with chronic lung disease in preterm infants. *Archives of Disease in Childhood* **66**: 776–779.

Costello, I., Powell, C. and Williams, A.F. (1995) Sodium glycerophosphate in the treatment of neonatal hypophosphataemia. *Archives of Disease in Childhood* **73**: F44–F45.

Fishbein, J.D., Friedman, H.S., Bennett, B.B. and Falletta, J.M. (1990) Catheter related sepsis refractory to antibiotics treated successfully with adjunctive urokinase infusion. *Pediatric Infections Disease Journal* **9**: 676–678.

Freeman, J., Goldman, D.A., Smith, N.E., Sidebottom, D.G., Epstein, M.F. and Platt, R. (1990) Association of intravenous lipid emulsion and coagulase negative staphylococcal bacteremia in neonatal intensive care units. *New England Journal of Medicine* **323**: 301–308.

Koo, W.W.K. and Tsang, R.C. (1992) Calcium, phosphorus, magnesium and vitamin D requirements of infants receiving parenteral nutrition. In: *Intravenous Feeding of the Neonate*, Yu, V.Y.H. and MacMahon, R.A. (eds). Edward Arnold, London and Melbourne, pp. 68–75.

Peters, O., Ryan, S., Matthew, L., Cheng, K. and Lunn, J. (1997) Randomized controlled trial of acetate in neonates receiving parenteral nutrition. *Archives of Disease in Childhood* **77**: F12–F15.

Raupp, P., von Kries, R., Schmidt, E., Pfahl, H-G. and Gunther, O. (1988) Incompatability between fat emulsion and calcium plus heparin in parenteral nutrition of premature babies. *Lancet* **i**: 700.

Silvers, K.M., Darlow, B. and Winterbourn, C.C. (1998) Pharmacologic levels of heparin do not destabilize neonatal parenteral nutrition. *Journal of Pediatric and Enteral Nutrition* **22**: 311–314.

Sosenko, I.R.S., Rodriguez-Pierce, M. and Bancalari, E. (1993) Effect of early initiation of intravenous lipid administration on the incidence and severity of chronic lung disease in premature infants. *Journal of Pediatrics* **123**: 975–982.

Teitelbaum, D.H. (1997) Parenteral nutrition associated cholestasis. *Current Opinion in Pediatrics* **9**: 270–275.

Yu, V.Y.H. (1999) Parenteral nutrition in the newborn. In: *Textbook of Neonatology*, 3rd edn, Rennie, J.M. and Roberton, N.R.C. (eds) Churchill Livingstone, Edinburgh, pp.349–358.

Yu, V.Y.H. and MacMahon, R.A. (eds) (1992) *Intravenous Feeding of the Neonate*. Edward Arnold, London and Melbourne, 68–75.

FURTHER READING

Yu, V.Y.H. (1999) Parenteral nutrition in the newborn. In: *Textbook of Neonatology*, 3rd edn. Rennie, J.M. and Roberton, N.R.C. (eds) Churchill Livingstone, Edinburgh, pp.349–358.

6

RESUSCITATION OF THE NEWBORN

- *Most babies do not need any resuscitation or suction.*
- *Most babies who are depressed at birth respond to bag and mask ventilation given properly.*
- *Babies who are not responding quickly to bag and mask ventilation (by 3 minutes) should be intubated, and help will be required.*
- *Babies <30 weeks gestation are at risk from RDS, and unless they are vigorous at birth should be intubated for resuscitation and given surfactant prophylaxis as early as possible.*
- *"Blind" drug therapy should not be given during resuscitation except in asystolic babies.*

Only a small percentage of newborn babies are not pink, vigorous and howling lustily by 1–2 minutes of age. About 5% of all babies born are apnoeic at 1 minute of age, and 0.5–1.0% will need intubation in the delivery room. In general, babies who need resuscitation fall into four groups:

1. those who make no respiratory effort at all;
2. those who make feeble and inadequate respiratory efforts, and remain cyanosed and bradycardic;
3. those who remain cyanosed despite vigorous respiratory efforts;
4. those with primary disorders of muscle or the CNS.

In about 70% of cases the birth of a baby who will require resuscitation can be predicted because there is a complication of pregnancy or labour. A neonatal paediatrician should always be present at such deliveries (Table 6.1). The workload generated by attending such deliveries, which are followed by about 78% of the total yield of one minute Apgar scores less than 7, is attendance at about 37% of all deliveries (Primhak *et al.* 1984). The corollary of this is that 20–30% of babies who require resuscitation are unexpectedly depressed. The implication of these data for those undertaking delivery in isolated maternity units or at home is clear.

Table 6.1 Deliveries which should be attended by a paediatrician with training and experience in neonatal resuscitation

Gestation less than 36 weeks
Instrumental or surgical deliveries (excluding "lift-out" forceps or elective caesarean section under epidural anaesthesia)
Malpresentations
Twins and higher multiple deliveries
Fetal distress and meconium staining (p. 180)
Antenatal diagnosis of fetal malformation
Antenatal diagnosis of blood group incompatability e.g. Rhesus
The accoucheur requests the presence of a paediatrician

Table 6.2 Factors other than asphyxia which may delay the onset of respiration after birth

Drugs depressing the CNS
Trauma — especially of the CNS
Prematurity — in particular surfactant deficient, stiff lungs
Sepsis — classically early onset group B streptococcal sepsis (p. 239)
Maternal hypocapnia from overbreathing
Muscle weakness, due to prematurity or primary muscle disease
Anaemia (e.g. fetal haemorrhage)
Previous neurological damage *in utero*
Congenital malformations affecting the airway or preventing lung expansion

CAUSES OF DELAYED ONSET OF REGULAR RESPIRATION

Many factors other than asphyxia can delay the onset of respiration after delivery (Table 6.2); several of these may be present in a single baby.

It is crucial to recognize that even if the delayed onset of respiration is *not* the result of asphyxia, adequate resuscitation must nevertheless be carried out at once, or else all of the biochemical and clinical consequences of asphyxia will develop very quickly.

PHYSIOLOGY OF ASPHYXIA

In order to understand the effects of asphyxia on both the fetus and the neonate, and in particular its role in delaying the onset of spontaneous respiration, it is helpful to consider chronic partial asphyxia and acute asphyxia separately.

CHRONIC PARTIAL ASPHYXIA

A frequent clinical problem is the previously normal baby who suffers recurrent episodes of partial asphyxia during labour. This can be due to declining placental function with postmaturity or just the contractions of labour. There may be oxytocin induced hypertonic and incoordinate uterine contraction, or recurrent episodes of umbilical cord occlusion due to entanglement round a fetal part. During such episodes the fetus initially increases his blood pressure, then becomes bradycardic, and the cardiac output is concentrated on the placenta, brain and myocardium. The fetal PaO_2 falls, and energy is produced by anaerobic metabolism of glycogen and glucose to lactate. Since the $PaCO_2$ also rises, a combined metabolic and respiratory acidaemia develops. These episodes may be transient and/or infrequent, in which case the fetus makes a complete "clinical" and biochemical recovery before the next episode, or before delivery. If such a baby is delivered at this stage, his respiration may be depressed, but he will usually respond promptly to resuscitation and have few if any sequelae.

If these episodes persist or are prolonged the fetus no longer recovers between each one, and he gradually becomes hypotensive and profoundly acidaemic. Damage to many organ systems, including the brain, will occur as a result of ischaemia. In this situation, severe neonatal illness and/or permanent neurological sequelae may result despite prompt resuscitation after delivery.

Obstetric data suggest that such changes have to persist for about an hour before the fetal defence mechanisms are overwhelmed, cardiac output falls and ischaemic brain damage occurs (Low 1993).

ACUTE ASPHYXIA

In clinical practice this is relatively rare, but study of acute total asphyxia in animals has been very useful in advancing our understanding of the pathophysiology of asphyxia and our management of it. In newborn monkeys delivered in good condition by caesarean section, and then asphyxiated before the onset of breathing by sealing their heads in a bag of saline, after a few shallow "breaths" without achieving any gas exchange, the animals stop "breathing". This period of "primary" apnoea may last 10 minutes. However, after 1–2 minutes in primary apnoea most animals start to gasp with increasing frequency and vigour, and then with decreasing frequency and vigour until they literally reach the last gasp. Gasping lasts for 5–10 minutes after which the animal is again apnoeic (Fig. 6.1). The whole process lasts about 20 minutes.

The heart rate falls rapidly after birth, rises slightly in primary apnoea and early in the phase of gasping, but then slows. Cardiac activity continues for 10 minutes or more after the last gasp. The period between the last gasp, and cardiac arrest, is known as

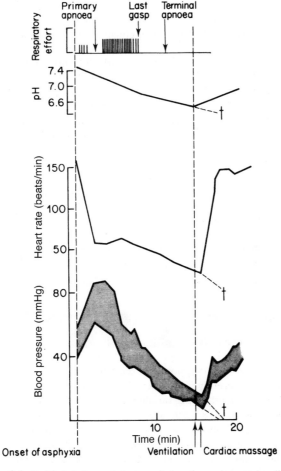

Figure 6.1 Physiological changes during resuscitation of a newborn monkey. (Adapted from Dawes *et al.*, 1963.)

secondary or terminal apnoea. The changes that occur in blood pressure are shown in Fig. 6.1. A severe mixed acidaemia develops; by the end of terminal apnoea in animals the $PaCO_2$ exceeds 13.5 kPa (100 mmHg), the H^+ exceeds 300 nmol/1 (pH <6.5) and the PaO_2 is unrecordable. Hyperkalaemia of more than 15 mmol/1 develops.

The neonatal primate can survive 20 minutes of complete oxygen deprivation. This is due to the large stores of glycogen in the brain, liver and myocardium which can produce energy by anaerobic glycolysis, and also to the ability of neonatal brain to metabolize lactate and ketones rather than glucose during hypoxia (Volpe 2001). Although primates can survive up to 20 minutes of anoxia, in the same experiments brain damage affecting primarily the basal ganglia and brainstem appeared within 10–12 minutes, probably due to anoxia before the heart fails and ischaemic organ damage occurs (Fig. 6.1).

The response to removing the bag of saline from the animal's head during the above experiment depends on the state of asphyxia. In primary apnoea, the apnoea will persist until some stimulus provokes gasping, when the animal will inhale air or oxygen, and soon develop regular respiration. If the animal is gasping when the bag is removed, air or oxygen enters its lungs and a regular respiratory pattern develops. If the bag is removed in terminal apnoea respiration will never occur. To resuscitate such an animal, positive pressure ventilation must be used. If the heart rate is very low (or has stopped), external cardiac massage will be necessary.

RELEVANCE OF ACUTE EXPERIMENTS TO CLINICAL NEONATAL CARE

There is no reason to suppose that the human neonate will respond to asphyxia differently to monkeys. The response of a human baby at birth will depend on the variables listed in Table 6.2, all of which will interact with the severity of the acidaemia. If, for example, there is some complication such as heavy sedation or prematurity, primary apnoea may be prolonged, or the gasping efforts may be too weak to establish alveolar ventilation. Severe intrapartum asphyxia can result in the delivery of a baby with an H^+ concentration above 100 nmol/1 (pH <7.0) who is limp, bradycardic and in terminal apnoea.

The animal experiments have provided other useful information, which help us to understand the behaviour and treatment of the human baby who is asphyxiated or apnoeic immediately after delivery. The main points are summarized below:

1. The onset of gasping, and therefore regular respiration, can be expedited in primary apnoea by peripheral stimuli, including rubbing the baby with a warm towel or giving him an intramuscular injection.
2. Drugs administered to the mother, including all commonly used sedatives, analgesics and anaesthetics, can pass to the fetus and may prolong primary apnoea to such an extent that the acidaemia becomes severe, and the phase of gasping may never occur.
3. In babies resuscitated from terminal apnoea, the time from the onset of artificial ventilation to either the first gasp or regular respiration is proportional to the severity of the asphyxia before ventilation was started (Fig. 6.2). If artificial ventilation started before the pH was depressed too far, the baby may be expected to gasp and start regular respiration after 3–4 minutes of IPPV. However, if resuscitation was started well into terminal apnoea when the H^+ concentration is likely to be above 150 mmol/l (pH

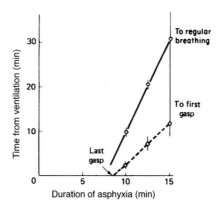

Figure 6.2 Time from beginning positive pressure ventilation with oxygen until first gasp (– – – –) and until the establishment of rhythmic breathing (———) in newly delivered rhesus monkeys asphyxiated for 10, 12.5 or 15 min at 30°C. The vertical bars indicate the standard errors of the means in each group of 5 or 6 monkeys. (From Adamsons *et al.*, 1964.)

<6.8) (Fig 6.1), gasping may be delayed for 20 minutes and regular respiration for over half an hour. Babies who have not started to breathe spontaneously 4–5 minutes after starting IPPV should, in the absence of other causes of neonatal respiratory depression, be assumed to have a very low pH.

4. Injections of Lobeline, Nikethamide or Vandid, or any other analeptic drug, are not only valueless but dangerous. Like immersion of the newborn alternately in hot and cold water, sealing him in a hyperbaric oxygen chamber, or stuffing a raven's beak in his rectum, they are unnecessarily painful and physiologically unsound methods of initiating respiration in primary apnoea. In terminal apnoea they cause a more rapid fall in blood pressure and heart rate, and thus earlier death, than would have occurred if the baby had been treated by masterly inactivity.

ASSESSMENT OF THE SEVERITY OF ASPHYXIA

THE APGAR SCORE

The traditional way of assessing the newborn is to use the score devised by Dr Virginia Apgar (1953). This grades five clinical features with scores from zero to 2 at one minute of age (Table 6.3).

Although the one minute score is not an index of asphyxia, it is undoubtedly an efficient measure of the overall condition of the baby, and the need for resuscitation. There are many causes for a baby having a low Apgar score at 1–2 minutes (Table 6.2) but whatever the cause, he requires active resuscitation as soon as possible.

The Apgar scores at 15 and 20 minutes are more strongly correlated with asphyxia and the likelihood of subsequent neurological deficits, and changes in the Apgar score from 0–20 minutes are an

Table 6.3 Apgar score

Score	0	1	2
A Appearance (colour)	Pale or blue	body pink but extremities blue	Pink
P Pulse rate	Absent	<100	>100
G Grimace (response to suction catheter)	Nil	Some	Cry
A Activity (muscle tone)	Limp	Some flexion	Well flexed
R Respiratory effort	Absent	Hypoventilation	Good

internationally understood shorthand for describing the success or otherwise of the resuscitative effort.

However, because of the limitations of the Apgar score, one should not merely state that the baby had an Apgar of 5 at one minute, but should also accurately describe the baby's condition. For instance:

> "At one minute the baby was apnoeic had blue hands and feet, a heart rate of 90 beats per minute and normal tone; he grimaced when sucked out."

or

> "At one minute the baby was pink with a heart rate of 120 bpm and gasped twice but he was limp and made no response to suction".

Both these situations equate to an Apgar of 5, but have entirely different clinical and physiological implications. The response to resuscitation should then be continued as a narrative in the baby's notes, ideally ending only with the information that the baby is pink, breathing normally and is active. Otherwise the narrative should end with an account that he is, at least, pink and stable and connected to a ventilator with a note of his blood glucose and blood gas result.

If the baby does not start to breathe, the crucial question is whether or not he is in primary or terminal apnoea. Babies in primary apnoea are usually in reasonable clinical condition with a heart rate near 100 beats/min, good peripheral perfusion and body tone, although centrally cyanosed and apnoeic (Apgar 5–7). Babies in terminal apnoea are more likely to be pale and apnoeic with little or no body tone or reflex response, and their heart rate is usually less than 60 (Apgar score 1–3).

However, in many babies this differentiation is not clear-cut, and if apnoea lasts for more than 2–3 minutes after delivery, active resuscitation is always indicated.

CORD BLOOD GAS ANALYSIS

Another way of assessing whether or not a baby is asphyxiated at the moment of birth is to measure the blood gases and pH in a sample drawn from the umbilical artery in a section of the umbilical cord clamped immediately after delivery. These data are usually available within 5–10 minutes, and then can be extremely useful in guiding the baby's subsequent management. Umbilical vein gases are less

Table 6.4 Normal cord blood results (From Helwig 1996)

	Mean	Standard deviation	2.5th centile
Artery pH	7.26	0.07	7.10
Artery base deficit (mmol/l)	4	3	11
Vein pH	7.34	0.06	7.20
Vein base deficit (mmol/l)	3	3	8

accurate than umbilical arterial pH. The umbilical vein pH is 0.01–0.1 pH points better than the umbilical artery result (Table 6.4); and in cord entanglement the umbilical vein pH may be normal, representing blood leaving the placenta, but the fetus distal to the cord obstruction may be severely acidaemic.

RESUSCITATION

PREPARATION

Do not be proud. If a very sick baby (or several babies) are expected, call for help. Do not wait for the baby to be born. In addition, ensure that you have adequate equipment and that it is in working order. Remember that a need for resuscitation in babies is primarily a respiratory problem; the heart continues to function long after breathing has ceased, and at worst needs a "bump start". The situation is very different from a cardiac arrest in an adult, which is usually due to heart disease. The strategy for resuscitation still follows the familiar A, B, C, D, which is taught for resuscitation at all ages, with the addition of E and F;

A airway
B breathing
C circulation
D drugs
E environment
F family

Equipment

The following equipment is needed:

1. An adequate shelf on which to lie the babies.
2. A supply of up to 5 1/min of air or oxygen for the face mask, bag

and mask, Y piece, or endotracheal tube. Whichever method of administering oxygen is used, the gas *must* be passed through a blow-off valve set at 30 cm/H_2O. Most babies can be resuscitated adequately with air. However oxygen is sometimes required and must always be available. Inevitably clinicians are at the mercy of the equipment manufacturing companies; ideally we should be able to vary the oxygen concentration between 20% and 100% at the turn of a knob. However if bag and mask systems are being used without modification they will give air. A bag and mask system with 5 l/min of oxygen attached delivers about 40% oxygen. Use of an oxygen reservoir hose increases the inspired oxygen to 60–70% (Hermansen and Prior 1993). This degree of variability is adequate for the vast majority of resuscitations. A Y piece resuscitation system attached directly to the oxygen supply via a pressure relief valve will deliver 100% oxygen.

3. Adequate suction with a soft end on the sucker. The suction should not exceed 200 mmHg and, for routine use, should be set at 100 mmHg ($\cong$ 136 cm H_2O) to prevent damage to the oropharyngeal mucosa. FG 3–4 suction tubes are needed to clear the ETT and FG 8–10 tubes to clear the airway and occasionally to empty the stomach.

4. An overhead radiant heat source, and sides to the resuscitation shelf to minimize the convective and radiant heat losses.

5. A clock with a second timer, since time passes very quickly in any emergency procedure.

6. A mask for blowing oxygen over the face of the cyanosed but breathing baby.

7. A bag suitable for attaching to the mask to give artificial ventilation in a non-breathing baby. A bag with a large reservoir is preferable; the Infant Laerdal bag has a reservoir of 500 ml which allows a long inspiratory time (Field *et al.* 1986). The bag and mask must be detachable in order that the mask can be replaced by a connector for an endotracheal tube. The bag and mask systems *must* be used in accordance with the manufacturer's instructions, otherwise dangerously high inflation pressures can be applied. The round, soft and flexible semi-transparent autoclavable silicone rubber "Laerdal" face mask is the most suitable (Palme *et al.* 1985). The hard, rigid moulded plastic Rendell–Baker masks are much less suitable.

8. An alternative to a self-inflating bag is to use a Y piece on the ETT or mask. This is connected to the oxygen supply via a suitable pressure control system with a manometer in the circuit

for pressure monitoring. A baby must *never* be connected directly to an unlimited pressurized oxygen or air supply. This can result in severe and possibly fatal lung damage.

9. A selection of baby-size oropharyngeal airways (sizes 00 and 000).

10. At least two laryngoscopes (since one may fail at the crucial moment). Which blade to have on the laryngoscope is a matter of individual preference, but generally speaking a straight-bladed one of the Wisconsin, Magill or Oxford Infant type is best.

11. A selection of endotracheal tubes (2.5, 3.0 and 3.5 mm), either oral or nasal. Oral tubes with a shoulder are easiest to insert. Endotracheal tube introducers are very occasionally needed.

12. Magill forceps for nasoendotracheal tubes.

13. Appropriate devices for connecting the ETT to the resuscitation bag, and for securing the tube to a hat or the baby's face.

14. A selection of syringes, needles and specimen bottles.

15. Adhesive tape and a large pair of scissors.

16. A stethoscope.

17. Equipment for emergency cannulation of the umbilical vessels and a thoracentesis set.

18. ECG monitor and pulse oximeter.

Drugs

Only the following drugs are required on the trolley:

Adrenaline 1:1000 (1mg/ml)	1 ml ampoules
and 1:10 000 (100 microg/ml)	1 ml ampoules
Sodium bicarbonate (4.2%, 7.5% or 8.4%)	10 ml ampoules
THAM 7%	10 ml ampoules
Normal saline	10 ml ampoules
10% dextrose	10 ml ampoules
Naloxone 0.4 mg/ml (Adult)	2 ml ampoules
Vitamin K	1 mg ampoules

A small box should be included containing the following drugs which are occasionally needed in emergencies – frusemide, calcium gluconate, atropine. Heparin (1000 units/ml) for anticoagulation of blood gas syringes and arterial or venous catheters should be kept in the labour ward fridge. There should be an emergency unit of universal donor O negative blood, also kept on the labour ward.

Checklist

When preparing for a resuscitation always run through the following checklist:

1. Introduce yourself to the mother and her partner; the sudden arrival of an unknown crowd of people into the delivery room after a long day in labour can be very unnerving for the mother.
2. Read the mother's notes and obtain a history from the midwife or obstetrician about her medical/obstetric past – including the reasons for any surgical delivery, and a list of all drugs she has received during pregnancy and labour.
3. Send for help straight away if you assess the situation as being likely to result in a severely depressed or malformed infant.
4. Ensure that the resuscitaire oxygen is turned on and working. Test bag, set the blow-off pressure to 30 cm H_2O. Ambu bags, in particular, have blow-off valves which can stick. Check Y piece pressure manometer setting, if applicable. Check that there are compatible connectors available for masks and endotracheal tubes.
5. Check that the clock is working (remember, some resuscitaire clocks are still clockwork and need winding up).
6. Check that the suction is working at pressure of 100 mmHg and that a good-sized sterile suction catheter is attached.
7. Go round and close all the doors and windows and turn off fans near the resuscitation trolley. The labour ward staff will hate you, but it is important to do this to prevent the baby becoming profoundly hypothermic, particularly if he is premature. The ideal room temperature for babies is 25°C, uncomfortable for most adults.
8. Make sure there are warmed dry towels to wrap the baby in during resuscitation and a hat for premature babies.
9. Wash your hands, put on gloves (goggles for high risk cases).

INITIAL ASSESSMENT OF THE BABY

Start the clock the moment the baby is free from the mother's body (not when the cord is clamped).

Receive the baby. Dry him, throw away any wet towels and cover him with a warm dry towel.

Assess the heart rate, respiration, colour and tone as soon as possible. For heart rate listen with a stethoscope – do *not* feel the cord, since all you feel is your own heart beat pounding away in your fingertips.

The baby will fall into one of four groups:

1. fit and healthy, bawling lustily;
2. not breathing too well, but no immediate need for panic (5–6%);
3. probable terminal apnoea – pale, limp and apnoeic, heart rate <60 (0.2–0.5%);
4. dead but resuscitatable (<0.1%).

Fit and healthy

Leave this baby alone! Do not suck him out, since this traumatizes the pharynx, and is a powerful vagal stimulus that provokes a reflex bradycardia. Vigorous suction is based on the frequently held misconception that what is coming out of the baby's mouth is inhaled liquor. It is not; it is pulmonary fluid which was in the lungs prior to birth, and it will do no harm if it stays there a few moments longer. If the upper airway is full of meconium, blood, antiseptic cream or some other extraneous material, the baby should be laryngoscoped and his mouth, larynx and trachea aspirated under direct vision.

The baby should be dried and wrapped in a warm blanket to minimize heat loss, given a dose of vitamin K, and *given to his mother who should be reassured that all is well and encouraged to put the baby to the breast.* Snatching him away for some arcane medical ritual at this point is cruel and unnecessary – even the vitamin K can wait. In the first hour babies are awake and alert, and this period is very important for establishing a close attachment between mother and baby. There is absolutely no need to bathe the baby at this time; it does him no harm to be covered in vernix or have some blood in his hair. Having a bath in a labour ward is a very efficient way of dropping even a healthy baby's body temperature to below 35°C.

Not breathing too well, heart rate >100 beats per minute – needs help but do not panic

For preterm babies (<30 weeks) at risk from RDS, there is no point procrastinating in this situation. Intubate them at once and get them pink and breathing as soon as possible, and give surfactant as prophylaxis (p. 144–146). Such babies should stay intubated and on IPPV until they are in the intensive care unit and base line blood gases and X-rays have been done (Chapter 7). For term babies, follow the diagram in Fig. 6.3.

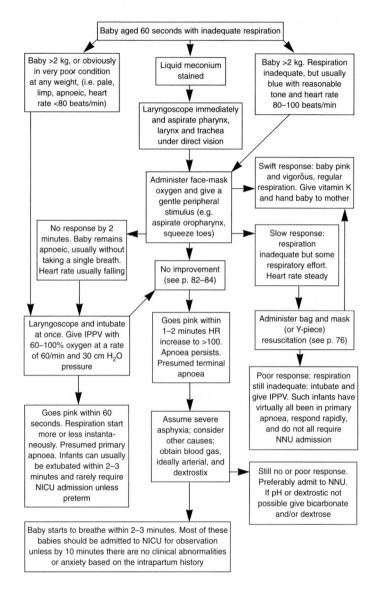

Figure 6.3 Resuscitation of the newborn.

In all infants, start the clock on the resuscitaire when the baby is separate from his mother's body; as soon as the baby is on the trolley dry him, and wrap him in warm towels; assess the features of the Apgar score at 60 seconds of age. Most babies will be pink, vigorous and breathing satisfactorily by this stage. If they are not, follow the flow diagram.

Most term babies will start to breathe spontaneously or will respond promptly to bag and mask resuscitation. For some, because they are premature, drug depressed and/or respond poorly to the bag and mask, resuscitation will need to be by intubation within the first 5 minutes. However, their clinical condition at birth, and their relatively prompt response to IPPV (see above), indicate that they are in primary apnoea. Babies who are active, breathing easily and pink by 10 minutes can go to the postnatal ward with their mother unless there was a long history of fetal distress or a very low cord pH, when a period of observation on NICU is wise in case hypoxic ischaemic encephalopathy develops (pp. 315–320). Early feeds and glucose monitoring are important.

Note the following.

1. Bag and mask ventilation is difficult to do effectively, and in the baby who has never breathed and cleared his lungs of liquid will not achieve effective gas exchange (Milner *et al.*, 1984). This technique should therefore only be used in those babies who have made some, albeit inadequate, respiratory effort. To perform bag and mask ventilation effectively, there must be a tight seal between the mask and the baby's face. Use the correct size of face mask and position it over the baby's mouth and nose (Fig. 6.4). Slightly extend his neck (chin lift), and hold his jaw forward (jaw thrust). An oropharyngeal airway may help but will not substitute for incorrect positioning.

2. There is much to be said for using a simple Y connector attached to the endotracheal tube. It is safe, easy to use and has the advantage that a long inspiratory time (>1 sec) can be used, which is

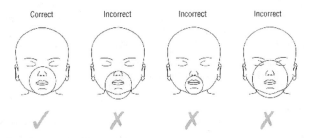

Figure 6.4 Positive pressure ventilation: correct position and size of face mask. (Adapted from Royal College of Paediatrics and Child Health (1997) *Resuscitation of Babies at Birth*. London: BMJ Publishing Group.)

important in establishing a functional residual capacity (Milner and Vyas 1985). This system does, however, give 100% oxygen (v.s.) unlike the bag and mask systems.

3. When resuscitating a baby by any method, make sure that the chest is moving and the lungs are being inflated. If this is not happening you are doing something wrong, and if you are giving bag and mask ventilation it is safest to progress to intubation.

4. To intubate a baby lie him flat or slightly extend his neck. Even moderate extension pushes the larynx into a very anterior position that makes it difficult to visualize. Insert the blade of the laryngoscope into the vallecula and pull the epiglottis forward to reveal the larynx. Press lightly on the cricoid cartilage (with the fifth finger of the hand holding the laryngoscope), and the view of the larynx is improved. See pp. 151–2, 487 for more detail.

5. Mouth-to-mouth (plus nose) resuscitation is satisfactory in an emergency, but it is important to put in an oral airway. Blow very gently – just enough to ensure that the chest is being inflated.

6. Naloxone is overused, and is only indicated in babies whose mothers received opiates within 2–5 hours of delivery. In any case, babies who are affected by opiate respiratory depression usually cry immediately and then become apnoeic. *Never* give naloxone to an apnoeic baby; it is not a substitute for resuscitation. Naloxone is a specific opiate antagonist and is of no value in babies in whom the respiratory depression is attributable to benzodiazepines or maternal general anaesthesia. Naloxone is best given intravenously because it takes 40 minutes to work when given IM. A dose of 100 microg/kg (0.1 mg/kg) should be given. This corresponds to 0.25 ml/kg of adult strength narcan which is 400 microg/ml of solution in the UK. The dose may be repeated if necessary. Since pushing 1.0 ml blind into the umbilical vein will probably not reach the systemic circulation, and giving a "chaser" of normal saline is unsafe, you either need to insert a venous catheter, find a peripheral vein, or use the intramuscular route and wait for an effect.

7. There is a tendency to give babies who respond slowly to resuscitation a few millimoles of bicarbonate or a push of albumin. This is bad practice and should not be done. Only give IV base after blood gases have been measured and the base deficit is >10 mmol/l or if the baby is failing to respond to resuscitative efforts (v.i.). Albumin should not be used in this situation at all. Infants who require resuscitation are not usually hypovolaemic; the rare

baby who has lost blood at, or just before, delivery can and should be identified.

Apparent terminal apnoea

About 0.2–0.5% of all deliveries are in this condition, and they represent about 5–10% of all babies who are apnoeic at 2 minutes of age. These babies are pale, floppy, not breathing and brady-cardic. Such a baby is usually severely asphyxiated, though other causes are possible. He will never breathe on his own unless you intubate and ventilate him, yet if you succeed it is likely that he will recover completely. The longer you delay, the more profound will be the biochemical and physiological abnormalities, and the greater the likelihood of brain damage (p. 64–66). Expeditious action is essential. Follow Fig. 6.3, starting with intubation and IPPV.

Note the following:

1. Most babies respond briskly to IPPV, increasing their heart rate and turning pink. However, if despite this they are not breathing by 3–5 minutes it can be assumed that they are probably severely asphyxiated and acidaemic and were, in fact, in terminal apnoea (Fig. 6.1).
2. Babies with marked bradycardia (<30–40) will benefit from a short period of ECM, and/or a dose of intratracheal adrenaline (*v.i.*). All you are trying to achieve is to move a small amount of oxygenated blood from the pulmonary veins a small distance to the coronary arteries. Once this is done the baby, who has had a respiratory and not a cardiac arrest, will "bump start" his heart without further action on your part.
3. Avoid injecting drugs directly into the umbilical vein. Insert a venous catheter. Direct injection may:
   (a) swill an umbilical vein clot into the systemic circulation;
   (b) not reach the systemic circulation, especially when small volumes are being given (e.g. naloxone, adrenaline);
   (c) traumatize the umbilical artery, causing haemorrhage and/or making subsequent arterial catheterization difficult;
   (d) go directly into the umbilical artery, causing spasm and ischaemia in the distribution of the iliac vessels.
4. Only give naloxone if indicated (*v.s.*).
5. With the exception of the baby who does not respond to IPPV and O_2 or is a fresh stillbirth (*v.i.*) treatment with bicarbonate or glucose should wait until appropriate measurements have been made.

Dead

If the obstetrician or midwife was certain that the fetal heart was heard up to 10 minutes before delivery, it is always worth attempting to resuscitate the fresh stillbirth. For one thing, some babies respond very dramatically to resuscitation and are vigorous and active by 5–10 minutes of age. These were either not stillbirths (i.e. they had very quiet and slow heart sounds not detected by the panicking paediatrician), or they had undergone sudden acute asphyxia without previous prolonged and potentially brain-damaging asphyxia. The neurological outcome for survivors is surprisingly good (Scott 1976, Casalaz *et al.* 1998).

When you are confronted with a fresh stillbirth, do the following:

1. Yell for help. *All cardiac arrest situations need more than one pair of expert hands.*
2. Give 6–8 beats of ECM. This must be given properly – prodding the sternum with two fingers is useless. The baby must be seized around the thorax with both hands. Then, with the fingers of both hands supporting the thoracic spine, the sternum is depressed with both thumbs placed just below the sternal angle (Fig. 6.5). Try to halve the distance between the sternum and the spine. It is virtually impossible with this technique to break ribs or rupture the liver. Give about 40–60 chest compressions/min.
3. Laryngoscope and aspirate under direct vision; intubate and give IPPV.
4. Intratracheal adrenaline (0.1 ml/kg (10 microg/kg) of 1:10 000) given at this point can be absorbed into the pulmonary circulation, and thus reach the heart.

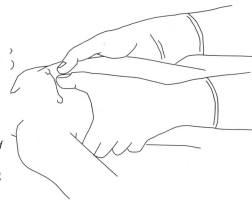

Figure 6.5
Technique of encircling the chest to give cardiac massage. (Adapted from Royal College of Paediatrics and Child Health (1997) *Resuscitation of Babies at Birth.* London: BMJ Publishing Group.)

5. Continue ECM and IPPV. There is good evidence that they can be given simultaneously, without pauses in the ECM to inflate the lungs. If operating a ratio with chest compressions, use a ratio of compression to ventilation of 3:1 or 5:1.

6. Attach ECG and pulse oximeter, if available. Insert a UVC.

7. Give 10 mmol of sodium bicarbonate through the UVC.

8. Assess the situation. The baby will now be 3–4 minutes old. If there are no signs of life, give a further 10 mmol of sodium bicarbonate, 10 ml 10% dextrose, and 0.1 ml/kg estimated weight of 1/10 000 adrenaline IV in that order. Do not continue with endotracheal adrenaline because there is some evidence that it is less effective than when given IV (Kleinman *et al.* 1999). If these fail, repeat the sodium bicarbonate, give a 3rd dose of 1 ml of 1/10 000 adrenaline (100 µg/kg) and consider intracardiac adrenaline.

9. If there is no response at all, with no cardiac output by 15 minutes, abandon resuscitation, providing the resuscitation procedure has been carried out without delay. If there are no regular respirations by 30 minutes the outlook is poor.

10. Once a heart beat is detected, the following drugs may be useful: naloxone (100 microg/kg IV) (if relevant); atropine (0.1 mg IV) for persisting bradycardia; calcium (1–2 ml of 10% calcium gluconate) slowly under ECG control for hyperkalaemia and poor cardiac output. Glucagon (0.5 mg IV as a bolus), and dopamine (5–20 microg/kg/min IV by continuous infusion) are useful in babies with a poor cardiac output, but are not usually started on the labour ward.

11. Admit the baby to the NNU continuing IPPV until base line blood gases, PCV, glucose, electrolytes and chest X-ray have been taken.

USE OF DRUGS IN RESUSCITATION

With the rapid availability of biochemical analyses, ECG, SpO_2 and BP monitoring, "blind" therapy on the labour ward is inappropriate other than with naloxone or in the baby who does not respond to resuscitation. Once the baby is pink and has a good heart rate, transfer him to the NNU, obtain base line data, and treat accordingly.

Bicarbonate/THAM

These should be considered in the baby with a H^+ >85 (pH <7.10) or a base deficit >20 mmol/l. Term babies who have responded well to IPPV and O_2, who by 10–15 minutes of age appear stable, rapidly and spontaneously correct their metabolic acidaemia. If base is indicated use the formula on p. 139 to calculate the dose once the blood gas results are available. Giving "just a touch" of bicarbonate – 1–2 mmol – is daft.

Glucose

If the glucose is <2 mmol/l give a push of 1 ml/kg of 10% dextrose whilst setting up an intravenous infusion. Aim for normoglycaemia (p. 284).

Adrenaline

Given intratracheally in very depressed babies 10 microg/kg (0.1ml/kg of 1:10 000 adrenaline) is beneficial. Thereafter it can be repeated in a ten fold larger dose (1 ml/kg 1:10 000) intravenously or as an intracardiac injection. The outcome for neonates, especially those born preterm who were so asphyxiated that they were given intravenous or intracardiac adrenaline on the labour ward is very poor.

Calcium

This has been overused in the past. However, there is a high likelihood of hyperkalaemia in asphyxiated neonates so if, following IPPV and O_2 there is poor cardiac output or the ECG suggests electromechanical dissociation, the response to an *i.v.* dose of 0.2 ml/kg of 10% calcium gluconate should be tried.

Albumin

Blind administration of 10 ml/kg of albumin during resuscitation has become the fashionable absurdity of neonatal resuscitation. It is completely unjustified. If the neonate is hypotensive after IPPV and O_2 (an unusual finding, see Fig. 6.1) consider the causes; if hypovolaemia is likely (cord occlusion, blood loss) give blood or saline. If not, volume overload may be harmful and thoughtful evaluation and treatment of the hypotension are then essential.

MECONIUM STAINING

The neonatologist's response to the cry from the labour ward of "meconium liquor – baby about to deliver" is a matter of controversy. If there is meconium staining plus other signs of fetal distress, or the recent appearance (within the last hour or two) of thick meconium then he should certainly attend the delivery. If the baby is depressed enough at birth to allow laryngoscopy and meticulous pharyngeal and even endotracheal toilet this should be done. If the baby fights you off, pursuing this course of action may do more harm than good and gently sucking out the upper airway is all that is required.

In situations where there is thin meconium staining of a copious amount of liquor and no fetal distress then it is doubtful whether routine attendance for "meconium-liquor" is justified. In many labour wards, there is a problem with achieving this distinction and most resuscitation protocols, like that of Table 6.1, require the attendance of a paediatrician for safety.

PROBLEMS WITH RESUSCITATION

THE BABY WHO TURNS PINK BUT DOES NOT START TO BREATHE

If, by 20 minutes of age, the baby has made no spontaneous respiratory effort – despite adequate oxygenation and correction of acidaemia and hypoglycaemia – then further therapy should be delayed until the baby is transferred to a NNU. Once there, further blood gas analysis, blood glucose measurements and a chest X-ray should be carried out. If these tests show some persisting abnormality, appropriate therapy can be given. If they are normal, yet apnoea persists, this suggests profound asphyxia with severe neurological damage and a grave prognosis. Alternatively, if the evidence for predelivery asphyxia is unimpressive, consider some underlying neurological disorder such as cervical cord transection; *in utero* neurological damage or a primary muscle disease (p. 332).

THE BABY WITH NO RESPONSE TO IPPV

A few babies will remain blue, apnoeic and bradycardic. In some cases the reasons will be obvious (e.g. severe skeletal abnormalities in thanatophoric dwarfism). However, in babies who look normal, the reason for the poor response is commonly some technical error in resuscitation. Therefore check the following:

1. If a bag and mask system is being used, is there a poor seal around the face, and is the baby's chest moving?
2. If the baby is intubated, is the endotracheal tube in the trachea and not in the oesophagus?
3. Is the endotracheal tube too small (a common mistake)? A 3.0 or 3.5 mm tube should always be used except in babies <1 kg. Smaller tubes have a high internal resistance, allow a big air leak, and can very easily get pushed in too far so that they lodge in a main-stem bronchus. This is not only bad for overall ventilation, but carries the risk of rupturing the lobe and causing a pneumothorax (p. 183).
4. Is an adequate inflation pressure being applied? The blow-off valve may have become inadvertently reset at a low pressure.
5. Is enough oxygen being given? Has the supply been disconnected or the reservoir removed from a bag and mask system? Should 80–100% oxygen be given by using a Y piece or connecting the baby to a ventilator or a CPAP device?

If technical errors can be excluded, check the following:

1. Is the asphyxia more severe than the initial clinical assessment suggested? Check blood gases and blood glucose. Give a few beats of external cardiac massage, 1 ml of intra-tracheal 1:10 000 adrenaline and 5–10 mmol of intravenous sodium bicarbonate plus 5 ml of 10% dextrose (if indicated), and continue IPPV. If possible transfer the baby to the NNU for further evaluation.
2. Is the baby premature and developing severe RDS, or could he have congenital GBS pneumonia (p. 239–241)? Increase the inflating pressure to 35 cm H_2O if possible, give high F_IO_2 and surfactant, and increase the ventilation rate. This virtually always improves the baby enough to allow transfer to the NNU (*v.i.*).
3. Has the baby developed a pneumothorax during the early resuscitation procedures (*v.i.*)?
4. Is the baby very pale? Consider fetal haemorrhage (p. 433–435). Such babies may have lost more than half their blood volume. If the history is suggestive and the pallor seems due to anaemia, give 15–20 ml/kg of fresh uncrossmatched O negative blood at once over 10 minutes; repeat this if necessary. Blood is much better than saline, because blood carries oxygen. This will usually improve the baby enough for him to be transferred to an NNU where a more accurate assessment of the anaemia can be made.

THE VIGOROUS BUT CYANOSED BABY

A few babies are fairly vigorous and active with a normal heart rate, often marked respiratory distress, yet remain very cyanosed. This situation strongly suggests some underlying structural problem in an (initially) unasphyxiated baby. Consider the following:

1. Is there a diaphragmatic hernia, suggested by mediastinal shift, poor air entry on the left side (the usual side of the hernia) and a scaphoid abdomen? Intubate the baby, transfer him to the NNU, and X-ray him (p. 195).
2. Is there a pneumothorax? This can be spontaneous, or the result of over-vigorous positive pressure respiration – especially with bag and mask systems or if too small an endotracheal tube has been pushed down into a segmental bronchus. The clinical signs are given on p. 183–184. There is rarely time to confirm the diagnosis radiologically, but a fiberoptic light source may help. If the baby is deteriorating quickly, insert a wide-bore needle into the second intercostal space in the mid-clavicular line. If you are wrong, surprisingly, it does not matter. If you are right, there will be a gratifying hiss of escaping air, the baby's condition will improve, and the needle can be followed by insertion of a chest drain.
3. Is there lung malformation or pulmonary hypoplasia? Airway, lung or cardiac malformations which make the baby unresuscitatable are rarely surgically correctable, and are, therefore, usually fatal.

THE HYDROPIC NEWBORN

Always attempt to resuscitate a hydropic neonate for the reasons outlined on p. 459.

REFERENCES

Adamsons, K., Behrman, R., Dawes, G.S., James, L.S. and Koford, C. (1964) Resuscitation by positive pressure ventilation and tris-hydroxymethyl-aminomethane of rhesus monkeys asphyxiated at birth. *Journal of Pediatrics* **65**: 807–818.

Apgar, V. (1953). Proposal for a new method of evaluation of newborn infants. *Anesthesia and Analgesia* **32**: 260–267.

Casalaz, D.M., Marlow, N. and Speidel, B.D. (1998) Outcome of resuscitation following unexpected apparent stillbirth. *Archives of Disease in Childhood* **78**: F112–F115.

Dawes, G.S., Jacobson, H.N., Mott, J.C., Shelley, H.J. and Stafford, A. (1963) Treatment of asphyxia in newborn lambs and monkeys. *Journal of Physiology* **169**: 167–184.

Field, D., Milner, A.D. and Hopkin, I.E. (1986) Efficacy of manual resuscitation at birth. *Archives of Disease in Childhood* **61**: 300–302.

Helwig, J.T. (1996) Umbilical blood acid–base state – what is normal? *American Journal of Obstetrics and Gynecology* **174**: 1807–1814.

Hermansen, M.C. and Prior, M.M. (1993) Oxygen concentrations from self-inflating resuscitation bags. *American Journal of Perinatology* **10**: 79–80.

Kleinman, M.E., Oh, W. and Stonestreet, B.S. (1999) Comparison of intravenous and endotracheal epinephrine during cardiopulmonary resuscitation in newborn piglets. *Critical Care Medicine* **27**: 2748–2754.

Low, J.A. (1993) The relationship of asphyxia in the mature fetus to long-term neurologic function. *Clinical Obstetrics and Gynecology* **36**: 82–90.

Milner, A.D. and Vyas, H. (1985) Resuscitation of the newborn. In: *Neonatal and Pediatric Respiratory Medicine*, Milner, A.D. and Martin, R.J. (eds). Butterworths, London, pp. 1–16.

Milner, A.D., Vyas, H. and Hopkin, I.E. (1984) Efficacy of face mask resuscitation at birth. *British Medical Journal* **289**: 1563–1565.

Palme, C., Nystron, B. and Tunell, R. (1985) An evaluation of the efficiency of face masks in the resuscitation of newborns. *Lancet* **i**: 207–210.

Primhak, R.A., Herber, S.M., Whincup, G. and Milner, R.D.G. (1984) Which deliveries require paediatricians in attendance? *British Medical Journal* **289**: 16–18.

Royal College of Paediatrics and Child Health (1997) *Resuscitation of Babies at Birth.* British Medical Association, London.

Scott, H.M. (1976) Outcome of very severe birth asphyxia. *Archives of Disease in Childhood* **50**: 712–716.

Volpe, J.J. (2001) Hypoxic ischaemic encephalopathy: Biochemical and Physiological aspects. Chapter 6 in *Neurology of the Newborn*, 4th edn. Volpe, J.J. WB Saunders Philadelphia, pp. 217–276.

FURTHER READING

Richmond S (ed.) for the Northern Neonatal Network(1996) *Principles of Resuscitation at Birth.* Hindson Print Ltd, Newcastle Upon Tyne.

Roberton, N.R.C. (1999) Resuscitation of the Newborn. In: *Textbook of Neonatology*, 3rd edn, Rennie, J.N. and Roberton, N.R.C. (eds). Churchill Livingstone, Edinburgh, pp. 241–265.

Royal College of Paediatrics and Child Health (1997) *Resuscitation of Babies at Birth.* British Medical Association, London.

Volpe, J.J. (2001) *Neurology of the Newborn*, 4th edn. WB Saunders, Philadelphia.

7

FIRST HOUR CARE, INCLUDING CARE
AFTER RESUSCITATION

A whole chapter is devoted to this area of neonatal intensive care in order to emphasize its importance. Even in the most sophisticated and well-run neonatal units, the care meted out to babies during this crucial hour is often inferior to that given at any other time.

Good first-hour care is of particular importance in the premature baby at risk from RDS, in whom failure to control clinical, biochemical and physiological abnormalities results in severe surfactant depletion and RDS by the mechanisms shown in Fig. 7.1. Put simply, sloppy first-hour care can convert mild RDS into severe, or fatal RDS, or a treatable case of septicaemia into a fatal one. Equally important is the immediate care of the baby who has required resuscitation for birth depression. Not all babies with low Apgar scores have suffered *in utero* hypoxia (Table 6.2, Chapter 6) but some will develop hypoxic ischaemic encephalopathy requiring close monitoring (p. 76, 315–320); others need investigation to exclude sepsis, myopathy or some other pre-existing CNS disorder.

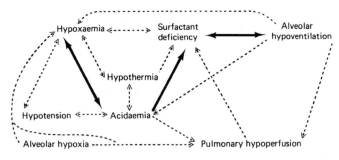

Figure 7.1 Interrelationships between factors that affect surfactant and other components of lung function.

PREPARATION

Good communication between obstetric and paediatric teams allows preparation to be made for an admission and prevents potentially life-threatening delays while appropriate staff and equipment are found. Most neonatal units are operating to capacity and do not have the luxury of an intensive care cot permanently kitted out and ready, ideal though that would be. Babies often have to be moved to create space and early warning helps. In many cases the optimum time for delivery – often by caesarean section – can be planned 12–24 hours in advance.

TRANSFER FROM THE LABOUR WARD

This is where the control and care of the sick neonate often starts to go awry. It is a grossly substandard level of care – but one that applies all too often – to transfer a sick baby with inadequate respiration from the labour ward to the NNU wrapped in a blanket and without supplementary oxygen. The baby arrives in the NNU cold, blue, limp and grunting (if you are lucky) or apnoeic and half dead (if you are unlucky).

After resuscitation, any baby who requires admission (Fig 6.3, p. 76) must be placed in a warmed transport incubator, and transferred in that from the labour ward to the NNU with appropriate oxygen supplementation and monitoring. If resuscitation by IPPV was necessary after delivery, it is sensible to keep such a baby intubated and ventilated during transport and until base line blood gases have been obtained after admission to the NNU. The neonatal resident responsible for resuscitation must accompany the baby from the labour ward with a trained neonatal nurse who will ensure the baby is labelled. A copy of the maternal notes or a good history is vital. This is another link in the chain which often breaks; there may be an important diagnosis such as maternal HIV or hepatitis infection for which immediate treatment is required.

ADMISSION ROUTINE

As soon as an ill baby arrives in the NNU, he should be weighed and placed in his own warmed incubator or under a suitable radiant heater. If he was ventilated during transfer, this should be continued. Unventilated babies with respiratory distress should be given warm humidified oxygen via a head box. Attach a pulse oximeter and give enough oxygen (by IPPV if necessary) to keep the SpO_2 >90%. Take arterial blood for blood gas analysis and check the blood glucose and PCV as soon as possible. Organize vitamin K if it was not given in the labour ward. Length measurements and bathing can be omitted at this stage; a little crusted blood on his scalp will not harm the baby but chilling will.

Next, quickly and accurately examine the baby; measure his head. Always take his blood pressure. Babies who may have suffered severe asphyxia should be assessed neurologically (p. 316–317). The baby should be connected to an ECG monitor, and if not being ventilated, to an apnoea monitor. The cuff of a blood pressure recording device should be left on, and frequent recordings taken. If there is any doubt about the accuracy of the oscillometric (Dinamap) BP recordings connect the arterial catheter (*v.i.*) to a pressure transducer as soon as arterial access is secured.

IMMEDIATE CARE

All ill babies admitted directly from the delivery suite should have the following investigations set in train within 30 minutes of admission:

1. arterial blood gases;
2. blood glucose;
3. haemoglobin (PCV), full blood count with differential WBC;
4. swabs from ear and throat;
5. blood culture;
6. group and crossmatch;
7. electrolytes, urea, creatinine.

A chest X-ray will be required but can wait, especially if arterial lines are to be inserted. Coagulation studies may be indicated. Think about collecting blood for chromosomes if you need to give a blood transfusion urgently.

An indwelling UAC of the type with an inbuilt PaO_2 transducer provides the most satisfactory way of monitoring sick babies with RDS (p. 101). Umbilical catheterization should be attempted in all VLBW babies who require ventilation, in any other ventilated baby who is requiring more than 30% oxygen and is not rapidly weaning, and in any shocked or very ill baby of any gestation. The risk of complications is low (p. 473). The catheter can always be removed later if it is not needed and the chance of success is high if you try whilst the cord is fresh. We insert an umbilical venous catheter in babies weighing less than 1 kg at the same time as the UAC. This helps minimal handling, and we replace it with a silastic "long" line after a day or two when the baby is more stable. If insertion of the UAC fails, then try peripheral arterial cannulation (p. 98, 481). If all attempts fail then obtain the first blood gas sample by arterial puncture; capillary blood gases from sick underperfused babies at any gestation are meaningless.

On the basis of the initial investigations, a working differential diagnosis must be made and appropriate treatment started without delay. If RDS is present surfactant should be given (p. 144–146). On the basis of the first set of blood gases appropriate changes in the ventilator settings or inspired oxygen concentration can be made. Although large vigorous babies have a considerable capacity for correcting metabolic acidaemia spontaneously, small sick babies do not, and acidaemia depresses surfactant synthesis and function. Base deficits above 8–10 mmol/l present in symptomatic babies less than 60 minutes old should almost always be corrected by infusing an appropriate dose of base (p. 139).

All sick babies should be started on 10% dextrose at once, either intravenously or through the UAC or UVC. Give 40–60 ml/kg/24 h and monitor the glucose. Anaemia should be corrected by transfusion, urgently if appropriate (p. 435).

Hypotension accompanied by poor capillary refill and/or an acidosis should always be treated. A useful rule of thumb is that the mean blood pressure roughly equates to the baby's gestational age in weeks, but what matters most is any evidence of poor tissue perfusion. If hypotension is accompanied by anaemia, fresh blood should be transfused (10–15 ml/kg). However, if the haematocrit is greater than 45%, then infuse 10–15 ml/kg of normal saline. If the hypotension persists despite correction of acidaemia and hypoxia, or if there are signs of heart failure, give dopamine (p. 142–143).

Since it is impossible to exclude serious infection – especially with group B streptococcus – as the cause of any illness presenting in the first hour, start the baby on antibiotics after taking cultures. Give penicillin and an aminoglycoside to all seriously ill babies, including any who require IPPV. Consider a lumbar puncture if there is a high index of suspicion of sepsis, for example prolonged rupture of membranes or known maternal infection.

The baby will now be an hour old. If the above routines have been carried out correctly, even the sickest baby should now be in the optimal condition possible. At this stage make detailed notes, see the parents, explain what is happening, and encourage them to visit the ward. If possible take a photograph of the baby for the mother to keep with her on her bedside table. For specific advice on the care of babies at risk of developing hypoxic ischaemic encephalopathy, see pp. 315–320.

8

MINIMAL HANDLING

This chapter is included to remind the reader that a basic tenet of neonatal intensive care is that handling and disturbing a sick neonate in any way may cause his condition to deteriorate, usually by making him hypoxic (Speidel 1978).

Anything that makes a baby cry, by making his respiration irregular, will compromise his ventilation (even if he is ventilated), increase his pulmonary artery pressure, increase the right to left shunt (pp. 117–118), and thus lower his PaO_2. Handling the baby involves opening the doors of the incubator, which lets the oxygen out. Complex manoeuvres – such as a chest X-ray or an LP, disconnecting the oxygen supply when sucking out the endotracheal tube, or giving chest physiotherapy – are other potent causes of hypoxia.

Many spontaneously breathing low birth weight babies, when handled or made to cry, start to writhe about, take a deep inspiration, stop breathing, remain apnoeic and become cyanosed with a bradycardia.

POINTS TO REMEMBER

The less you touch a baby the less likely you are to transmit infection to him from your own hands, or to transfer his infection to another baby. Always wash your hands before and after handling a neonate.

Heel pricks, venous and arterial punctures are painful and make babies cry. This not only gives incorrect results for blood gases (p. 101), but also causes clinical deterioration. If blood sampling for biochemistry, blood gases or haematology is going to be frequent, an intra-arterial sampling line is essential.

ECG, respiration, temperature, blood pressure, and blood gases should be monitored continuously by electronic means (Chapter 10).

Continuous monitoring is, in any case, always superior to intermittent monitoring.

Putting arterial lines and monitors in place does involve one period of intense activity and interference immediately after admission (p. 88–89). Do these procedures within the incubator or under a radiant heat source, and ensure that the baby's oxygenation is sustained throughout.

Use local anaesthetics or boluses of analgesic for painful procedures; there is no doubt that neonates feel pain. For advice on a suitable choice and the dose, see Chapter 9.

Oropharyngeal suction, and in particular suction down an ETT during assisted ventilation is notorious for causing deterioration. ETT suction is overused, and with rare exceptions is not indicated at all in the first 24 hours of ventilation, and then not more than 12 hourly unless there is infection or bronchorrhea. If the PaO_2 falls below 6.6 kPa (50 mmHg), *stop* suctioning at once and reconnect the IPPV.

If a lumbar puncture needs to be done or an intravenous line resited, do it as expeditiously as possible without moving the baby from his incubator and interfering with oxygen administration.

If anyone fails on any procedure more than twice, *stop*. Let the baby recover, and then get someone else to try.

X-rays involve major man-handling of the baby if the incubator does not have a film cassette. A member of the medical or nursing staff must always help the radiographer. Take great care to sustain oxygenation during the procedure.

If you are taking an X-ray to exclude pneumothorax or to ensure that an endotracheal tube is properly sited – and if the X-ray gives you that information even if it is blurred, rotated, expiratory or over penetrated – do not repeat it. A surfeit of technically poor films may stop the X-ray department sending inexperienced staff to take X-rays on very sick babies!

Does the baby's incubator really need a spring clean, and does he really mind a small amount of meconium in his nappy or crusted blood on his scalp? The nursing staff may feel that a clean baby in a clean incubator is a healthy baby, but he will not share their enthusiasm if they make him hypoxic and apnoeic.

Does the baby perhaps need a rest? Studies have shown that babies in intensive care are never left alone for more than a few minutes. They certainly do not get the chance to sleep without someone stuffing a suction tube up their nose, a thermometer into their rectum or a needle into their skin (Korones 1976, Barker and Rutter 1995).

REFERENCES

Barker, D.P. and Rutter, N. (1995) Exposure to invasive procedures in neonatal intensive care unit admissions. *Archives of Disease in Childhood* **72**: F47–F48.

Korones, S. B. (1976) Disturbance and infant's rest. In: *Iatrogenic Problems in Neonatal Intensive Care.* 69th Ross Conference. Ross Laboratories, Columbus, Ohio, pp. 94–96.

Speidel, B. P. (1978) Adverse effects of routine procedures on preterm infants. *Lancet* **i**: 864–866.

9

ANALGESIA AND SEDATION

In the past it was thought that neonates did not feel pain, and even major surgery was carried out without analgesia. It is only in the last 10 years that this situation has been recognized to be unsatisfactory and anaesthetists now ensure that appropriate intraoperative and postoperative analgesia is given (Wolf 1999).

For babies on IPPV, appropriate sedation and/or analgesia are required. An infusion of a sedative such as midazolam (10–60 microg/kg/h) with bolus doses of morphine (100–200 microg/kg over 15 min) or a low-dose background infusion of morphine (1–5 microg/kg/h) works well in our hands. If bolus doses of morphine are given to self-ventilating babies they must be given much more slowly, over 30–60 min. Fentanyl (1–2 microg/kg as a bolus with 1–2 microg/kg/h) is an alternative, and was considered more effective in one RCT (Saarenmaa *et al.* 1999). Fentanyl has a much more potent effect on the respiratory reflex with the potential for respiratory depression and loss of the protective airway reflexes. The onset of action is more rapid than morphine, making fentanyl more suitable for procedure related analgesia. Prolonged infusions of opiates can produce a withdrawal syndrome.

Adequate control can be assessed by the nursing staff using one of the "pain scores". Signs that a ventilated baby is experiencing pain include the following:

- tachycardia;
- increasing oxygen requirements;
- increased blood pressure;
- high glucose levels;
- facial expressions of brow furrowing, eye squeezing;
- swiping (?defensive) movements of the limbs;
- jitteriness (p. 311).

Local anaesthetic infiltration with lignocaine 1–2 mg/kg should be used (except in dire emergencies) for all the following procedures:

- inserting chest/pericardial/abdominal drains
- cut downs (aterial or venous)
- incision of local abscess.

For the following procedures it is arguable whether the needle prick and stinging from local anaesthetic application is more painful than the procedure alone. We would not use local anaesthetic unless the procedure seemed likely to be difficult, in which case we would certainly consider it.

- Lumbar and ventricular puncture
- Arterial puncture and arterial line insertion
- Peripheral long line or venous line insertion
- Heel prick for blood sampling
- Suprapubic puncture.

One problem is that topical local anaesthetics (e.g. EMLA cream) seem to be ineffective when used on the heel although they appear to work on thinner skin elsewhere (Stevens 1996, Rushforth *et al.* 1995). Amethocaine (ametop) may work better than EMLA (Jain and Rutter 2000). Sucking a sweet solution during the procedure reduces the behavioural response and can help. The use of a spring-loaded lancet for heel-prick sampling is less painful for babies and obtains blood more reliably and is strongly recommended.

REFERENCES

Jain, A. and Rutter, N. (2000) Local anaesthetic effect of topical amethocaine gel in neonates: randomised controlled trial. *Archives of Disease in Childhood* **82**: F42–F45.

Rushforth, J.A., Griffiths, G., Thorpe, H. and Levene, M.I. (1995) Can topical lignocaine reduce behavioural response to heelprick? *Archives of Disease in Childhood* **72**: F49–F51.

Saarenmaa, E., Huttunen, P., Leppaluto, J., Meretoja, O. and Fellman, V. (1999) Advantages of fentanyl over morphine in analgesia for ventilated newborn infants after birth: a randomized trial. *Journal of Pediatrics* **34**: 144–150.

Stevens, B. (1996) Management of painful procedures in the newborn. *Current Opinion in Pediatrics* **8**: 102–107.

Wolf, A.R. (1999) Analgesia in the neonate. In: *Textbook of Neonatology,* 3rd edn, Rennie, J.M. and Roberton, N.R.C. (eds). Churchill Livingstone, Edinburgh, pp. 435–441.

10

MONITORING THE ILL NEONATE

- *Respiration (apnoea), heart rate (ECG), BP and blood gases should be monitored continuously in critically ill neonates on IPPV.*
- *Arterial PO_2 is the only acceptable and safe way to avoid hyperoxaemia and minimize the risk of ROP; capillary samples and intermittent arterial puncture are useless.*
- *Fluid balance must be monitored by daily weighing, continuous records of fluid input and output and frequent estimations of the serum sodium and creatinine.*
- *In VLBW babies in intensive care blood electrolytes, creatinine, and full blood count should be monitored daily with more frequent estimations in ELBW.*
- *Until a baby is stable on ventilation with less than 30% inspired oxygen, daily CXR should be considered.*
- *Close liaison with the bacteriology laboratory is essential with frequent monitoring of blood cultures, tracheal aspirate and surface swabs.*

PHYSIOLOGICAL MONITORING

Even the most sophisticated monitor is no substitute for a good intensive care nurse. The equipment outlined in this chapter is there to assist minimal handling (Chapter 8). Equipment can only achieve this if it is maintained and used properly.

RESPIRATION MONITORING

Apnoea monitoring

Various systems are available for monitoring respiration. They all have the problem that if the baby gasps or moves when apnoeic they fail to alarm. Nevertheless, some form of apnoea monitor should be attached to all spontaneously breathing babies at risk of apnoea.

The most widely used device (Valman *et al.* 1983) consists of a pressure sensitive capsule (Graseby monitor) which is attached to the baby's abdominal skin, close to the umbilicus or on the lower abdomen. The movements of the abdominal wall distort a membrane which covers the capsule, producing pressure changes.

Modern multichannel monitors have built-in impedance monitors and detect respiration by using a high frequency oscillator to send a small current across conventional ECG electrodes on the chest wall. The volume alterations during breathing produce tiny changes in electrical resistance, which are detected and recorded electronically.

The other devices are now rarely used but respiratory inductive plethysmography has proved to be a useful research tool.

Dual monitoring of heart rate and oxygen saturation for apnoea

The best and most widely used method to detect apnoea in routine clinical care is to use the Graesby monitor plus heart rate (recorded by ECG), or oxygen saturation plus heart rate measured with a pulse oximeter. This allows detection of the two consequences of apnoea which may be harmful, namely bradycardia and hypoxaemia.

Respiratory pattern and waveform

A large number of devices are now commercially available which, in addition to detecting apnoea, display the baby's respiratory rate and combine this with a visual display of the respiratory waveform and trend recording.

Blood gases

The target range for PaO_2, $PaCO_2$, and pH, and the physiological justification for the tight control required is given in Chapter 11.

In order to monitor blood gases adequately it is necessary to have an indwelling arterial line and ideally some device for continuous oxygen (and occasionally CO_2) monitoring. It must be emphasized that only arterial blood gases can be relied on to give accurate analysis of the baby's oxygenation, particularly in those babies at risk from ROP. An indwelling arterial line also enables the neonatologist to take frequent samples without contravening the minimal handling rule (Chapter 8).

Arterial blood gases must be measured at least 4–6 hourly during the acute phase of any respiratory illness even in the presence of continuous oxygen monitoring. Arterial sampling is also necessary to calibrate the continuous PaO_2 or $TcPO_2$ device and to measure the $PaCO_2$ and acid–base status. If continuous PaO_2 catheters or $TcPO_2$ monitors are being used, are found to be accurate in an individual baby, and the neonate is otherwise stable, the frequency of direct blood gas sampling can be reduced to 6–8 hourly after 4–5 days of age or sooner if the baby is in less than 30% oxygen.

UMBILICAL ARTERIAL CATHETERS

The umbilical arteries are easily cannulated for 4–5 days after birth (Ch. 33). The catheter should be 3.5 or 4.0 French gauge for babies <1500g and 5.0 for larger ones. In general end hole catheters are preferred because they may cause less injury to the endothelium of the aorta wall (p. 473, Wesstrom *et al.* 1979). Where to position the catheter tip is a matter of controversy, but all agree that the area of D12-L3/4 should be avoided (Fig. 10.1, Phelps *et al.* 1972), as this is where the renal, coeliac and mesenteric vessels arise from the aorta. Positioning the catheter tip above this level still carries the theoretical risk of embolization but avoids the considerable problems with arterial obstruction to the legs seen when the tip is in the lower aorta (Mokrohisky *et al.* 1978).

Once a UAC is *in situ*, blood can be taken from it as required for PaO_2, $PaCO_2$ and acid–base estimations as well as other laboratory investigations: even blood cultures can be taken from it under appropriate circumstances (Pourcyrous *et al.* 1988). Only coagulation studies present a problem; because of heparinization of the fluid infused through the catheter, more accurate data are obtained from a peripheral venous sample. Blood pressure can be measured continuously via a transducer connected to the catheter. The risk of bleeding should be minimized by using only Luer lock connections and careful observation. Never cover the umbilical stump when a UAC is in place.

PERIPHERAL ARTERIAL CANNULAE

If a UAC cannot be inserted (and the success rate is over 90% in experienced hands) then a peripheral artery should be cannulated to enable frequent arterial sampling without disturbing the baby. These cannulae can be used for continuous measurement of blood pressure, and for withdrawing samples for biochemical and haematological monitoring but they must not be used for infusions, other than

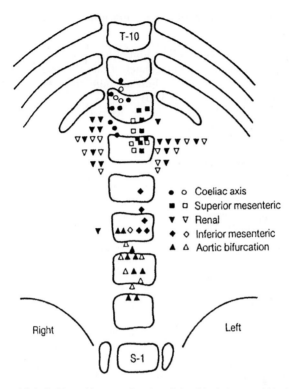

Figure 10.1 Positions of important branches of the abdominal aorta which should be avoided by umbilical artery catheter tips. (Reproduced with permission from Phelps *et al.*, 1972.)

the 0.5–1.0 ml/h of heparinized saline used to keep them patent. The preferred arteries are the radial and posterior tibial since they have good collateral supplies. The ulnar artery should not be cannulated unless the radial artery is patent (and vice versa) (p. 479).

COMPLICATIONS

Horrific complications of arterial cannulation have been reported (Chapter 32). The complication rate with UACs is no greater than that with peripheral arterial lines. Umbilical catheters **can** be left *in situ* for at least two weeks, whereas peripheral arterial lines rarely last for more than 6–7 days. The complications of either type of cannula can be reduced to a minimum if the following rules are observed:

- infuse 1 ml/hr of saline with 1 unit of heparin/ml;
- remove all arterial lines immediately if they show signs of partial or complete blockage (i.e. if there are other than transient vascular changes in the area supplied);
- remove all central lines (venous or arterial) if septicaemia is not responding rapidly to treatment.

INTERMITTENT ARTERIAL PUNCTURE

If none of the available arteries can be cannulated, but arterial blood is required, there is no alternative other than to use peripheral arterial puncture. Any artery can be used for this, and although in theory end arteries should be avoided in order to prevent distal ischaemia secondary to spasm, in practice this is not only extremely rare but can probably always be reversed by vasodilators (Wong *et al.* 1992).

Nevertheless, it must be emphasized that taking samples by direct puncture from a peripheral artery, albeit backed up by continuous transcutaneous blood gas or SpO_2 monitoring, is a sub optimal way of monitoring the ill VLBW neonate with RDS. There are two main drawbacks. First the number of available sites, and the number of times each can be used, is limited. Secondly, and more importantly, frequent direct puncture contravenes the minimal handling rule in a way that is not only generally bad for the baby but is specifically bad in this situation since the disturbance of the baby lowers his PaO_2. This makes the PaO_2 measurement on a sample obtained by direct puncture valueless for either calibrating a transcutaneous PaO_2 monitor or preventing retinopathy of prematurity. However, in babies with mild disease who are too mature to be at high risk from ROP, arterial stabs backed up by $TcPO_2$ monitoring or oximetry can be adequate, if second-best. In the ELBW neonate who requires ventilation for months, peripheral arterial stabs may be all that is available after the sites for arterial cannulation have been rendered unusable. If one is forced into this situation in the neonate who is still at risk from ROP, great care should be taken to minimize the trauma of arterial puncture by, for instance, using local anaesthetic. Changes in the transcutaneous PO_2 monitors or oximeters should be watched carefully during the puncture attempt and if there are significant falls the procedure should be abandoned and re-attempted 20–30 minutes later after the baby has stabilized.

CAPILLARY BLOOD GASES

These have no place in the early management of the critically ill VLBW baby at risk from ROP. Capillary PO_2 can never be relied upon to detect hyperoxaemia, and in the first few days after birth capillary acid–base values are also unreliable, tending to read high for $PaCO_2$ and low for pH. However, after 48–72 hours of age, capillary samples can be useful for pH and PCO_2.

Capillary gas analysis is of greatest value in babies with chronic lung disease. In such babies, who are usually sufficiently mature not to be at risk from ROP, oxygenation is effectively monitored by oximetry (*v.i.*). However it is important to know the degree of carbon dioxide retention in such cases and capillary blood gas analysis achieves this.

CONTINUOUS BLOOD GAS MONITORING

Continuous PaO_2 catheters

These are miniaturized PaO_2 electrodes built into the tip of an FG4 or FG5 double lumen side hole UAC. One lumen contains the wiring for the electrode, and the other is a sampling lumen which can be used in exactly the same way as a normal UAC.

Our preference is to insert a continuously recording FG4 or FG5 PaO_2 catheter during the first hour of life into all neonates with severe respiratory disease, especially very low birth weight babies with RDS. These catheters are very reliable, reduce the number of blood gas analyses required by about half (thereby reducing the transfusion requirement), give instantaneous information on the baby's PaO_2 which provides prompt and early warning of deterioration in the baby's oxygenation (Fig 10.2) and indicate when procedures on the baby are causing an unacceptable degree of hypoxaemia. The accuracy of the PaO_2 transducer deteriorates over a period of days due to blood and protein coating the tip. This means that the accuracy of the PaO_2 readout must be checked against an arterial sample 3 or 4 times per day.

Continuous transcutaneous monitoring

Transcutaneous monitoring for PO_2 and PCO_2 is possible using appropriately adapted electrodes accurately applied to the skin. Transcutaneous devices work on the principle that the partial pressure of oxygen and carbon dioxide diffusing from the capillaries

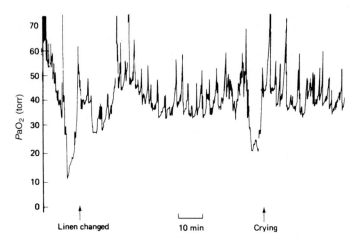

Infant N. M.51227 Birth weight 3.8 kg IRDS on CPAP

Figure 10.2 Marked variation in arterial PaO_2 recorded from continuous intra-aortic PaO_2 catheter.

through skin heated to 44°C is very close to the true arterial PO_2. Great care has to be taken with the *in vitro* calibration of these devices, and with how they are attached to the skin. To ensure accuracy, and to prevent skin damage from prolonged exposure to the temperature of 44°C the electrode site should be changed every 4 hours. With the advent of oximetry, which is much easier to use, transcutaneous monitoring is being used less.

Transcutaneous devices give an instantaneous measure ($\pm15\%$) of PaO_2 in most babies (American Academy of Pediatrics 1989). However, in routine clinical use they are not predictably accurate particularly at higher PaO_2 values (Wimberley *et al.* 1985), or in ill hypotensive neonates following vasodilator therapy, or in mature babies with a thick skin, or in preterm babies with thin skin and protruding ribs. It is for these reasons that the accuracy of $TcPO_2$ monitors must always be checked by intermittent arterial blood gas analysis; initially this should be done 4 hourly but once the baby is stable this can be reduced to 2–3 times per day (American Academy of Paediatrics 1989). Continuous $TcPO_2$ monitoring, used in conjunction with 3–4 hourly blood gas analyses on blood drawn from an indwelling arterial line, is an acceptable way of monitoring the critically ill neonate. However the use of TcPO$_2$ monitors as the sole means of monitoring to prevent ROP is not safe.

TcPCO$_2$ monitors consistently over-read by about one third. The true arterial value is 70–75% of the TcPCO$_2$ (Wimberley et al. 1985, Rennie 1990). The error is systematic and can be allowed for by deliberately calibrating the monitor to under-read against the calibration gas. In addition monitors are subject to considerable drift over time. However, they are useful when adjusting ventilator settings in critically ill ventilated babies, and they may give early warning of a blocked ETT or pneumothorax.

Continuous pulse oximetry

The correct shorthand for a pulse oximeter reading is SpO$_2$. Oximetry estimates the percentage oxygen *saturation* of haemoglobin in arterial blood (SpO$_2$), not the partial *pressure* of oxygen (PaO$_2$); it is not the same as true saturation (SaO$_2$) measured *in vitro* with a co-oximeter.

The technique of oximetry is dependent on the differential absorption of red (c. 660 nm) and infra-red (c. 940 nm) light by deoxyhaemoglobin and oxyhaemoglobin respectively. In routine clinical practice pulse oximetry is used without an *in vivo* calibration.

The SpO$_2$ values measured by pulse oximeters have a standard error of about ±2–3% from true SaO$_2$ in the range of saturation between 70–100%. Thus at a SpO$_2$ read out of 92%, the true saturation (SaO$_2$) could be anywhere between 88% and 96% (±2 standard errors). Hay has shown that at a SpO$_2$ of 92% the arterial oxygen tension can be anywhere between 5.3 and 13 kPa (Hay et al. 1989). The errors get bigger with underperfusion (Clayton et al. 1991), or during dopamine infusion. Anaemia and polycythaemia can also affect the result. The results are not influenced by racial pigmentation of the skin or staining from bilirubin, but extraneous light can affect the reading. When all these potential inaccuracies are translated into PaO$_2$ values the potential error is huge.

The relative inaccuracy, especially in the 90–100% range, has major implications for neonatal intensive care, since it means that to avoid dangerous hyperoxaemia with the risk of ROP the target SpO$_2$ should be 90–91% with the alarm set to go off at 95–96%. The practical problem is that if the alarm is set at 95–96% babies who are normally oxygenated with PaO$_2$ levels in the range 8–10 kPa often have these saturation levels. This leads to a high number of nuisance alarms with the possibly disastrous consequence that the alarm is switched off. Pulse oximetry must never be relied upon to prevent hyperoxaemia in at risk babies (Dear 1987, Moyle 1996) since PaO_2 values may be unacceptably high even at a saturation of 95%.

Oximeters are popular because they are easy to use. They do not require calibration, rarely injure the skin, are not subject to drift and give virtually instantaneous results when correctly attached. This latter feature is of benefit during resuscitation immediately after birth, during transport, and during the initial period of stabilization after admission to the neonatal unit. Oximetry can be very helpful for confirming or refuting hypoxia in babies with suspected cyanotic congenital heart disease. The non-invasive sensors mean that two can be applied easily to measure pre and post-ductal oxygen saturation in pulmonary hypertension (p. 191). Oximetry is of great value in the long term survivor with chronic lung disease (Chapter 12) who is too mature to be at risk from ROP, has a thick skin (which makes $TcPO_2$ monitoring less accurate), but who nevertheless has severe lung disease and a high oxygen requirement which needs careful monitoring.

HEART RATE MONITORING

As part of intensive care an ECG should be continuously recorded and displayed. Small pre-gelled electrodes suitable for use in the preterm neonate are widely available. Some thought should be given to the positioning of the electrodes to minimize the effect of the inevitable shadow they will cause on a CXR. The pattern of the ECG may alert the clinician to electrolyte disturbances (p. 375); myocardial hypoxia (p. 319) or even a pneumothorax. Regularity of the heart rate is a sign of severe respiratory disease. A fixed slow heart rate is a sign of central nervous system depression. Tachycardia can be an early warning sign of haemorrhage, inadequate analgesia or drugs (e.g. methylxanthines). Bradycardia can be an early sign of a blocked ETT or raised intracranial pressure.

BLOOD PRESSURE MONITORING (normal ranges in Appendix C).

This is an essential part of the care of ill neonates of all birth weights and gestation. Older methods such as the flush method have been superseded by invasive or oscillometric monitoring. For a summary of normal blood pressure ranges, see Appendix C.

Oscillometry

Oscillometry detects movement (oscillations) within the limb caused by the inflow of blood. A small plastic sphygmomanometer type cuff is inflated and automatically deflated at regular intervals. When the air pressure within the cuff is above systolic pressure no movement is detected; when the cuff pressure is reduced blood enters the limb, increasing the limb volume and compressing the cuff thereby oscillating the pressure within it. These devices can only be relied upon if a suitably sized cuff is carefully applied (2/3 of the length of the upper arm), the baby weighs more than 1 kg, and the blood pressure is reasonable. In the shocked ELBW baby these devices overestimate systolic blood pressures in the range 35–45 mmHg (Diprose et al. 1986) by as much as 5–10 mmHg.

Invasive blood pressure monitoring

Direct recording from an indwelling arterial cannula is the preferred method of monitoring blood pressure in sick very low birth weight neonates. It is important to avoid common mistakes when using pressure transducers – in particular ensuring that the apparatus is at the same level as the neonates' heart, and that there is no damping due to bubbles in the connecting lines. Having a visual display of the blood pressure waveform which should show a good pulse pressure and a dichrotic notch provides a check on the presence of damping, as well as on the state of the cardiac output in the patient.

CENTRAL VENOUS PRESSURE MONITORING

Although widely used in babies and older children CVP monitoring has not caught on in neonatology. Yet it is clear that ventilated neonates with low CVP do badly (Skinner et al. 1992). It is very difficult to pass a central line of sufficient diameter from a peripheral site to give an undamped trace. Passing the catheter through the ductus venosus into the right atrium has been used, but it is often impossible to get the UVC to pass through the ductus venosus and leaving it in situ may result in serious venous thrombosis in the liver or air embolism. However the pressure in the IVC does give clinically useful information (Lloyd et al. 1992). To monitor CVP the transducer should be attached to the end of the UVC and the techniques used are identical to those of blood pressure monitoring.

TEMPERATURE MONITORING

Temperature can be monitored either by four hourly use of a rectal or axillary thermometer, or by the use of a rectal or skin thermistor which is left in place to minimize handling. The use of mercury in thermometers and sphygmomanometers is no longer permitted because of the risk of breakage with mercury contamination of the surrounding area. Measuring the central/peripheral temperature difference with two probes e.g. axilla and foot can provide useful information about the state of the circulation and/or early warning of infection (p. 11, 230), particularly circulating blood volume. Continuous skin or core temperature monitoring will need to be used if the incubator or radiant heat cradle is used in servo mode. The advantages, disadvantages and dangers of this type of control of the thermal environment compared with air control mode are outlined in Chapter 2.

CLINICAL AND LABORATORY MONITORING

FLUID BALANCE

A fluid balance chart is an integral part of the monitoring of all ill babies, although it is difficult to record accurately all the fluid infused including that given as drugs or for flushing catheters after sampling. Boluses of saline, blood and bicarbonate must always be included. Urine output should be checked regularly. Critically ill neonates should have an absolute measure of urine output daily, together with urinalysis for protein, blood and electrolyte concentration (Chapter 3). Because catheterization carries the risk of infection, and adhesive urine bags frequently damage the thin frail skin of preterm newborns, the most effective way to measure urine output is by weighing disposable nappies (or cotton wool balls placed within them). These items must be weighed as soon as possible after voiding to avoid evaporative loss.

Weighing is the single most important investigation in the assessment of fluid balance in the critically ill neonate, and should be done at least once a day. In very preterm babies who have an enormous transepidermal water loss; 12 hourly weighing is indicated.

It is possible to weigh the intubated ventilated neonate with an indwelling arterial catheter by transiently disconnecting the infusion and quickly putting him, still ventilated, on electronic scales beside the incubator. Alternatively, within-incubator scales are available on which the baby can be nursed.

BACTERIOLOGICAL MONITORING

As part of the work-up to exclude infection all neonates with respiratory distress will have a full set of swabs and a blood culture taken (p. 137). Thereafter we find culture of ETT aspirates 2 or 3 times per week useful. Such surveillance enables identification of colonization of the respiratory tract with serious pathogens, and can help to target therapy should such babies develop a deteriorating chest X-ray, a rise in CRP and/or white cell count, or other symptoms suggesting pneumonia.

BIOCHEMICAL MONITORING (Table 10.1)

It is impossible to predict hypo- or hyperglycaemia, hypo- or hypernatraemia, hypo- or hyperkalaemia, hypocalcaemia or hypoalbuminaemia in ill babies despite meticulous attention to the content and volume of the intravenous fluid therapy. It is more difficult

Table 10.1 Routine monitoring of the ill neonate

Four hourly
TPR
Glucose*
Bilirubin*
Blood gases (see pp. 97–98)

Daily
Haemoglobin, PCV, WBC platelets
Na, K, creatinine, calcium, phosphate, glucose^
CXR

2–3 times per week
Albumin
ETT aspirate culture
CRP

Weekly
Liver enzymes (when on TPN)
Triglycerides (when on TPN)
Alkaline phosphatase (for osteopenia)
Reticulocytes (for anaemia of prematurity)

* in babies with appropriate diagnoses. In stable babies glucose need only be checked daily. Bilirubin need not be measured in the absence of clinical jaundice.
^ Electrolytes should be measured 2–3 times per day in all babies <1 kg in the first 3–4 days until fluid balance stabilizes.

when TPN is used (p. 56–58). Bilirubin must be checked frequently in jaundiced babies.

HAEMATOLOGICAL MONITORING (Table 10.1)

Ill babies, especially those weighing <1.5 kg, tolerate anaemia badly (Alverson 1995) and are also subject to large blood loses from monitoring. These babies should have a daily haemoglobin and packed cell volume estimation.

The white cell count should always be checked as part of the initial evaluation when a baby is admitted to the NNU. Thereafter daily white cell counts in acutely ill babies can help in the detection of early sepsis and in the evaluation of antibiotic therapy in established sepsis.

MONITORING INFUSION PRESSURES

Modern infusion pumps are fitted with devices which continuously monitor the pressure required to deliver the infusion, and these can be set to alarm. Accurate delivery of small volumes is now taken for granted, but there is little information available on which to base a decision about the settings of pressure alarm limits for infusions in NNUs. The UK Department of Health standard of 300 mmHg is well above the operating pressure of most neonatal infusions. For peripheral venous infusions and silastic "long lines" 40 mmHg is a suitable choice for general purposes. This represents an acceptable compromise between the number of nuisance alarms from self-clearing occlusions and the rapid detection of genuine blockages. A suitable setting for an UAC is 100 mmHg.

X-RAY MONITORING

In the critically ill ventilated newborn, clinical signs and routine monitoring frequently fail to detect the development of pneumonia, small pneumothoraces and in particular PIE (p. 181), and misplaced endotracheal tubes which predicate immediate alterations in therapy. For this reason we routinely perform daily CXRs in seriously ill ventilated babies, and of course if there is any deterioration (sudden or otherwise) which is not readily explained by clinical findings.

Although there is justified anxiety about the irradiation dose received, the doses are small. Fifty neonatal CXRs provide no more radiation than living for a year surrounded by the uranium-rich granite of Aberdeen.

REFERENCES

Alverson, D.C. (1995) The physiologic impact of anemia in the neonate. *Clinics in Perinatology* **22**: 609–25.

American Academy of Pediatrics (1989) Task force on transcutaneous oxygen monitors. *Pediatrics* **83**: 122–126.

Clayton, D.G., Webb, R.K., Ralston, A.C., Duthie, D. and Runciman, W.B. (1991) A comparison of the performance of 20 pulse oximeters under conditions of poor perfusion. *Anaesthesia* **46**: 3–10.

Dear, P.R.F. (1987) Monitoring oxygen in the newborn. *Archives of Disease in Childhood* **62**: 879 – 891.

Diprose, G.K., Evans, D.H., Archer, L.N.J. and Levene, M.I. (1986) Dinamap fails to detect hypotension in very low birth weight infants. *Archives of Disease in Childhood* **61**: 771–773.

Hay, W.W., Brockway, J.M. and Eyzaguirre, M. (1989) Neonatal pulse oximetry: accuracy and reliability. *Pediatrics* **83**: 717–722.

Lloyd, T.R., Donnerstein, R.L. and Berg, R.A. (1992) Accuracy of central venous pressure measurement from the abdominal inferior vena cava. *Pediatrics* **89**: 506–508.

Mokrohisky, S.T., Levine, R.L., Blumhagen, J.D., Wesenberg, R.C. and Simmons, M.A. (1978) Low positioning of umbilical artery catheters increases associated complications in newborn infants. *New England Journal of Medicine* **299**: 561–564.

Moyle, J.T.B. (1996) Uses and abuses of pulse oximetry. *Archives of Disease in Childhood* **74**: 77–80.

Phelps, D.L., Lachman, R.S., Leake, R.D. and Oh, W. (1972) The radiologic localization of the major aortic tributaries in the newborn infant. *Journal of Pediatrics* **81**: 336–339.

Pourcyrous, M., Korones, S.B., Bada, H.S., Patterson, T. and Baselski, V. (1988) Indwelling umbilical arterial catheter: A preferred sampling site for blood culture. *Pediatrics* **81**: 821–825.

Rennie, J.M. (1990) Transcutaneous carbon dioxide monitoring. *Archives of Disease in Childhood* **65**: 345–346.

Skinner, J.R., Milligan, D.W.A., Hunter, S. and Hey, E.N. (1992) Central venous pressure in the ventilated neonate. *Archives of Disease in Childhood* **67**: 374–377.

Valman, H.S., Wright, B.M., and Lawrence, C. (1983) Measurement of respiratory rate in the newborn. *British Medical Journal* **286**: 1783–1784.

Wesstrom, G., Finnström, O. and Stenport, G. (1979) Umbilical artery catheterization in the newborn I. Thrombosis in relation to catheter type and position. *Acta Paediatrica Scandinavica* **68**: 575–581.

Wimberley, P.D., Frederiksen, P.S., Witt-Hanson, J., Helberg, S.G. and Friis-Hansen, B. (1985) Evaluation of a transcutaneous oxygen and carbon dioxide monitor in a neonatal intensive care department. *Acta Paediatrica Scandinavia* **74**: 352–359.

Wong, A.F., McCulloch, L.M. and Sola, A. (1992) Treatment of peripheral tissue ischemia with topical nitroglycerine ointment in neonates. *Journal of Pediatrics* **121**: 980–3.

ACUTE DISORDERS OF THE RESPIRATORY TRACT

- *Fetal lung liquid is produced throughout the second half of pregnancy and must be cleared rapidly from the lungs at birth for normal gas exchange to start.*
- *The lung of a normal term baby has only a fifth of the final number of alveoli and preterm babies have no alveoli at all.*
- *By 15 minutes of age major changes in blood gases, lung mechanics and pulmonary perfusion have already taken place, and by 60 minutes lung function is close to normal.*
- *Normal arterial blood gases at 60 minutes of age are pH 7.4; PaO_2 11 kPa; $PaCO_2$ 4 kPa.*
- *Right to left shunts are common in the neonate; the true shunt is estimated from the preductal PaO_2 after breathing 100% oxygen for 15 minutes.*
- *Surfactant is a complex mixture of phospholipids, neutral lipids and protein. Surfactant appears in the lung during the third trimester and is present in adequate amounts when the L:S ratio in liquor is >2:1.*
- *The oxygen affinity of fetal and early neonatal blood (P_{50}) is increased, in part due to a reduced effect of 2,3-DPG in red cells when haemoglobin F is present.*

RESPIRATORY PHYSIOLOGY

FETAL LUNG FLUID

This has a composition which is completely different to that of amniotic fluid and plasma (Table 11.1). It is produced by active transport mechanisms, the dominant one being the transfer of chloride from plasma into the lung fluid. In human fetuses lung fluid first appears during the second trimester, and by full term alveoli contain approximately 30 ml/kg.

Table 11.1 Composition of lung liquid, liquor amnii and fetal plasma (sheep)

	Plasma	Lung liquid	Liquor amnii
Na (mmol/l)	150	150	113
Ca (mmol/l)	3.3 (0.62)*	0.8 (0.22)*	1.6
K (mmol/l)	4.8	6.3	7.6
Cl (mmol/l)	107	157	87
HCO₃ (mmol/l)	24	2.8	19
Osmolarity (mosmol/kg H₂0)	291	294	265
pH	7.34	6.27	7.02
Protein (g/100 ml)	4.09	0.03	0.10
Glucose (mg%)	152	113	304

* Ionized calcium in brackets.

In the term fetal lamb, about 250–300 ml of lung fluid are produced per day. The fluid spills into the amniotic fluid from the trachea, mainly during fetal breathing. This outward flow carries surfactant out into the amniotic fluid, where its presence can be detected using tests of surface tension (p. 121). Obstruction to the flow of lung fluid leads to an increase in lung volume (Plug the Lung Until it Grows).

THE ONSET OF RESPIRATION

The first breath

The following are all important in initiating breathing:

1. Physical stimuli. In newborn animals delivered into a bath of warm saline or on to a warm bench beside the mother, physical stimuli such as cold or touching the fetus can initiate respiration. If, however, the baby is kept warm and has an intact umbilical circulation, breathing is rarely sustained. Newborn babies are suddenly exposed to light, gravity, sound and cold – an immense sensory input.
2. Chemoreceptors. An important factor in the initiation of breathing is stimulation of the central chemoreceptors by the changes in blood gas concentrations which follow cord clamping. The role of the peripheral chemoreceptors remains controversial, since if they are denervated, respiration still starts after the cord is clamped.

3. CNS activity. Respiratory centre activity may also be involved in the onset of respiration. In animals, this area becomes much less electrically active if the sensory input to the CNS is removed.

Aeration of the lungs

When aerating the lungs at birth the neonate generates an opening pressure of at least 20 cm H_2O to overcome the viscosity of the fluid in the airway, the surface tension within the fluid-filled lung, and the elastic recoil and resistance of the tissues of the chest wall, lungs and airways. Large positive end expiratory pressures above 30 cm H_2O are also generated, which help to squeeze the liquid out of the lungs.

Clearance of lung liquid

By the time of delivery, the lungs contain about 30 ml/kg of fluid. Shortly before the onset of labour the production of fetal lung liquid is reduced by β-adrenergic stimulation, which may also serve to activate the epithelial sodium ion pumps. Some fluid drains from the mouth during a vaginal delivery. Lung epithelial cells switch from chloride-secreting to sodium-absorbing at birth, a function which they then retain throughout life. Activation of sodium absorption across the alveolar epithelium at birth moves alveolar liquid into the lung interstitium from where it is rapidly removed via the lymphatics and the pulmonary capillaries. The lungs appear lucent on X-rays within 2–3 breaths, and a normal FRC is established within 60 minutes (Fig. 11.1). The role of surface active phospholipids in this rapid "dewatering" process is under debate.

Pulmonary perfusion

All the factors involved in the onset of respiration – lung expansion, the fall in $PaCO_2$ and the rise in PaO_2 each have an independent effect to increase pulmonary blood flow immediately after delivery (Fig 11.2). Thereafter, pulmonary vasodilatation is maintained by powerful endothelium derived vasodilators including endothelin 1, prostacyclin, and nitric oxide, the release of which is stimulated by the expansion and ventilation of the lung (Ziegler *et al.* 1995).

MECHANICS OF RESPIRATION IN THE NEWBORN

(See Table 11.2.)

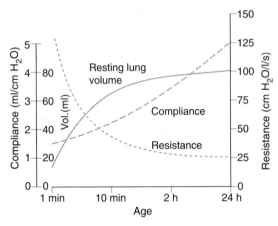

Figure 11.1 Changes in the mechanical properties of the lungs expressed on a logarithmic scale during the first day of life (from Godfrey 1981).

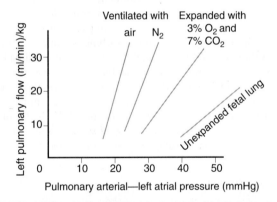

Figure 11.2 Effect of expansion of lung with 3% oxygen and 7% CO_2 in nitrogen (equivalent to ventilation without change in blood gases), ventilation with nitrogen (equivalent to blowing off CO_2) and ventilation with air on pulmonary vascular resistance in mature fetal lambs. (From Dawes, 1966.)

Rate

The normal newborn baby breathes 30–50 times/min when asleep at all gestations. This is the respiratory rate at which the calculated work of breathing is minimal. When awake the normal respiratory

Table 11.2 Lung function in the newborn

Measurement	Full-term	Preterm (if different from term)	Adult
Thoracic gas volume TGV (ml/kg)	30–35	35–45	30
Functional residual capacity FRC (ml/kg)	27–30	20–25	30
Total lung capacity (ml/kg)	55–70		80–85
Vital capacity V_C (ml/kg)	35–40		60
Tidal volume V_T (ml/kg)	5–7		7
Alveolar volume V_A (ml/kg)	3.8–5.8		4.8
Dead space V_D (ml/kg)	2.0–2.5		2.2
V_D/V_T	0.3		0.3
Alveolar ventilation $\dot{V}_A$ (ml/kg/min)	100–150		60
Minute ventilation $\dot{V}_E$ (ml/kg/min)	200–260		90
Lung compliance C_L (ml/cm H_2O)	5–6	0.5–3.0	200
Specific compliance C_L/FRC (ml/cm H_2O/ml)	0.04–0.06	0.012–0.05	0.04–0.07
Total pulmonary resistance R_L (cm H_2O/l/s)	40–45		1.7–2.6
Airway resistance (nose breathing) R_{AW} (cm H_2O/l/s)	25–30	60–80	3.5
Airway resistance (mouth breathing) R_{AW} (cm H_2O/l/s)	15	25–30	1.3
Specific conductance SG_{AW} (cm H_2O/l/s/ml FRC) nose breathing	0.31	0.35–0.5	0.1
Work of breathing (g.cm/min)	1500	500	16 000–50 000
Diffusion capacity for CO, DL_{CO} (ml/CO/min/mmHg)	0.8–3.0	0.3	15–25

rate is up to 60 breaths/min. The normal newborn breathes irregularly, with apnoeic pauses of up to 10 seconds.

Functional residual capacity and thoracic gas volume

Normally these two measurements of resting lung volume are similar, but in the newborn, the TGV may be 30–35 ml/kg compared with an FRC of only 20–25 ml/kg. Whether this represents genuine air trapping or is a methodological artefact remains uncertain.

Dead space (V_D), tidal volume (V_T), minute volume (V_E), and vital capacity (V_C)

These are similar in premature and full-term babies, when expressed per kilogram of body weight.

Lung compliance (C_L)

This is the change in volume (expressed in ml) for unit change in pressure (expressed in cm H_2O). Compliance measured in the spontaneously breathing baby is the dynamic compliance, and is inversely proportional to the respiratory rate. Static compliance is measured (in adults) by the subject voluntarily holding his breath at different points during inspiration and expiration, an experiment which it is difficult to reproduce in babies. To compare compliance at different lung volumes, specific compliance is used which is the compliance divided by the FRC. During the first few days of life, compliance increases up to the normal value of 5 ml/cm H_2O (Fig. 11.1).

Airways resistance (R_{AW})

Pulmonary resistance (R_L) is calculated by measuring inspiratory and expiratory flow (in l/s) using a pneumotachograph, and dividing this into the pressure difference between the mouth and the oesophagus (equivalent to the intrapleural pressure). To measure R_{AW} the alveolar pressure has to be estimated, and this can only be done with a plethysmograph. Alveolar pressure can then be substituted for oesophageal pressure in the calculations. If the flow measurements are made using a face mask, rather than a mouthpiece or ETT, the nasal resistance will be included in the measurement. Half of the airways resistance in the neonate is in the nose.

The reciprocal of the resistance is conductance, which can be expressed as specific airways conductance (SG_{AW}), i.e. conductance per ml of FRC. Normal values are given in Table 11.2, and the rapid postnatal fall is shown in Fig. 11.1.

The abnormal stiffness of the lung in RDS results in a change of the pressure–volume curve. Normally air is retained until low volumes are reached (hysteresis). In RDS large pressure changes are needed to achieve a small increase in volume and during deflation the lung volume follows a similar track to the inflationary curve (Fig. 11.3).

Work of breathing

This can be derived from the formula $W = 0.6PV$, where P is the pressure swing during respiration in cm H_2O, and V is minute volume in ml. A wide range of normal values have been obtained in

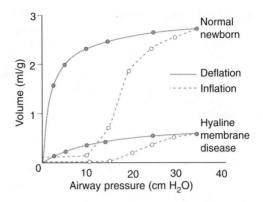

Figure 11.3 Pressure volume loops in excised lungs of neonates dying with and without RDS. In RDS the deflation curve follows the inflation curve and little air is retained at zero pressure. In normal lungs much more air is retained on the deflation limb of the loop (the phenomenon of hysteresis). Reproduced with permission from Gribetz *et al.* 1959.

the newborn, averaging around 1500 gcm/min. This represents about 1% of the total metabolism of the full-term baby.

PULMONARY GAS EXCHANGE

Ideally the ratio of alveolar ventilation ($\dot{V}_A$) in ml/min to pulmonary capillary blood flow ($\dot{Q}_C$) in ml/min – the ventilation:perfusion ratio – is one. In the normal adult lung the value is 0.8–0.9, and in the normal newborn the value is lower, particularly during the first few hours of life.

A right to left shunt is blood passing from the right to the left side of the heart without being oxygenated. There are four shunt sites in the newborn:

1. cardiac veins draining into the left side of the heart and anastomoses between the bronchial and pulmonary circulations;
2. the foramen ovale and ductus arteriosus during postnatal circulatory adaptation;
3. intrapulmonary shunting owing to pulmonary arterial blood going through the lung without passing a ventilated alveolus – this is a true intrapulmonary shunt with a $\dot{V}_A/\dot{Q}_C$ of 0;
4. intrapulmonary shunting owing to partially ventilated alveoli

having a lower P_AO_2 than elsewhere in the lungs. This results in $\dot{V}_A/\dot{Q}_C$ ratios that are lower than normal, but greater than 0. This component of the shunt can be eliminated by breathing pure oxygen for 15–20 minutes, which eventually washes all the nitrogen out of even poorly ventilated alveoli, and equalizes the P_AO_2 throughout the lung. This procedure is known as the hyperoxia test. If the PaO_2 does not exceed 20 kPa (150 mmHg) in 100% oxygen there is a right to left shunt due to congenital heart disease (Chapter 22), very severe respiratory disease, or PPHN (p. 191).

These four shunts constitute the total venous admixture – but if the fourth site is eliminated by inhaling pure oxygen, then what is left is the true right to left shunt.

A measurement of the size of the shunt is provided by the A-aDO$_2$ (alveolar-arterial oxygen difference in mmHg). This is normally less than 2 kPa (<15 mmHg). The bigger this value, the bigger the shunt (Appendix B). When breathing pure oxygen, the A-aDO$_2$ indicates the true right to left shunt.

REGULATION OF RESPIRATION

The central neural control of respiration is modulated by the chemoreceptors and mechanoreceptors.

Central control

The "respiratory centre" sited in the dorsal and ventral respiratory group of neurones within the medulla, generates the central respiratory rhythm. Afferents from many parts of the brain, in addition to those from chemoreceptors and mechanoreceptors, act on these neurones. Excitatory neurotransmitters in this region include glutamate, serotonin, substance P and catecholamines; inhibitory agents include GABA, glycine, endorphins, adenosine and the E prostaglandins.

Chemoreceptor function

Central chemoreceptors on the ventral surface of the medulla and the peripheral chemoreceptors in the carotid and aortic bodies modulate respiratory control in the neonate. The latter are relatively unimportant in the early neonatal period, as they are in the onset of respiration at birth (*v.s.*).

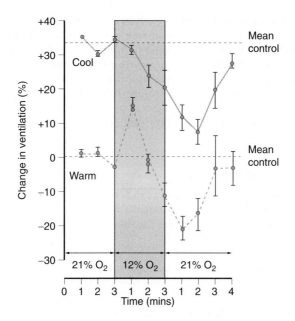

Figure 11.4 Percentage change in ventilation while breathing air and 12% oxygen in normal term babies in cool and warm temperatures. (From Ceruti 1966.)

Oxygen chemosensitivity When a baby is in a cool environment his responses to hypoxaemia are different from those obtained when he is in the neutral thermal environment (Fig. 11.4), and are different from those of older babies and adults.

In a thermoneutral environment, hypoxia (10–12% oxygen) causes hyperventilation for 1–2 minutes. The baby then hypoventilates, and premature babies in particular develop periodic breathing or even apnoea. In a cool environment, respiratory depression is the only response to hypoxaemia (Fig. 11.4).

The reason for this unusual response to hypoxia is not understood, but by 5–7 days of age hypoxia causes a sustained increase in minute and tidal volumes.

Breathing 100% oxygen for 30–60 seconds decreases ventilation by 10–15% in all neonates; in premature babies this may cause apnoea.

Carbon dioxide chemosensitivity Both premature and full-term babies have a lower $PaCO_2$ than adults. The reason for this is uncertain.

At term the central chemoreceptors are functional at the low $PaCO_2$, and the CO_2 response curve is left shifted compared to that of adults. Premature babies, however, when they are having apnoeic attacks, have a flattened CO_2 response curve, and the response curve may be right-shifted (i.e. they are less sensitive to increases in $PaCO_2$). Well-oxygenated premature babies have a steeper CO_2 response curve.

Raising the F_ICO_2 in preterm and term babies stimulates respiration.

Mechanoreceptors

Vagal afferents from the lung, as well as mechanoreceptors in the muscles of respiration, are stimulated by the distortion of respiratory movement, and the greater the distortion, the more they act to inhibit the drive to inspiration.

During rapid-eye-movement sleep, when resting muscle tone is minimal, the distortion of the rib cage caused by diaphragmatic activity results in major activation of this feedback loop, with a shortening of the inspiratory time, irregular breathing and even apnoea. This is probably a manifestation of the Hering-Breuer inflation reflex (cessation of the inspiratory drive with lung inflation). The reflex is also active in term babies. Head's paradoxical reflex or the inspiratory augmenting reflex in which lung inflation provokes a further major inspiratory effort, is also present in the neonate. It may be important at birth in helping to expand the lung and establish a FRC.

SURFACTANT

The lungs of all animals are lined with a layer of lipoprotein which keeps the pressure constant within the alveoli irrespective of their diameter. Lipoproteins which lower surface tension *in vitro* to less than 10–15 dyne/cm are known as surfactants. Surfactant is synthesized in the Type II or granular pneumonocytes of the alveolar epithelium, and is stored in the lamellar bodies of these cells. It is released by fusion of the lamellar body membrane with the cell wall. Surfactant is composed of 90% lipid and 10% protein (Table 11.3).

There are four surfactant proteins namely SP-A, SP-B, SP-C and SP-D. SP-A is the largest and most abundant and is involved in the regulation of surfactant metabolism. SP-B and SP-C play an important role in the surface tension lowering activities of the surfactant complex. SP-D interacts with SP-A and has anti-infection properties.

Table 11.3 Surfactant data: percentage composition of lipids

	Babies with RDS	Mature babies
Phosphatidylcholine	61.7	80.9
Sphingomyelin	11.0	2.0
Phosphatidylglycerol	0.9	3.7
Phosphatidylethanolamine	11.7	4.5
Phosphatidylinositol	4.9	–
Phosphatidylserine	5.3	–
Lysophosphatidylcholine	2.0	–
Neutral lipid	Approx 10%	Approx 10%

About 85% of the lipid is phospholipid, the remainder consisting of neutral lipid, cholesterol and sphingomyelin. The major phospholipids of surfactant are phosphatidylcholine (lecithin), phosphatidylglycerol and phosphatidylinositol. The phosphatidylcholine from alveolar surfactant is primarily dipalmitoyl phosphatidylcholine (dipalmitoyl lecithin; DPL), which comprises 50–60% of all surfactant phospholipid.

DPL alone does not reduce surface tension, and phosphatidylinositol or phosphatidylglycerol must be present. These appear one after the other in the neonatal lung, and until at least one of them has appeared the lungs remain unstable. *In vivo* the proteins SP-B and SP-C are important for effective surfactant function, but successful artificial surfactants have been produced which contain no protein (p. 145).

Surfactant and Type II pneumonocytes appear in the human lung at about 20 weeks gestation. The amount present increases slowly until, following a surge at about 30–34 weeks, the lungs are mature, and the baby should not develop RDS when delivered. Prenatally, the amount of surfactant in the lungs can be assessed by analysis of the liquor amnii, since surfactant is constantly washed up into the liquor in the lung liquid. In the human newborn, the surfactant content of the lung can be assessed by analysis of the pharyngeal or gastric aspirates.

The amount of surfactant present in any fluid is usually measured by comparing the ratio of lecithin to sphingomyelin – the L:S ratio – although many other techniques are used. Maturity of the lung surfactant system is indicated by a L:S ratio >2:1.

Many agents increase the amount of surfactant in babies' lungs. These include drugs which have been used therapeutically such as steroids (p. 132), agents of theoretical interest but which have raised little practical interest such as aminophylline, oestrogens, β-mimetics and bromhexine, and addictive drugs including heroin and cocaine. Babies born to mothers who have abused heroin or cocaine have a lower incidence of RDS than gestation matched controls. TRH works experimentally but the clinical results have been disappointing.

At birth, surfactant is released from the pneumonocytes. The most important factor in this process appears to be distension and ventilation of the lungs, though adrenergic agents and prostaglandins may well play a part.

Postnatally, surfactant synthesis is sensitive to cold, hypoxaemia and acidaemia. Postnatal exposure to temperatures less than 35°C, and pH less than 7.25, causes a rapid fall in the amount of surfactant in pharyngeal aspirates (Greenough 1999).

Surfactant, once released, has a half-life of about ten hours. Some is washed up the bronchial tree with normal fluid movement, some is ingested by alveolar macrophages which contain phospholipases, and some is broken down by tissue phospholipases. However, the majority (probably 90%) is taken up by the Type II pneumonocytes and recycled into the alveolus as fresh surfactant. The rate of breakdown is increased when breathing pure oxygen, and by over-ventilation.

BLOOD GASES

Table 11.4 gives average blood gas values for normal full-term and premature babies during the first month of life, and includes values obtained from babies less than 1 hour old in whom particular care was taken to avoid asphyxia and early neonatal hypothermia.

Measurement of SpO_2 shows that this is usually >90% by 10–15 minutes of age, though values recorded in the feet remain below this for longer.

OXYGEN TRANSPORT

The position of the oxyhaemoglobin dissociation curve is controlled by pH, temperature, the intracellular concentration of 2,3-DPG, and the interaction between these three factors and the haemoglobin present in the red cells. A decrease in pH and a rise in temperature and 2,3-DPG move the curve to the right, decreasing the affinity for oxygen (more oxygen being given up at the same

Table 11.4 "Normal" blood gas values in the newborn

	PaO$_2$				PaCO$_2$				H$^+$			
	kPa	mmHg	kPa	mmHg	kPa	mmHg	kPa	mmHg	nmol/l	pH	nmol/l	pH
15 minutes	11.6	87			3.7	28			48	7.32		
30 minutes	11.4	86			4.3	32			43	7.37		
60 minutes	10.8	81			4.1	31			40	7.40		
1–6 hours	8.0–10.6	60–80	*8.0–9.3*	*60–70*	4.7–6	35–45	*4.7–6*	*35–45*	46–49	7.31–7.34	*42–48*	*7.32–7.38*
6–24 hours	9.3–10.0	70–75	*8.0–9.3*	*60–70*	4.4–4.8	33–36	*3.6–5.3*	*27–40*	37–43	7.37–7.43	*35–45*	*7.36–7.45*
48 hours–1 week	9.3–11.3	70–85	*10.0–10.6*	*75–80*	4.4–4.8	33–36	*4.3–4.5*	*32–36*	42–44	7.36–7.38	*40–48*	*7.32–7.40*
2 weeks					4.8–5.2	36–39	*5.1*	*38*	43	7.37	*48*	*7.32*
3 weeks					5.3	40	*5.1*	*38*	42	7.38	*49*	*7.31*
1 month					5.2	39	*4.9*	*37*	41	7.39	*49*	*7.31*

The values at 15, 30 and 60 minutes are from our own unpublished observations on full-term babies. Data from 1 hour to 1 week are drawn from the literature on arterial samples. Data beyond 1 week are on capillary samples. Values in italics are those for premature babies; those not in italics are for full-term babies.

PaO_2). A rise in pH or a fall in body temperature and 2,3-DPG have the reverse effect.

The blood of the neonate has a left-shifted oxyhaemoglobin dissociation curve, due to the fact that within the cell haemoglobin F reacts poorly with 2,3-DPG.

The position of the oxyhaemoglobin dissociation curve, and thus the oxygen affinity of whole blood, is expressed as the P_{50}. This is the partial pressure of oxygen at which the haemoglobin molecule is 50% saturated. For adult blood the P_{50} is 27 mmHg, and for fetal blood it is 19.5 mmHg.

The fact that the newborn baby's blood has a high affinity for haemoglobin (low P_{50}) makes it more difficult to assess hypoxaemia clinically, since cyanosis occurs at a lower PaO_2 than in the adult (*v.s.*). Furthermore, since high-affinity fetal blood is reluctant to release oxygen to the tissues, in pulmonary diseases with hypoxaemia, tissue oxygenation may be more effective if the circulating blood is of adult (i.e. transfusion) origin.

LUNG GROWTH AND DEVELOPMENT

The term baby has 50 million alveoli, a number which increases to 250 million by adult life. Most of this increase occurs during the first 18 months, the surface area of the lung increasing from 3 to 70 m^2. This growth potential is important during the treatment of babies with chronic lung disease (Chapter 12). The growth factors involved are still under study. The canalicular stage of lung development occurs between 17 and 27 weeks of gestation. During this phase capillaries begin to appear and gas exchange can occur when the capillaries approximate to the air spaces. This enables gas exchange to commence and determines extra-uterine survival. During the canalicular stage bronchioles terminate in acinar units, not alveoli.

DIFFERENTIAL DIAGNOSIS OF NEONATAL RESPIRATORY DISEASE

RESPIRATORY ILLNESS STARTING WITHIN FOUR HOURS

Almost all the lung diseases which affect the neonate *can* develop within the first four hours of life. Indeed, the development of symptoms before four hours of age is an essential diagnostic prerequisite for surfactant-deficient RDS (*v.i.*). Differentiating this condition from all the other causes of early neonatal dyspnoea is usually easily done on the basis of a history, simple clinical examination, chest X-ray and the fact that most of the other problems usually occur in mature babies (Table 11.5).

The most difficult diagnostic problem at all gestations is differentiating RDS from congenital or intrapartum pneumonia. Furthermore, since these types of pneumonia and surfactant-deficient RDS can co-exist, it is impossible to exclude pulmonary infection as a component of the respiratory distress in any given baby – hence the need to put all breathless neonates on antibiotics (p. 166–167, 241). However, the following features greatly increase the likelihood that infection is responsible for some, if not all, of the baby's respiratory illness:

- prolonged rupture of the membranes
- maternal fever
- positive culture on high vaginal swabs before delivery
- purulent vaginal discharge
- offensive liquor.

Clinical signs in the baby that suggest pneumonia rather than RDS are pyrexia or persisting hypothermia, unusual hypotonia, jaundice before 12 hours of age, profound hypoxaemia without hypercapnia, early onset of apnoeic attacks, and persisting hypotension.

A low WBC (total $<6 \times 10^9/1$) with neutrophils below $2 \times 10^9/1$ is very suggestive of infection within the first 24 hours (p. 233). Other laboratory tests are rarely helpful. CRP takes several hours to rise and Gram stain of various secretions or gastric aspirate is a poor discriminator. GBS antigen detection tests have a high false positive rate.

Differentiating RDS from cyanotic congenital heart disease in the first few hours of life is less difficult now that echocardiography is readily available. The types of congenital heart disease presenting so early in life usually produce abnormal physical findings, an abnormal ECG, a very large heart and either very oligaemic or hyperaemic lung fields on CXR. Differentiating PPHN from RDS is rarely a problem and may be purely semantic since pulmonary hypertension is common in babies with RDS (p. 136). Differentiating isolated PPHN (p. 190) from cyanotic congenital heart disease or ascertaining whether a baby who undoubtedly has surfactant-deficient RDS also has co-existing CHD (cyanotic or otherwise) requires echocardiography. However, it is extremely unusual for babies with cyanotic CHD to be able to achieve a PaO_2 above 20 kPa (150 mmHg) in 100%

Table 11.5 Differential diagnosis of respiratory symptoms and signs in the newborn

Condition	Gestation	History	Examination[a]
RDS	Preterm		
TTN	Term >preterm	Often CS delivery	
Meconium aspiration	Term[d]	Meconium liquor, post-maturity	Meconium stained baby
Pneumothorax or pneumomediastinum	Term >preterm	Can be high pressures used at resuscitation	
Massive pulmonary haemorrhage	Preterm >term	Asphyxia, heart failure, bleeding tendency. Artificial surfactant	Crepitations, pallor. Blood in endotracheal tube. Often associated with patent ductus
After perinatal hypoxia-ischaemia	Term[e]	Birth depression, fetal distress	Other features of HIE (p. 315–320)
Infection (Pneumonia)	Any	Maternal pyrexia, PROM	Rarely helpful
Congenital lung malformation	Term >preterm	Usually normal. May have antenatal USS diagnosis	Rarely helpful
Congenital heart disease	Term >preterm		Murmurs, heart size, signs of heart failure
Pulmonary hypoplasia	Any	Prolonged rupture of membranes. Dwarfs (p 309)	Potter's facies (p. 379).
Persistent pulmonary hypertension	Term >preterm	May have had antenatal hypoxia	May hear murmur of tricuspid incompetence
Inhalation of feed	Any	Usually obvious	
Inborn error of metabolism	Term >preterm	May be positive FH or FH of unexplained neonatal deaths	No evidence of lung disease. Tachypnoea driven by acidaemia
Primary neurological disease	Term >preterm	May be positive FH or FH of unexplained neonatal deaths. Polyhydramnios	Hypotonia. Areflexia, myopathic facies, deformities. No lung disease
Upper airway obstruction	Term >preterm	May be typical in choanal atresia (p. 196–197)	Stridor. Problems resolve on intubation. Laryngoscopy may be diagnostic

a) mentioning features other than cardinal features of respiratory disease (p. 133).
b) most conditions cause hypoxaemia and hypercarbia; only if the blood gas patterns differ from this is it noted here.
c) frequency of presentation graded + to +++; rarely and never.

Gases[b]	Presentation[c]		Chest X-ray	Comments
	<6 hours	>6 hours		
	+++	Never	Diagnostic but see p. 135	Working diagnosis in all preterm neonates unless CXR suggests alternative. Always consider infection
Mild hypoxaemia rarely needing >40% F_1O_2	+++	Rarely	Diagnostic but see p.242	Commonest cause of breathlessness in term babies. By definition a mild disease
	+++	Never	Streaky	Diagnosis usually obvious on history. Infection may co-exist
	++	Rarely[f]	Diagnostic	
	+	+++	Unhelpful; usually a whiteout	Diagnosis based on clinical findings
Metabolic acidaemia with respiratory correction	++	Never	Unhelpful	Respiratory correction of a metabolic acidaemia
Often severe acidaemia and easy to reduce $PaCO_2$ without increasing PaO_2	++	+++	Unhelpful in most, may show patchy changes	Impossible to exclude in any baby with respiratory distress. Working diagnosis in the absence of specific CXR findings in babies older than 6 hours
May be profound hypoxaemia with raised CO_2	+++	+	Can be diagnostic	Diaphragmatic hernia, cysts, effusions, agenesis present this way. TOF should not present this way (p. 395)
CO_2 normal or reduced. In cyanotic CHD PaO_2 rarely >13.5 kPa even in 100% oxygen with IPPV	Rarely	+++	May be helpful or diagnostic	The alternative common diagnosis in babies presenting after 6 hours of age, and particularly after 24 hours. Echocardiogram usually diagnostic
Profound hypoxaemia and hypercapnia	+++	Never	Diagnostic, very small lungs	Virtually always rapidly fatal
Marked hypoxaemia with normal or reduced CO_2	+++	+	Usually normal or nearly normal	Can be difficult to exclude CHD unless echocardiogram available
	Rarely	+++	Unhelpful	Should not happen; normal term babies rarely inhale, so seek alternative diagnosis such as infection
Severe metabolic acidaemia, with respiratory correction; low $PaCO_2$	Rarely	+++	Often normal	Diagnosis based on blood changes, plus ketonaemia in many cases
Gases normal, unless apnoeic	++	++	Often normal	Usually easy to identify as a group
Gases normal when intubated; $PaCO_2$ raised beforehand	++	++	Often normal	

d) if preterm consider *listeria*.
e) severely asphyxiated premature babies get RDS.
f) usually a complication of pre-existing severe lung disease especially HMD.

oxygen, whereas this can usually be achieved in both severe RDS and PPHN with a 10–15 minute period of vigorous hand bagging using 100% oxygen through an ETT (p. 118).

RESPIRATORY ILLNESS STARTING *DE NOVO* AFTER FOUR HOURS

In essence there are only five possibilities:

- pneumonia – bacterial and viral
- congenital heart disease with pulmonary oedema
- congenital malformation
- the dyspnoea of acidaemia due to underlying metabolic disease
- rare, late-onset lung disease of the VLBW baby (e.g. Wilson-Mikity syndrome, CPIP) (p. 212–214).

Differentiating these conditions rarely poses any problems, since typical clinical, radiological or ECG changes are virtually always present.

RESPIRATORY DISTRESS SYNDROME; HYALINE MEMBRANE DISEASE

- *Surfactant deficient RDS is the commonest cause of morbidity and mortality in neonates.*
- *RDS is due to surfactant deficiency as a result of prematurity and/or asphyxial lung damage.*
- *All women with threatened preterm delivery between 23 and 34 weeks of gestation should be considered for antenatal steroids, which reduce the risk of RDS.*
- *The treatment of RDS involves artificial ventilation, surfactant and intensive care support.*
- *Preterm babies of less than 30 weeks gestation should receive surfactant as soon as possible after birth (prophylaxis). Other babies should be given surfactant if they require ventilation and the diagnosis of RDS is confirmed (rescue treatment).*
- *The choice of surfactant preparation is largely a matter of individual preference. There is evidence to support natural surfactant preparations but their rapid mode of action means that good monitoring is essential. Two doses are better than one, but more doses are not usually necessary.*
- *All babies at risk of RDS should be closely monitored for evidence of respiratory failure. Artificial ventilation should be instituted early if the*

blood gases deteriorate or the baby has persistent apneoic attacks, and continued from birth in babies intubated for resuscitation.

- *Any ventilator designed for babies can be used, and the settings tailored to minimize asynchrony. On the whole, synchrony is achieved at ventilator rates of around 60 breaths/min with inspiratory times of about 0.3 seconds. There is at present no evidence that any method of ventilation is better than conventional ventilation for the treatment of neonatal RDS. There is evidence that fast rates (60–80 breaths/min) are associated with fewer pneumothoraces.*

- *Randomized trials comparing different levels of blood gas control in RDS have not been done. There is consensus that ventilation should be adjusted to maintain the following:*
  pH above 7.25
  PaO_2 in the range 6–10 kPa (45–75 mmHg)
  $PaCO_2$ in the range 5.0–7.5 kPa (37.5–56.0 mmHg). The upper limit depends on the pH.

- *Successful treatment of RDS requires careful monitoring of blood gases, electrolyte levels and blood glucose concentrations in addition to monitoring of body weight, heart rate, respiration and blood pressure. Total parenteral nutrition may be required.*

- *Failure to respond to surfactant is rare, and advice from an experienced neonatologist should be sought if a baby remains in >60% oxygen and requires high peak ventilator pressures (>26 cm water) after two doses of surfactant.*

AETIOLOGY

Four factors are important in the aetiology of surfactant-deficient RDS:

- prematurity;
- perinatal asphyxia;
- maternal diabetes;
- caesarean section.

Prematurity

Since surfactant does not appear in the lungs until the second trimester, and not in large amounts until the third trimester, gestational age is the major determinant of RDS (Fig. 11.5). However, not all premature babies will develop the disease and it can occur at term. Around 80% of fetuses with an L:S ratio just before delivery of <1.5:1 develop RDS; some do not, because they

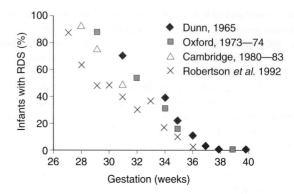

Figure 11.5 Incidence of RDS at different gestations. The lower incidence in the Robertson series may represent a genuine fall in recent years or different nomenclature; some American studies use the term respiratory insufficiency for severe lung disease in the ELBW neonate.

have a mature L:S ratio at alveolar level. About 20% of babies with L:S ratios measured just before delivery in the range 1.5:1–2.0:1 may develop RDS, and the incidence is higher if they are asphyxiated. Babies with L:S ratios >2:1 rarely get RDS, except if they are infants of diabetic mothers or suffering from Rhesus haemolytic disease when phosphatidylglycerol may be absent. The further the L:S ratio is above 2:1, the less likely is RDS to develop.

Perinatal asphyxia

Asphyxia predisposes to RDS in various ways. Hypoxaemia and acidaemia reduce surfactant synthesis (p. 122), and the asphyxiated preterm baby may make such feeble respiratory efforts that he cannot release what surfactant he does possess from the pneumonocytes.

Much more important, however, is the fact that asphyxia damages the pulmonary vasculature, allowing protein-rich fluid to leak out on to the alveolar surface where it inhibits surfactant activity. In term babies with surplus surfactant this is of no consequence, but in preterm babies with small surfactant reserves, it results in lungs that are rapidly rendered surfactant deficient, and thus non-compliant and atelectatic.

The association between asphyxia and RDS has major clinical implications. With premature babies every effort must be made to avoid asphyxia during labour, using CTG and pH measurements, and delivering by caesarean section if there is evidence of fetal compromise. The prognosis for such babies is also improved if they are promptly and vigorously resuscitated after birth by IPPV to establish FRC, release surfactant and control the baby's oxygenation and acid–base status enabling the normal postnatal fall in pulmonary artery pressure to occur (p. 86).

Maternal diabetes

Maternal diabetes is associated with an increased incidence of RDS. In part, this is due to elective, pre-labour delivery by caesarean section, but it is also due to delay in surfactant maturation, in particular the appearance of phosphatidylglycerol. In recent years, with first class antenatal control of maternal diabetes allowing delivery to be delayed until 38–40 weeks gestation, RDS is less often seen in this situation.

Caesarean section

Caesarean section carried out pre-labour in women beyond 32 weeks gestation is associated with an increased incidence of both RDS and TTN in babies, presumably because they have been denied the β-adrenergic mediated surfactant release and reduction in fetal lung liquid which occurs in the 24–48 hours before spontaneous labour (p. 113). However, in babies of less than 32 weeks gestation caesarean section has minimal effect on the incidence of RDS, and anxieties on this score should not influence the decision whether or not a very preterm baby should be delivered vaginally or by caesarean section.

PREVENTION OF RDS

Avoiding the four problems listed above will help to reduce the incidence of RDS, and of these the most important are the prevention of prematurity and asphyxia. However, there are two other ways in which the incidence and the severity of neonatal RDS may be reduced, namely the administration of steroids antenatally to the mother, and the prophylactic administration of surfactant to the baby at resuscitation and, ideally, both (p. 144–146).

Antenatal steroids

It is now recognized that giving these drugs antenatally has many beneficial effects (Table 11.6) in addition to influencing surfactant synthesis.

An overview of the results of 18 trials enrolling over 3700 babies provide clear evidence that corticosteroids reduced the risk of RDS with a typical odds ratio for RDS of 0.35 (95% confidence intervals 0.26–0.45), and for death from RDS of 0.6 (95% confidence intervals 0.48–0.76) (Crowley 1997). The greatest benefit against RDS is seen when the time interval between the start of treatment and delivery is more than 48 hours and less than seven days. The Royal College of Obstetricians and Gynaecologists in the UK recommended that two doses of 12 mg of betamethasone should be given 24 hours apart. The value of repeated courses is doubtful. Antenatal betamethasone should be considered for all women who threaten to deliver at less than 34 weeks.

Experiments in preterm lambs suggested synergism between TRH and glucocorticoids, and clinical trials followed. Crowther's most recent meta-analysis of trials evaluating the addition of TRH to antenatal corticosteroid therapy in women at risk of preterm delivery showed no evidence of benefit (Crowther 1997).

Prophylactic surfactant – see p. 144–146

Table 11.6 Benefits of antenatal steroids

Improved Apgar scores
Maturation of lung structure
Initiation of surfactant apoprotein synthesis
Improved nitric oxide mediated pulmonary venous relaxation
Reduced pulmonary capillary leakiness
Interaction with postnatal exogenous surfactant therapy
Increased resistance to high oxygen exposure
Higher blood pressure in the neonatal period
Higher neonatal white cell counts
Less patent ductus arteriosus
Less GMH-IVH
Less NEC
Less handicap in the survivors

CLINICAL SIGNS OF RDS

RDS presents within four hours of birth with:

- sternal retraction, intercostal and sub costal recession
- an expiratory grunt
- tachypnoea above 60/min.

Babies with these signs are said to have respiratory distress. There are many other causes of respiratory distress presenting by four hours of age (Table 11.5), but these can usually be excluded comparatively easily on the basis of history, clinical signs and chest X-ray (Figs 11.6 and 11.7). The baby can then be diagnosed as having "respiratory distress syndrome" (RDS), with the implication that the lungs are surfactant-depleted. If the lungs were examined histologically they would show HMD. If one is being semantic, the term HMD should only be used if there is histological proof of the diagnosis.

Since respiratory distress may be transient, the definition of RDS usually includes some statement about the duration of symptoms. However, common to all definitions of the disease is that the signs should be present *before* four hours of age, should still be there *at* four hours of age, and should persist for some period *beyond* four hours of age.

Without supplementary inspired oxygen, the baby becomes cyanosed (cyanosis is not a sign of RDS but a sign of a baby in whom

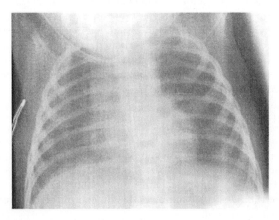

Figure 11.6 The chest X-ray in mild RDS.

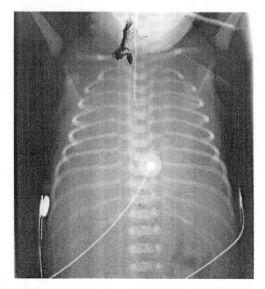

Figure 11.7 The chest X-ray in severe RDS "Whiteout".

the treatment of the RDS is out of control). Listening to the lungs reveals that the air entry is reduced and there may be a few crepitations. The baby's heart rate tends to be fixed at 120–130/min, with little beat to beat variation, and the blood pressure is 20–25% lower than normal for his gestation (see Appendix C). The baby is inactive, tends to lie in the frog position, and has moderate generalized subcutaneous oedema owing to increased capillary leakiness and delayed onset of the normal postnatal diuresis. He passes only small amounts of urine, has an ileus, and may not pass meconium until the third or fourth day of life.

NATURAL HISTORY OF RDS

In uncomplicated RDS, surfactant begins to reappear in the lungs (and laryngeal aspirate) at about 36–48 hours of age. The illness therefore gradually worsens over the first 24–36 hours as the baby tires. His condition then stabilizes for 24 hours, and from 60–72 hours of age he steadily improves. By the end of the first week he has usually recovered.

HISTOPATHOLOGY

The earliest histological changes in RDS are interstitial oedema and congestion of the alveolar walls leading to desquamation of the Type II alveolar epithelial cells. The alveolar ducts dilate, but the alveoli become atelectatic because of the surfactant deficiency. There is exudation of plasma into the alveoli and airways, and this further compromises surfactant function. The proteins in this exudate coagulate to form the characteristic hyaline membranes which line the respiratory bronchioles and alveolar ducts.

RADIOLOGY

There is a reticulogranular pattern due to the atelectasis, and the air-filled major airways stand out as radiolucent areas – the so-called "air bronchogram" (Fig. 11.6). In severe cases the lungs cannot be clearly separated from the cardiac border (Fig 11.7). To some extent the severity of the X-ray changes reflects the severity of the disease; but if assisted ventilation or CPAP is being used or surfactant has been given, atelectasis is reduced and the chest X-ray changes may appear surprisingly mild.

PATHOPHYSIOLOGY OF RDS

Once the baby's lungs have become depleted of surfactant, the alveoli collapse and the lungs become very stiff. This causes the following changes in pulmonary physiology (Table 11.7):

Table 11.7 Respiratory function tests in babies with RDS

	Normal	**RDS**
Compliance (ml/cm H_2O)	5–6	<1.0
Airway resistance (cm H_2O/l/s)	40–45 (total)	55–95 (inspiratory)
		140–200 (expiratory)
FRC (ml/kg)	30	5–20
V_T (ml/kg)	5–7	3–7
$\dot{V}_E$ (ml/kg/min)	200	250–350
$\dot{V}_A$ (ml/kg/min)	150	50–90
V_C (ml/kg)	35–40	20–25
V_D/V_T	0.3	0.55–0.6
Work of breathing (g.cm/kg/min)	500	2500–3500

- lung compliance falls to about 25% of normal; there is a decreased FRC, TGV, crying V_C, and an increased dead space and dead-space/tidal-volume ratio, with a comparatively normal R_{AW};
- increased work of breathing;
- increased intrapulmonary shunting (p. 117–118) and severe hypoxaemia;
- hypoventilation, causing a respiratory acidaemia.

Many of the other features of RDS are secondary to hypoxaemia. They include:

- pulmonary artery and right heart pressure at or above systemic level (pulmonary hypertension), facilitating right to left shunts through the ductus arteriosus and the foramen ovale.
- vascular damage, causing transudation of fluid on to the alveolar surface (p. 130–131) and into the subcutaneous tissues.
- hypotension. The baby may have a low blood volume dating from the time of delivery, and as a result of the capillary leak; in addition hypoxaemia depresses the myocardium and prevents peripheral vascular responsiveness. Acidaemia has similar effects.
- severe metabolic acidaemia, partly the aftermath of birth asphyxia, and also from lactic acid accumulation during the anaerobic glycolysis of hypoxaemia. The lactic acidaemia and hypoxaemia are also aggravated by the hypotension so that a vicious cycle develops which perpetuates surfactant deficiency (p. 86).
- decreased perfusion and/or oxygenation of other tissues, impairing their function: e.g.
  a) the kidney – poor water and $(H)^+$ excretion (Table 23.1);
  b) the gut – ileus and mucosal injury with NEC (p. 386);
  c) the CNS – intracranial haemorrhage (p. 324–328).

INVESTIGATION OF RDS

Within an hour of admission basic investigations should be requested on all babies suspected of having RDS. This is both to confirm the diagnosis and to exclude other possibilities, as well as establishing base line values for monitoring the progress of disease (Chapter 7). These investigations include:

- Hb, WBC and platelets (? need to transfuse or ? evidence for infection);
- electrolytes, creatinine, calcium (establishing base line);

- blood gases (initiating treatment);
- group and cross-match (in preparation for transfusion);
- deep ear and throat swabs (p. 232) (? infection);
- blood culture (? infection);
- CXR (diagnostic and noting position of UAC, ETT).

There is normally no need to do a LP (p. 233). Subsequent investigation is described in the section on monitoring (Chapter 10).

TREATMENT OF RDS

The aim of treatment is to keep the baby alive and in good condition until he starts to synthesize his own surfactant 36–48 hours after birth. This means avoiding hypoxaemia, acidaemia and hypothermia, which inhibit surfactant synthesis, and achieving complete control of the baby's cardiorespiratory, electrolyte and renal homeostasis. In addition the baby should receive synthetic surfactant to tide him over until endogenous synthesis is effective (p. 144–146).

MONITORING

See Chapter 10 for more information on intensive care monitoring techniques. The following should be monitored continuously in all babies with RDS:

1. ECG;
2. PaO_2: we prefer continuously recording arterial catheters (p. 101), but if these are not available intermittent arterial gases backed up by continuous transcutaneous oxygen tension ($TcPO_2$) or oximetry (SpO_2) should be used (p. 101–104). The latter two techniques are not suitable alone for monitoring of arterial oxygen tension because they cannot reliably detect hyperoxaemia;
3. F_IO_2;
4. blood pressure, ideally from the arterial catheter;
5. respiratory activity/apnoea monitor.

The following should be monitored 3–4 hourly and more frequently if necessary:

1. TPR;
2. $PaCO_2$, arterial pH and base deficit.

The following investigations should also be carried out routinely:

1. PCV 2 or 3 times daily;
2. electrolytes, calcium and albumin daily or twice daily;
3. chest X-ray daily or every other day in the acute phase.

TEMPERATURE CONTROL

(See also Chapter 2.)

Essentially, the baby must be kept in the environmental temperature appropriate for his weight (Fig. 2.2). If the baby remains cold, carry out the procedures suggested on p. 14.

ACID–BASE HOMEOSTASIS

It is important to keep the baby's H^+ below 65 nmol/l (pH >7.25), because surfactant synthesis is inhibited below this value. Furthermore, at somewhat lower pH values, body functions such as cardiac output are impaired. Acidaemia has an effect on the oxygen-dissociation curve too.

Metabolic acidaemia

A base deficit of more than 5 mmol/l (i.e. a base excess of more than –5 mmol/l) indicates a metabolic acidaemia. There has been much argument about whether correction of metabolic acidaemia is more dangerous than the persisting acidaemia. There can be no doubt that over-enthusiastic correction of metabolic acidaemia is harmful. Rapid infusions of hypertonic base cause big surges in the intravascular volume, which may cause intracranial haemorrhage; THAM may cause apnoea, and sodium bicarbonate can cause hypernatraemia. There can equally be no doubt that many sick, collapsed acidaemic babies improve when base is infused. Improvements in PaO_2, blood pressure, peripheral perfusion and physical activity follow correction of their acidaemia.

The most important reaction to the presence of a metabolic acidaemia is not how to treat it, but to find out why it developed. Is it due to the baby developing some complication such as hypotension, hypoxaemia, sepsis, anaemia or a metabolic error? Babies given early total parenteral nutrition tend to develop a hyperchloraemic acidaemia which can be reduced by replacing some of the sodium chloride with sodium acetate. The obvious solution to the arguments about whether or not to correct metabolic acidaemia is to prevent these complications from occurring. If this is done, metabolic acidaemia will be very rare except in the immediate post-birth asphyxia period, or following episodes of sudden collapse such as a blocked ETT or a tension pneumothorax.

Base therapy should be considered in all babies whose base deficit exceeds 10 mmol/l. If the baby is stable, well perfused, normotensive and mature and the degree of acidaemia is between 5 and 10 mmol/l, spontaneous correction is common, and it is reasonable to withhold therapy and measure the base deficit again after 2–3 hours. In sick babies, particularly those of less than 32 weeks gestation, base deficits above 10 mmol/l should always be corrected. Sodium bicarbonate should usually be used, and the rate of infusion should never exceed 0.5 mmol bicarbonate/min.

THAM has two major theoretical advantages: it is sodium-free and does not raise the $PaCO_2$. However, it stops premature babies breathing. It should therefore only be used in babies who are being ventilated. The dose of intravenous base is calculated from the formula:

Dose in mmol of sodium bicarbonate =
Base deficit (mmol/l) × body weight (kg) × 0.4

(8.4% sodium bicarbonate contains 1 mmol of bicarbonate/ml, and 1 ml of 7% THAM is approximately equivalent to 0.5 mmol bicarbonate.)

This calculated dosage will always undercorrect the acidaemia, and the blood gases should always be checked within an hour, or sooner if the baby's condition does not improve. Despite the fact that many babies have a coexisting respiratory acidaemia, the infusion of bicarbonate to correct metabolic acidaemia rarely causes a rise in $PaCO_2$ of more than 0.6–1.3 kPa (5–10 mmHg).

Metabolic alkalaemia

This may be seen following excessive use of bicarbonate but is also seen in babies with severe chronic lung disease who have CO_2 retention and chloride depletion due to vigorous diuretic therapy. An induced metabolic alkalaemia may be useful as an adjunct to the treatment of PPHN (p. 192).

RESPIRATORY ACIDAEMIA AND ALKALAEMIA

A respiratory alkalaemia, i.e. a $PaCO_2$ below 4 kPa (30 mmHg) may occur if hyperventilation is stimulated by acidaemia, or brain damage. However, it is commonly iatrogenic, due to over-vigorous IPPV. It should be avoided, since preterm babies with $PaCO_2$ values below 3 kPa (approx 20 mmHg) have an increased incidence of PVL (p. 300–301). An induced hypocarbic alkalaemia was formerly often used in the treatment of term babies with PPHN (p. 192). Now nitric oxide has become more widely available over-ventilation, with its attendant risks, is not necessary. Liberal administration of base should be used to keep the pH at normal levels in PPHN.

$PaCO_2$ is raised (respiratory acidaemia) in all but the mildest cases of RDS, and may reach 13.3 kPa (100 mmHg) or more if untreated. Cerebral blood flow increases by about 10% for each rise of 1 kPa in $PaCO_2$. Because of the role of increased CBF in the aetiology of GMH-IVH (p. 324) it is prudent to keep the $PaCO_2$ below 7.0–7.5 kPa (52.5–56.0 mmHg) in very preterm babies at risk from this complication.

$PaCO_2$ measurements in RDS are of value in the following situations:

1. A steadily rising $PaCO_2$ at any stage in the disease is an indication that ventilatory assistance is likely to be needed.
2. A sudden rise in $PaCO_2$ may be an indication of acute changes in the baby's condition – e.g. pneumothorax, collapsed lobes, misplaced endotracheal tube.
3. A swift rise in $PaCO_2$ (often accompanied by hypoxaemia) during an attempt to wean a baby off IPPV or CPAP indicates that the time was not appropriate for that change in therapy.
4. A gradual rise in $PaCO_2$ at the end of the first week in a low birth weight baby on a ventilator who has previously been stable, may herald the development of a PDA (p. 355–356) or CLD (p. 203).

FEEDING

In babies with RDS, oral feeding should be omitted for the first 2–3 days of life, because virtually all babies have a paralytic ileus. Hydration should be maintained by glucose-electrolyte infusions through the UAC or intravenously. By the third day, many babies, although still quite ill or receiving assisted ventilation (CPAP or IPPV), will have passed meconium and bowel sounds will be present. In such babies 0.5–1.0 ml of milk, preferably breast milk, can be given hourly through a nasogastric tube – minimal enteral nutrition (p. 43–44), and gradually increased along the lines suggested in Chapter 4. The IV fluids should be cut back appropriately as the enteral feeding is tolerated.

If by 3–4 days of age (or at any subsequent time) oral feeding is not tolerated, then either supplemental or total parenteral feeding should be considered (Chapter 5).

FLUID AND ELECTROLYTE BALANCE

(See also Chapter 3.)

Great care must be taken to prevent excessive fluid administration in babies with RDS since:

- In the presence of hypoalbuminaemia and increased capillary leakiness, excessive fluid intake may aggravate interstitial pulmonary oedema and worsen the hypoxaemia.
- Fluid overload predisposes the baby to complications of RDS, including PDA, NEC and CLD.

For these reasons use fluid restriction, aiming to give insensible losses plus urine output only, with no added sodium. A good starting point is to give 60 ml/kg/24 h in the first 24 hours. Thereafter fluid intake should be guided by the principles laid down on p. 30–32. However, since fluid overload is so damaging be prepared to restrict the intake to 50–60 ml/kg/24 h for several days if the baby is oedematous, oliguric and not losing weight. Pancuronium paralysis often aggravates problems with oedema and fluid retention.

Sick babies are very prone to both hypernatraemia and hyperkalaemia in the first few days. Controlling sodium and potassium balance is described on p. 24–27.

Hypocalcaemia is also common in the first 48 hours of life, with levels at or below 1.5 mmol/l. The baby's plasma calcium can be kept within the normal range by adding 5–10 ml of 10% calcium gluconate every 24 hours to the infusion fluid. This can usually be discontinued by 5–6 days of age.

Premature babies are often hypoalbuminaemic, since they have low levels at birth, and liver synthesis may be compromised if they are very ill. There is a poor correlation between serum albumin and oedema in babies. Recent work suggests that albumin may have detrimental effects when given to older children and adults in intensive care units. As yet there are very few data specific to the newborn, but frequent infusions of albumin are best avoided. If hypovolaemia is suspected saline will increase the circulating volume. Infusion of albumin to correct hypoalbuminaemia is not helpful when the baby still has leaky capillaries.

During the first 24–48 hours most babies with severe RDS are oliguric. Recovery from RDS is heralded by a spontaneous diuresis and resolution of subcutaneous and pulmonary oedema. Diuretic treatment has not been shown to hasten this process when used routinely in RDS. However, confronted by a profoundly hypoxaemic oedematous oliguric preterm baby with severe RDS, no harm can come from a trial of frusemide (2 mg/kg), which can be repeated if there is a diuresis and improvement in the baby's blood gases.

BLOOD VOLUME AND BLOOD PRESSURE

In ill babies, blood pressure is easily and safely monitored with one of the automated oscillometric devices such as the Dinamap. This method may overestimate blood pressure, especially in VLBWI (p. 105), and direct recording of arterial BP from indwelling cannulae is preferable. Normal BP values are given in Appendix C.

Babies with severe RDS are often hypotensive during the first few hours of life. In some cases the hypotension is due to hypovolaemia, while in others it is due to depression of cardiac and vascular function by severe metabolic disturbance and hypoxaemia. Whatever the cause, hypotension must be corrected as a matter of urgency in sick infants, particularly if there is reduced capillary filling and oliguria. There is no universally agreed definition of neonatal hypotension, which in any case relates to gestational age. A good general rule is to aim to keep the mean BP above the baby's gestational age in weeks, with the systolic pressure being at least 10 mmHg higher than this. If the hypotensive baby's PCV is less than 40%, then he should be given a blood transfusion; but if his haematocrit is at least 45%, then normal saline (0.9%) should be used, otherwise polycythaemia may develop.

Initially give 15–20 ml/kg of saline or blood, but 30–40 ml/kg may be needed to achieve a satisfactory blood pressure especially if the initial hypotension was due to blood loss.

Larger transfusions than this should only be given if there is clear evidence that the hypotension is hypovolaemic (i.e. no signs of heart failure, but persisting anaemia and low central venous pressure). If hypotension persists in the absence of signs of hypovolaemia, the correct treatment is to give inotropic support.

Two inotropes are widely used, dopamine and dobutamine. Dopamine at doses of <8–10 microg/kg/min has a direct inotropic β-adrenergic effect on the heart, while at the same time causing renal vasodilatation by dopaminergic mechanisms. Because of its beneficial effect on renal blood flow, dopamine is widely used during the first 24–48 hours in babies with severe RDS, even in those whose hypotension is only borderline. Clear evidence that this is beneficial is lacking. At doses above 15 microg/kg/min dopamine is an α-adrenergic constrictor of all vascular beds (including the pulmonary bed), and such high doses should probably be avoided.

Dobutamine has primarily a β-adrenergic inotropic effect on the myocardium. It has few peripheral actions, and no specific effects on the renal vasculature. If the BP is not adequate after volume replacement and dopamine up to 15 microg/kg/min, give dobutamine up to 20 microg/kg/min. If, after volume replacement, dopamine and dobutamine a VLBW baby remains hypotensive the prognosis is poor. Other inotropes including isoprenaline, adrenaline and the newer agent dopexamine can be tried. Success has also been reported with hydrocortisone 2.5 mg/kg 6 hourly for 48 hours, the dose being subsequently tailed off (Bourchier and Weston 1997). Dexamethasone is also effective. Remember to ask about maternal labetalol therapy; this can cause persistent neonatal hypotension and glucagon acts as a specific antidote. Use a bolus of 0.2 mg/kg and repeat 12 hourly.

Blood loss into the laboratory

The frequent blood sampling of intensive care causes chronic iatrogenic hypovolaemia, anaemia and hypotension. Some neonatal units note all blood sampled and transfuse when 10% of the blood volume has been removed. Others wait until the PCV is below 40% or the baby becomes hypotensive before transfusing. Whichever method is used, small sick babies may require several top-up transfusions of 10–15 ml/kg of blood. Donor exposure can be reduced by using blood prepared as pedi-packs, where a single unit is divided into up to eight small satellite bags. This system is now widely used, and no harm results from the use of older blood for top up transfusions (see p. 454 for more detail regarding blood transfusions).

DRUG THERAPY IN RDS

In general the pharmacy has little part to play in the routine management of RDS, apart from supplying surfactant. Other drugs may be used (Table 11.8), and antibiotic therapy is routine (p. 166–167, 241).

Table 11.8 Drugs occasionally required in babies with RDS

General indication	Drugs available	Page
Analgesia for intubation, chest drains, infusions	Morphine, fentanyl, paracetamol, sucrose	94
To assist intubation and ventilation	Pancuronium, vecuronium; Atracurium for intubation	151
Treatment of PDA	Indomethacin	356
Prevention of infection	Immunoglobulin??	237
To assist extubation	Dexamethasone, aminophylline, caffeine	174, 176
To prevent/treat CLD	Dexamethasone	209–210
To treat pulmonary hypertension	Nitric oxide	192–193
To treat hypotension	Dopamine, dobutamine, adrenaline, dopexamine	143
To correct acidaemia	Bicarbonate, THAM	138–139

SURFACTANT THERAPY

Exogenous surfactant has now been in use for over a decade and it has had a dramatic impact on the incidence and severity of RDS. Surfactant is even more effective when combined with antenatal steroids; the treatments have independent effects (Jobe *et al.* 1993). Surfactant reduces the neonatal mortality from RDS by about 40% and reduces air leaks by up to 60% (Morley 1997). However, surfactant treatment has little or no effect against complications such as CLD, GMH-IVH and PDA.

The questions which remain are whether prophylaxis is better than rescue treatment, which natural surfactant is best (Table 11.9), and whether there is a role for surfactant in the treatment of other neonatal respiratory illnesses such as meconium aspiration. Recent meta-analyses favour prophylactic natural surfactant, and in a head-to-head trial natural surfactant was associated with a lower mortality than the artificial surfactant ALEC, which is now no longer available in the UK (Ainsworth *et al.* 2000). Our current practice is to give prophylactic natural surfactant to babies less than 30 weeks gestation who require intubation for resuscitation. We do not apply a lower gestational age "cut-off" for prophylaxis, although in very tiny babies it is sometimes advisable to give a half dose on the labour ward and the rest an hour later in view of the large volume. In more mature babies surfactant should be given as rescue therapy as soon as the baby is intubated. If, after prophylactic therapy in the labour ward, the baby continues to

Table 11.9 Surfactants used in clinical studies

Surfactant (Manufacturer)	Animal source (if natural)	Composition/additives (natural)	Dose in mg/kg (natural)	Availability	N doses/vol each dose
Surfactant TA	Cow	DPPC, palmitic acid	120	Not available in UK	
Beractant/Survanta (Abbott)	Cow	DPPC, palmitic acid, tripalmitin	100	Available in UK	4 doses 4 ml/kg
Infasurf: CLSE	Cow		100	Not available in UK	
Curosurf (Serono)	Pig		100	Available in UK	3 doses 1.25–2.5 ml/kg
Alveofact	Cow		100	Not available in UK	
Exosurf/Cofosceril (Glaxo Wellcome)	Artificial	DPPC, tyloxapol and hexadecanol	5 ml/kg	Available in UK	2 doses 5 ml/kg

have significant RDS we give a further dose at 12 hours. Two doses are better than a single dose, and if the baby remains very ill further doses, up to a maximum of four, can be given (Table 11.9).

OXYGEN THERAPY

This is the most complex, important and difficult part of the treatment of RDS. In general, we aim to keep the PaO_2 in the range 6.0–10.0 kPa (45–75 mmHg). The lower limit is chosen to allow some leeway before the PaO_2 falls to the dangerously hypoxic levels at which acidaemia develops, the ductus arteriosus opens, and surfactant synthesis decreases. The upper limit is chosen to minimize the risk of retinopathy of prematurity (p. 269–271).

Although this aim appears simple, it is difficult to achieve because in addition to the severe lung disease there are other clinical problems, most of which are unique to the neonate. The different methods of oxygen monitoring are described in Chapter 10.

Breathing pure oxygen is toxic because it activates surfactants and promotes atelectasis. Use 95% concentration as a maximum (p. 158).

Oxygen administration by headbox

Many babies with mild to moderate RDS can be successfully managed in an oxygen enriched atmosphere for 48–72 hours, when their disease improves and the inspired oxygen concentration can be reduced. These babies should receive oxygen which is warmed and humidified, and which should be given into a headbox to prevent rapid falls in the F_IO_2 when the incubator portholes are opened. If the baby needs more than 60% oxygen, not only is it difficult to keep the concentration steady within a headbox, but also it suggests that his disease is severe, and that alternative forms of therapy are indicated.

Oxygen administration by nasal cannulae

For babies in long-term oxygen, typically those with CLD, oxygen can be administered by nasal cannulae. These allow the baby to sit up, bottle feed and play while still receiving oxygen. An estimate of the oxygen concentration received is shown in Fig. 11.8.

Continuous positive airways pressure

Arguing teleologically, the grunt in RDS is a marker of the sudden

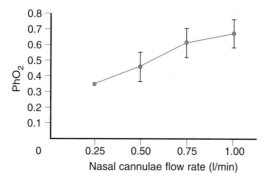

Figure 11.8 Hypopharyngeal oxygen concentration (PhO$_2$) at different nasal cannulae oxygen flows (from Vain *et al.* 1989 with permission).

opening of the glottis which had been held closed in an attempt to increase intrapulmonary pressure, blow open collapsed alveoli, reduce the atelectasis and the size of the right to left shunt, and thus improve oxygenation. CPAP attempts to mimic this effect on the baby's lungs by splinting the alveoli open with applied pressures of up to 8–10 cm H$_2$O. Furthermore, splinting the alveoli open and reducing the shearing forces in them helps to preserve alveolar surfactant.

Lung function The effects of CPAP on lung function are surprising. The FRC increases, respiration becomes regular, though the rate may increase or decrease, and the airways resistance falls. However, compliance, minute volume and tidal volume all fall, and the work of breathing may actually increase due to the effort required to overcome the resistance of the ETT or the nasal prongs used to administer CPAP. Despite this the A-aDO$_2$, V/Q ratio and right-left shunt all usually improve, and most important of all the PaO$_2$ usually rises. The PaCO$_2$ rarely rises unless pressures greater than 10 cm H$_2$O are used.

Cardiovascular effects In normal babies, 50% of the applied CPAP reaches an oesophageal pressure balloon, whereas in babies with RDS, less than 30% of the pressure is transmitted. In babies with RDS the central venous pressure rises by 10–20% during the application of CPAP, and the pulse pressure falls slightly.

Techniques for giving CPAP CPAP was first described using an endo-tracheal tube. In an attempt to avoid the problems of intubation, a headbox with a tight neck seal, or a tightly fitting face mask were then used. Boxes of various sorts traumatize the baby at the neck seal, make the baby very inaccessible, and involve him in a lot of handling. The survival rate with face masks is lower than with any other technique for delivering CPAP.

Single or double nasal prongs are now the most widely used and safest techniques for administering CPAP. We prefer a single nasal prong which is a cut-down 3.0 or 3.5 mm soft nasoendotracheal tube, since this leaves the mouth free for suction and to act as an extra safety "blow-off" valve, and leaves a free nostril for the naso-gastric feeding tube. Most neonatal ventilators now have a CPAP mode, and can be used to administer the CPAP since this makes it easier to warm and humidify the inspired gas. The ventilator is instantly available should IPPV be necessary. An alternative is to use equipment dedicated to CPAP. One such is that manufactured to give continuous pressure with a "fluidic flip" mechanism via double nasal prongs (the Electro Medical Equipment Infant Flow Driver). A comparison of the EME Flow Driver with single nasal prong CPAP showed no benefit for this system once the fact that the flow driver delivers a slightly higher concentration of oxygen had been taken into account (Ahluwalia *et al.* 1998). The tight seal required has been known to produce nasal deformities.

Complications of using prong CPAP include the following:

1. nasal trauma leading to nostril deformity;
2. feeding problems because the gas flow distends the stomach;
3. pneumothorax;
4. failure, with a need for IPPV (50% in babies below 1.5 kg).

Many of these complications can be avoided by careful nursing, and by inserting an open-ended nasogastric tube to drain gas out of the stomach. CPAP should not be undertaken in units without facilities for the rapid recognition and treatment of pneumothorax, or the ability to give IPPV. A major drawback of CPAP is that since the baby is not intubated surfactant cannot be given. The proven benefits of prophylactic surfactant therapy place significant constraint on the early sole use of CPAP in babies with RDS.

Indications for using CPAP in babies include the following:

1. PaO_2 <8 kPa (60 mmHg) in 60% oxygen;
2. recurrent apnoea with or without RDS (p. 221);

3. mild hypercapnia or mild hypoxaemia in infants who have recently been extubated (p. 175).

CPAP is of no benefit in babies with infection or meconium aspiration.

The earlier CPAP is started in babies with RDS, the more effective it is. Scandinavian groups and others have reported remarkable success with early CPAP and a "minitouch" technique. So far our experience in the UK is less impressive. We consider that if CPAP is required within 1 or 2 hours after birth in a baby weighing less than 1.5 kg who needs more than 30–40% oxygen, such a baby should be treated with surfactant. The correct course of action is therefore to intubate him, give him surfactant and put him on IPPV from the start. The evidence in favour of prophylactic surfactant is such that we strongly recommend elective intubation in the delivery suite for babies of 29 weeks gestation or less, who should then be given surfactant and transported to the neonatal unit, still ventilated, for further assessment. Many larger babies tolerate CPAP badly, thrashing around in irritation when prongs are shoved up their noses. The two main early applications of CPAP are:

1. to keep the lungs stable and expanded in babies weighing more than 1.5 kg with mild RDS or TTN who need 30–40% oxygen in the first 24 hours of life;
2. in bigger babies 36–72 hours old who are breathing well but are beginning to tire and need more than 60–70% O_2.

The management of babies on CPAP

Babies on CPAP require all the biochemical and physiological monitoring described in Chapter 10. Initially 5–6 cm H_2O CPAP should be applied. It is very difficult to get CPAP pressures higher than 8 cm H_2O using nasal prongs. Once the baby's condition improves reduce the CPAP pressure 1–2 cm at a time to 5–6 cm H_2O, then cut the oxygen to 30–40% in 5 or 10% steps. Finally reduce the CPAP to 2 cm H_2O. Always check the PaO_2 after each change. Once the PaO_2 has been satisfactory at 2 cm H_2O for 4–6 hours discontinue the CPAP. Within 1–2 hours of discontinuing the CPAP the baby's blood gases must be checked. If these have deteriorated, the CPAP should be restarted.

Stop all feeding after starting CPAP, since there is a danger that, if the baby regurgitates, the CPAP will blow the milk into his lungs. However, if prolonged CPAP is being used for recurrent apnoea, tube feeding by the nasogastric route is usually tolerated.

MECHANICAL VENTILATION: INTERMITTENT POSITIVE PRESSURE VENTILATION

The indications for starting IPPV in RDS are as follows:

1. sudden deterioration with apnoea or irregular gasping respirations;
2. failure to establish satisfactory respiration after resuscitation in the labour ward (preterm babies who are intubated for resuscitation and given prophylactic surfactant are best continued on artificial ventilation from birth);
3. deteriorating blood gases (*v.i.*).

The third category is the most difficult to define, particularly as neonatologists become ever more confident in their use of ventilators. The criteria outlined here are those for babies in the first 24–48 hours of life who are suffering from RDS and are usually deteriorating. For babies with chronic lung disease (p. 207–208), a relative hypoxaemia and quite marked hypercapnia are acceptable and safe prices to pay for not putting the baby back on the ventilator. The same blood gases would be an indication for starting ventilation in a baby with acute RDS.

Watching for a deteriorating trend is the key to avoiding a situation where the baby collapses with hypoxaemia which is difficult to reverse. This means that frequent blood gases must be taken from a reliable source, ideally an indwelling arterial line. Two blood gases in the first 24 hours in a VLBW baby receiving oxygen is simply not an acceptable level of monitoring (p. 97–98). Optimal care for a baby with RDS involves anticipating the need for artificial ventilation well before a disaster arises.

In general, PaO_2 values should be kept above 5.5–6.0 kPa (40–45 mmHg). If a VLBW baby cannot reliably maintain a PaO_2 above 5.5 kPa in 40–45% oxygen in the first few hours he should be intubated and given artificial ventilation and surfactant. In bigger and more mature babies, IPPV should be considered if more than 60% oxygen is needed to keep the PaO_2 >5.5 kPa (40 mmHg). These criteria apply whether oxygen is given by headbox or by CPAP. Tight control of the $PaCO_2$ is also important. There is a clear link between hypercarbia and GMH-IVH, mediated via an increased cerebral blood flow. Low $PaCO_2$ has been associated with PVL, and levels below 3 kPa (20 mmHg) must be avoided (p. 331). We aim to keep the $PaCO_2$ between 5.0 and 7.5 kPa (37–56 mmHg) in the first 48 hours in VLBW babies, and the $PaCO_2$ should not be allowed to rise above 8 kPa (60 mmHg) until these babies are more than 72 hours of age. In bigger babies, the rate of rise of $PaCO_2$ and the baby's overall condition should be considered before starting IPPV on the basis of a raised $PaCO_2$ alone. Hypercarbia associated with a pH of less than 7.2 is an indication for ventilation.

Intubation

(see also pp. 77, 487)

Although in theory there should always be a leak around an endotracheal tube (to provide reassurance that the fit is not too tight), in practice with a leaky tube and very stiff lungs all the inflating air leaks out! Use a 3.5 mm ETT for babies above 3.0 kg birth weight, and a 3.0 mm ETT for those of 1.0–3.0 kg. In babies of birth weight <1.0 kg who are a few days old it is worth trying to insert a 3.0 mm tube, since this makes it easier to ventilate the baby and to aspirate secretions, but a 2.5 ETT can be used in the early days.

There is no real evidence that oral tubes are better than nasal tubes, or that straight ETT are better than shouldered ones. Shouldered ETT are supposedly easier to place correctly, but one recent study showed that they were more often inserted too far. Introducers should be avoided wherever possible.

Note the following points:

1. Awake intubation is painful and associated with a stress response which is detrimental to the baby. We use fentanyl 2–5 microg/kg, atropine 10 microg/kg and suxamethonium 1 mg/kg for elective intubation, although we are still in a minority in the UK (Whyte *et al.* 2000). Alternatives are 10–50 microg/kg of morphine and 0.5 mg/kg of atracurium. Fentanyl is a better choice of analgesic than morphine because the time to onset is quicker. We use paralysis and analgesia for all intubations except those on the labour ward and in a dire emergency. The main difficulty is the time taken to obtain and draw up the drugs, particularly in view of the fact that fentanyl has to be kept in the controlled drugs cupboard.

2. The length of the ETT measured from the nostril or lips of babies of different weights is given in Fig 11.9. Always mark the tube at the nostril so that displacement will be noticed. Record the length on the X-ray which is taken to check the position. The tip of the tube on the X-ray should be at the level of the body of the first

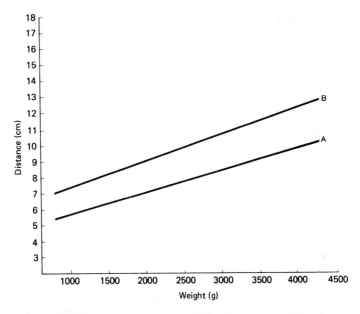

Figure 11.9 The distance required to insert endotracheal tubes into babies of different body weight. For oral tubes the lower line (A) is used for the lips to mid-tracheal position. For nasal tubes the upper line (B) is used for the nose to mid-tracheal position. (From Klaus and Fanaroff, 1979.)

thoracic vertebra (Blayney and Logan 1994). This is consistently 1–2 cm above the carina, which is at T3-4. The vertebral column is a more consistent radiological landmark than the clavicles.

3. Do not change tubes unnecessarily. Intubating babies never does them any good. Therefore only inflict reintubation on them if the tube is dislodged or blocked.

4. Immobilization of the tube at the nose or mouth is important to prevent it slipping out, or traumatizing the larynx by sliding up and down. One method of fixation involves tying an umbilical cord ligature tightly around the ETT, and then strapping the loose ends of the ligature to the baby's face using adhesive tape (Fig. 11.10). An alternative is to use a special ETT holder to grip the tube and tie the holder to a hat.

5. Try to keep the baby's head in a constant degree of slight extension on his trunk. Flexing and extending his neck causes vast

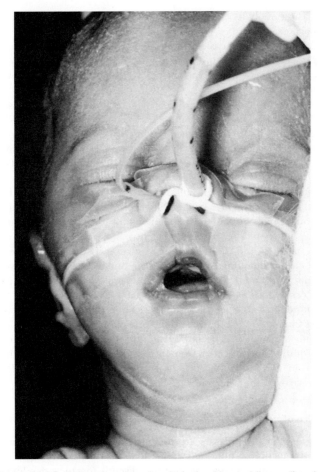

Figure 11.10 Fixation of a nasal endotracheal tube with a cord ligature. Note the redundant 3 cm of endotracheal tube.

differences in ETT position, and traumatizes the laryngeal mucosa.

6. Ensure that there is as small a dead space as possible between the ventilator circuit and the baby. However, we find that allowing an extra 2 cm of ETT is not a problem, and we favour this arrangement since it considerably reduces nasal trauma and allows much

greater mobility for the baby without using a complex head harness.

7. A good humidifier is essential, the aim being to keep the inspiratory gas temperature at 37.0°C, to achieve levels of humidification at least as high as 38 mg H_2O/l of air (100% relative humidity).

8. RDS is not a disease in which airway secretions are increased. There is no need to suck out the ETT routinely in babies with RDS during the first 36–48 hours. Sucking the baby out causes hypoxaemia, hypercapnia, hypertension and bradycardia, all of which are bad for him, and predispose him to GMH-IVH (pp. 324–326). Suction should not be done for at least 4 hours after surfactant is given unless the ETT is blocked. After the first 48 hours the frequency should be tailored to the amount of secretions, usually sucking the tube out once or twice per day. The sucking out should be swift and efficient. 0.5 ml of normal saline can be instilled into the ETT prior to suction if secretions are tenacious but should not be routine. The nurse needs to keep a very close watch on the baby; if he becomes cyanosed, if the reading of a continuous PaO_2 machine falls to 6.6 kPa (50 mmHg), or the saturation falls below 85% she must stop. Suctioning time should be limited to 15 seconds, and the procedure is ideally carried out with a system which allows continuous ventilation rather than requiring disconnection from the ventilator. If the baby is attached to an ECG monitor, suctioning should be stopped and IPPV restarted if the heart rate falls below 80 beats/min.

Choice of ventilator

Most neonatal ventilators are designed as pressure-limited, time-cycled machines, although improvements in technology have recently enabled suitable volume-limited ventilators to be developed. Experience with these is limited, but they are attractive because "volutrauma" may be as important as "barotrauma" in the genesis of CLD. Many modern neonatal ventilators offer high frequency oscillation and the facility for continuous on-line monitoring of pressure, volume, flow and compliance. Patient triggered ventilation is also an option, with the stimulus used for the trigger varying from an in-line flow or pressure sensor to an external respiration detector. Some ventilators can trigger in inspiration and expiration.

The ventilators currently available in the UK are listed in Table 11.10. They offer precise gas delivery with monitors and alarms for

Table 11.10 Summary of neonatal ventilators in the UK in 2000, with the different modalities available (developed from Sinha and Donn 1996)

Ventilator	Manufacturer	Modes (in addition to IPPV)	Trigger signal	Comments
Babylog 8000	Dräger (Germany)	PTV; SIMV; HFO (add on) Volume support	Airway flow via hot wire anemometer	Extensive graphic displays available
Sechrist	Sechrist Industries, Anaheim CA	PTV	Thoracic impedance	Real time analogue output
SLE HV2000	SLE Surrey UK	PTV, SIMV, HFO	Airway pressure/airway flow via airway pressure transducer	Graphic display
VIP-BIRD	Bird Products, California USA	PTV, SIMV, PSV	Airway pressure	Offers volume cycled or time cycled ventilation. On-line graphic display available

safety, trigger options, and a choice of ventilatory modalities including time cycled and volume cycled ventilation, pressure support and oscillatory ventilation (Sinha and Donn 1996). The mainstay of successful treatment for the average baby with RDS remains a good, safe, well-maintained ventilator correctly assembled, connected to a well humidified and warmed gas supply and used in conventional time-cycled pressure-limited mode. All those who care for acutely ill babies should be entirely comfortable with use of a ventilator this way, whilst keeping abreast of newer developments which may be shown to offer advantages.

Choosing and adjusting conventional ventilator settings in RDS

Key points about ventilation

- Effective ventilation is only likely to be achieved when the chest wall moves, ideally moving in phase with the ventilator.
- The PaO_2 is directly related to the MAP. MAP is dependent in turn on PIP, PEEP and the duration of inspiration (see Fig 11.11).
- Carbon dioxide tension is mainly affected by the rate and the difference between PIP and PEEP, that is the tidal volume. Slow rates, short expiratory times and high levels of PEEP are more likely to cause CO_2 retention.
- The blood gases in a ventilated baby are likely to be better if he is breathing synchronously with the ventilator (or if he is making no spontaneous respiratory effort).
- In addition to achieving better blood gases and synchrony at fast

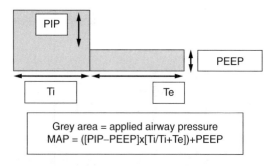

Grey area = applied airway pressure
MAP = ([PIP–PEEP]x[Ti/Ti+Te])+PEEP

Figure 11.11 Diagram to show relationship of ventilator settings to mean airway pressure.

rates, there is now clear evidence that the incidence of PIE and pneumothorax is also less in babies ventilated at rates of 60–80/min with a T_I of 0.3–0.5 seconds.

- $PaCO_2$ values below 3 kPa (approx 20 mmHg) must be avoided in preterm babies as this predisposes them to PVL (p. 330).
- Artificial ventilation damages the lungs. Use the lowest settings compatible with achieving satisfactory blood gases. The most important determinants of lung injury are the degree and the duration of PIP. Whenever possible, try to reduce the PIP and avoid long inspiratory times. In particular avoid an inspiratory time which is longer than the expiratory time (a reversed I:E ratio).

Initial ventilator settings in RDS

The following settings need to be considered:

- flow rate of gases through the ventilator circuit;
- inspired oxygen concentration (F_IO_2);
- peak inspiratory pressure;
- positive end expiratory pressure;
- duration of inspiration and expiration which determines the rate in breaths/min.

As a general guide start VLBW babies on:

- flow of 6 l/min
- inspired oxygen concentration of 50%
- PIP of 15 to 18 cm of H_2O
- PEEP of 3 cm of H_2O
- inspiratory time of 0.4 seconds, a rate of 60 breaths/min ($T_I:T_E$ = 1:1.5).

For larger babies born near term start with a PIP of 18 to 25 cm H_2O. Watch for chest movement and synchrony between the baby's respiratory effort and the ventilator. Use the minimum level of PIP which is required to move the baby's chest. Check a blood gas 20 minutes after starting ventilation and adjust the settings according to the guidelines in the next section.

Changing ventilator settings in RDS   Aim to keep the blood gases in the range PaO_2 6.0–10.0 kPa (45–75 mmHg) and $PaCO_2$ 5.0–7.5 kPa (37–56 mmHg) with a pH above 7.25. Vigorous high-pressure ventilation to keep the $PaCO_2$ in the normal range (Table 11.4) is not necessary, and is associated with a higher incidence of chronic lung disease.

Gentler ventilation is "kinder" to immature lungs (so called "permissive hypercarbia"). If oxygenation is poor, an improvement may be achieved by an increase in the PEEP, the F_IO_2 or the duration of inspiration instead of increasing the PIP. However, even in the era of antenatal steroids and postnatal surfactant the occasional baby remains hypercarbic and hypoxic unless a PIP of up to 35 cm H_2O is used. Do not be afraid to try higher pressures in order to avoid the baby remaining too long with unsatisfactory blood gases. There is no need to use more than 95% oxygen (p. 146), but it is better to leave the FiO_2 at 95% rather than increase the ventilator pressure.

Achieving synchrony

We strongly believe that achieving synchronous ventilation is the best way to ventilate an awake baby. By synchrony we mean that the ventilator inflation and deflation cycles coincide with the baby's cycles. There is some evidence that synchronous ventilation gives better oxygenation and fewer pneumothoraces (Greenough *et al.* 1998). Synchrony reduces the need for paralysis, and as pancuronium has several disadvantages including muscle wasting, ileus, hypotension and increased extracellular fluid volume we prefer to avoid it.

In general, synchronous ventilation uses a rate of >60 breaths/ min, because that is what the baby does. Babies of 26 weeks gestation breathe even faster, at rates of up to 100 breaths/min. In order to synchronize the ventilator with the baby, stand by the baby and alter the PIP so that there is adequate chest wall expansion. In addition, watch the baby's chest wall movements whilst listening to the ventilator; if the baby is synchronous the chest wall should move up in time with the ventilator inflation. To try and synchronize the baby's respiratory efforts with ventilator inflation the following manoeuvres can be undertaken:

- Increase ventilator rate to approximately the baby's breathing rate on CPAP.
- Shorten the inflation time in 0.05 second steps, but not below 0.2 seconds as that impairs delivered volume.
- Trigger ventilation can be used.

Babies who remain asynchronous despite rate and inspiratory time manipulation should be more heavily sedated and given an analgesic (use morphine and/or midazolam). If this is unsuccessful then trigger ventilation may succeed (usually in bigger babies) or the baby should be paralysed.

Trigger ventilation

One alternative that can be used to deal with the problem of asynchrony during IPPV is to use patient-triggered ventilation. In American textbooks this mode of ventilation is often referred to as assist/control ventilation. In PTV the machine-delivered breath is initiated in response to a signal derived from the baby's own inspiratory effort. Four signals have been used to provide PTV to the newborn; airway pressure, airway flow, measuring the baby's own activity via a Graesby capsule respiration monitor (p. 97) or using an impedance monitor. The latter two methods have a considerable "trigger delay". This means that the time it takes for the signal from the baby's own effort to start the ventilator cycling is so long that the baby has already taken much of his breath in before the ventilator starts to cycle. A recent large multicentre trial, enrolling almost 1000 babies, failed to show any advantage for PTV as the primary mode of ventilation in neonatal RDS using any of the SLE 2000, Draeger babylog or Sechrist ventilators (Baumer et al. 2000). This trial used a very short inspiratory time of 0.2 seconds (see below) in trigger mode. The main use for PTV may be weaning.

In PTV the neonatologist determines PIP, PEEP and inspiratory time. The baby sets his own rate. When starting PTV

- Leave the PIP, PEEP, and flow rate unchanged from conventional ventilation.
- Reduce the inspiratory time to about 0.4 seconds. If the baby has a very fast respiratory rate of over 60 breaths/min the inspiratory time should be reduced further, but not below 0.2 seconds.
- Set the back-up rate in conventional mode. This determines the number of breaths the baby will receive per minute should he become apnoeic. For example at a back-up rate of 30 breaths/min the baby who does not breathe for 2 seconds will then receive a ventilator breath.

Check arterial blood gases within 20 minutes of starting PTV. If the blood gases have not improved compared to conventional ventilation and/or the baby is still asynchronous, PTV will not be of benefit. Return to conventional mode and consider paralysis. Small babies tend to tire on PTV, which has not proved suitable for babies with acute RDS. Larger babies tend to breathe very fast and reduce their $PaCO_2$.

Synchronous intermittent mandatory ventilation

SIMV can facilitate weaning in VLBW babies who have normal blood gases on low pressure, low rate ventilation but cannot sustain adequate respiration. SIMV is an alternative to PTV for weaning, the idea being to avoid the adverse effects of prolonged apnoea while the baby "learns" to make some spontaneous respiratory effort. This mode of ventilation is a combination of trigger ventilation and IPPV. The baby can trigger breaths in the usual way (via an airway or body sensor), and these breaths are supported by the ventilator so that the baby achieves a full inspiration from a little effort. In between the triggered, supported breaths the ventilator is effectively operating in CPAP mode, with a supply of fresh gas from which the baby can take a spontaneous unsupported breath. There is a window of time during which the baby can trigger breaths and then a refractory window during which breaths, if detected, will not trigger a ventilator breath. The sensitive and refractory period is altered by the back-up rate chosen. For example, if the back up rate on the Dräeger ventilator is set to 30 breaths/min, the ventilator divides up the minute into 30 two second epochs. This ventilator remains sensitive for the whole of the epoch until a breath is taken and triggered, after which the rest of the epoch is refractory. Any more breaths taken by the baby will not be "trigger" breaths, but they are supported by CPAP. If no breath at all is taken for 2 seconds the ventilator will put in a ventilator breath. This elegant method would seem to be ideal for weaning, but research studies have not shown it to be better than PTV alone. Nevertheless the option is available on many modern ventilators and can be useful for some babies. SIMV is of no benefit in the acute phase of RDS.

Solutions to unsatisfactory blood gases in RDS

1. To improve oxygenation when the $PaCO_2$ is normal. In this situation, with the $PaCO_2$ 5.0–6.5 kPa (37–56 mmHg), there are three alternatives;
   - increasing the inspired oxygen concentration;
   - increasing the respirator rate (particularly if the baby is not breathing in synchrony);
   - increasing the MAP without increasing the peak pressures (by increasing T_I or the level of PEEP).

Try increasing the F_IO_2 first (not beyond 95% – *v.s.*), and next or at the same time adjust the rate to achieve ventilator/patient synchrony. If the baby is already in synchrony then it is acceptable to gradually increase the T_I towards 0.5–0.6 seconds, but never let the $T_I:T_E$ ratio exceed 1.5:1 nor the baby get out of phase with the ventilator. These manoeuvres increase the MAP. If they fail, increase the PIP and accept the lowish $PaCO_2$ as long as it is not below 3 kPa (p. 331). Increasing the PEEP to above 7 cm H_2O is rarely of any benefit.

2. To improve oxygenation when the $PaCO_2$ is low <4.5 kPa (34 mmHg). Consider;
   - **wrong diagnosis.** The baby has compliant lungs, so there may be another cause for hypoxaemia (e.g. congenital heart disease (p. 361 et. seq.), sepsis (pp. 239–41), PPHN (pp. 189–191);
   - **gross over-ventilation.** Over-ventilation prevents adequate pulmonary perfusion and reduces the PaO_2. The CXR in such babies shows lung fields which are black, with low flat diaphragms and a small heart shadow.

   If none of these diagnoses apply the baby probably has severe RDS. To improve oxygenation try to sustain the MAP, but change other things in ways that might increase the $PaCO_2$ (e.g. increase the PEEP or decrease the rate).

3. To lower a high carbon dioxide concentration ($PaCO_2$ >8–9 kPa (60–68 mmHg) with an acceptable level of oxygen. There are several alternatives;
   - increasing the rate but to no more than 90–100 min;
   - reducing the PEEP, but not to below 3 cm H_2O, since PEEP preserves surfactant;
   - reducing the inspiratory time (but not to less than 0.2 seconds);
   - lengthen the expiratory time.

4. After a change in ventilator settings always check the blood gases 1–2 hours later to confirm improvement.

These options are summarized in Table 11.11.

Failure to respond to ventilator manipulation

Confronted with a baby who fails to respond to these manipulations and remains hypoxic in 95% oxygen at pressures of 30/6 cm H_2O and a rate of 60–80 breaths/min, always check the CXR and consider the following possibilities:

Table 11.11 Summary of adjustments to ventilator settings on the basis of blood gas results

Oxygen	Carbon dioxide	Action
Low PaO_2	High $PaCO_2$	Increase PIP — which will increase MAP. In spontaneously breathing babies an increased rate may work
Low PaO_2	Normal $PaCO_2$	Increase F_iO_2; ↑ MAP but maintain PIP (i.e. ↑ PEEP or ↑ T_i)
Low PaO_2	Low $PaCO_2$	Consider alternative diagnoses to RDS; over ventilation
Normal PaO_2	High $PaCO_2$	↓ PEEP; ↑ rate; keep MAP constant
Normal PaO_2	Normal $PaCO_2$	Sit tight! unless weaning (p. 173–175)
Normal PaO_2	Low $PaCO_2$	↓ rate; maintain MAP
High PaO_2	High $PaCO_2$	Rare. Check for mechanical problems e.g. blocked tube. ↓ PEEP: ↓ T_i; ↑ rate
High PaO_2	Normal $PaCO_2$	↓ MAP (usually by ↓PIP): ↓F_iO_2
High PaO_2	Low $PaCO_2$	Over ventilated — ↓ Pressure ↓ rate ↓F_iO_2

1. There may be mechanical problems such as a blocked ETT, a leak around the ETT or ventilator failure. Check all machinery for leaks, try hand-ventilating with a bag and mask and insert a larger ETT.

2. The baby may have only moderately severe RDS but has uncorrected acidaemia*, hypotension* or hypoglycaemia*. Check pH, blood pressure, PCV, glucose and treat accordingly.

3. There may have been an incorrect diagnosis, or a complication of RDS may have developed:
   (a) pneumothorax or PIE (pp. 181–187);
   (b) congenital heart disease* (mature > premature) (Chapter 22);
   (c) pulmonary haemorrhage (pp. 188–189);
   (d) pulmonary oedema/fluid overload/patent ductus arteriosus (pp. 355–356);
   (e) persistent pulmonary hypertension* (mature > premature) (pp. 189–192);
   (f) over ventilation* (see above);
   (g) pneumonia and septicaemia* (p. 244); especially GBS sepsis (p. 239);
   (h) intracranial haemorrhage* (p. 324–326);
   (i) pulmonary hypoplasia (after very prolonged rupture of membranes with oligohydramnios).

   *these conditions will usually have a reduced or normal $PaCO_2$ whereas in the others it will be considerably raised.

A baby with a chest X-ray which shows RDS who remains hypoxic (PaO_2 <5.5 kPa, 42 mmHg) in spite of two doses of surfactant, high oxygen concentrations, and ventilator settings which achieve synchrony at a pressure of more than 30/6 cm H_2O is now unusual. Values for PaO_2 of 5.3–6.6 kPa (40–50 mmHg) and $PaCO_2$ of 7–8 kPa (52–60 mmHg) may be acceptable in a baby with very severe lung disease for a time if the pH remains above 7.25. The blood pressure should be supported and any acidaemia corrected. The advice of an experienced neonatologist must be sought.

High frequency oscillatory ventilation (HFOV)

The strategy of HFOV is to inflate the lungs and recruit "lung units" by applying a continuous distending pressure which keeps the lung at the optimal place on its hysteresis curve (Fig. 11.3). Oxygenation and carbon dioxide removal occurs via an oscillating pressure waveform superimposed on the MAP. High frequency oscillators are essentially airway vibrators (a piston pump or vibrating diaphragm) that operate at frequencies at around 10 Hz (1 Hz = 1 cycle/s, 60 cycles/min) (Table 11.12). During HFOV, inspiration and expiration are both active. A continuous flow of fresh gas rushes past the vibrating source that generates the oscillation and a controlled leak or low-pass filter allows gas to exit the system. Pressure oscillations within the airway produce a "tidal volume" of 2–3 ml around a constant mean airway pressure, which maintains lung volume in a manner equivalent to using very high levels of CPAP. The volume of gas moved in the "tidal volume" is determined by the amplitude of the airway pressure oscillation (ΔP). The following settings need to be considered for oscillatory ventilation:

Table 11.12 Summary of available neonatal oscillators in the UK 2000

Oscillator	Manufacturer	Modes apart from HFO	Comments
3100A	SensorMedics	None	Only oscillator used so far in RCTs. I:E ratio 1:2 recommended
Babylog 8000	Dräeger (Germany)	IPPV, PTV, SIMV	I:E ratio 0.2–0.8 adjusted by the machine, not the operator
SLE HV2000	SLE Surrey UK	IPPV, PTV, SIMV	I:E ratio fixed at 1:1

- flow rate of gases through the ventilator circuit (usually fixed around 6–8 l/min)
- inspired oxygen concentration
- mean airway pressure
- oscillatory frequency
- oscillatory pressure amplitude – ΔP
- inspiratory: expiratory ratio or percentage of cycle as inspiratory time.

Oscillators are powerful tools, and in "rescue" mode HFOV can save some babies with severe RDS who have failed to respond to conventional ventilation and surfactant, although the only RCT of rescue HFOV published to date showed no benefit in reduced mortality (HiFo study group 1993). HFOV is particularly effective in the management of hypercarbia. What is less certain than rescue is the role of HFOV used as the primary mode of ventilation in RDS in today's population of very small babies who have received antenatal steroids and postnatal surfactant. A meta–analysis of four trials of high frequency ventilation revealed no difference in mortality or the incidence of chronic lung disease (Cools and Offringa 1999). At the present time HFOV is reserved for rescue in most UK neonatal units, although a MRC sponsored trial of HFOV as the primary mode of ventilation in RDS has recently finished recruitment at over 800 babies.

There was concern in the early studies about a high incidence of GMH-IVH (HiFi study group 1989) but this complication has not been seen in the more recent HFO studies which have used a high volume/low FiO_2 strategy. This strategy harnesses the ability of HFOV to maintain alveolar recruitment by using a higher MAP with a lower peak airway pressure than conventional ventilation.

Although oscillators can generate a ΔP as high as 90 cm H_2O, this high pressure is not transmitted to the alveolus, and is attenuated. Only 10–20% of the proximal airway pressure is transmitted to the end of the endotracheal tube, depending on the size of the tube. Oscillation works best on homogeneous lung diseases in which the volume is reduced, such as severe RDS, bilateral PIE (p. 187), pneumonia, early meconium aspiration syndrome. HFOV does not work well in cases with patchy involvement or unilateral air leak. The cardiac effects of "mega-CPAP" mean that it is contra-indicated in babies with poor myocardial function who are already very dependent on inotropic support.

Indications for HFOV   These include the following:

- failure of RDS to respond to surfactant and IPPV;
- primary mode of ventilation for RDS (not proven; *v.s.*);
- meconium aspiration syndrome with homogenous disease, without pneumothorax;
- pneumonia failing to respond to conventional ventilation;
- severe bilateral uniform PIE with hypercarbia.

Relative contra-indications for HFOV – use with care   These include the following:

- hypotensive baby dependent on inotropic support;
- inhomogenous lung disease;
- pre-existing pneumothorax – need to use a high FiO_2/low volume strategy.

Starting oscillation from birth   The following settings should be used:

- F_IO_2 60%
- Frequency 10 Hz
- I:E ratio 1:2 (percentage of inspiratory time 33%) – SensorMedics only
- MAP 6–8 cm
- Oscillatory amplitude – increase until the chest wall is just perceptibly "bouncing" – usually about 18 cm H_2O

Changing to oscillatory ventilation from conventional ventilation

- Keep the F_IO_2 the same as that which the baby is already receiving;
- Set the frequency to 10 Hz;
- Set the inspiratory fraction to 0.3% – 0.5%. This is only relevant for the SensorMedics as the I:E ratio is either fixed or determined by the machine on the other oscillators;
- Amplitude (power, ΔP) – increase until the chest wall is bouncing, usually about 18 cm H_2O;
- Use the same MAP as when on IPPV to start with, then increase by 0.5–1.0 cm every 10–15 minutes until no further improvement in PaO_2 – at that point do a CXR to check the level of the diaphragms.

Ventilator changes during HFOV   **Oxygenation** is dependent primarily on:

- MAP
- F_IO_2
- Blood pressure.

As mentioned above, MAP should be increased by 0.5–1.0 cm every 10–15 minutes until there is no further improvement in PaO_2. At that point take a CXR to check the level of the diaphragms; over ventilation is present if the lung margin is below the 9th rib. If oxygenation decreases whilst on oscillation, assess whether the baby is hypovolaemic or hypotensive and perform a CXR. Persisting hypoxaemia may respond to a combination of NO (p. 192–193) and HFOV. There is now no place for systemic vasodilator therapy in RDS.

Carbon dioxide elimination is mainly dependent on the amplitude; if the $PaCO_2$ increases the amplitude should be increased. There is also an effect of frequency, but most oscillators operate at a fixed frequency. Start by altering the amplitude, and alter the frequency only as a last resort.

Weaning from HFOV   The aim during weaning is to maintain optimum lung volume: therefore reduce F_IO_2 before MAP. Once the F_IO_2 is down to 30% then reduce MAP by 2 cm steps monitoring the blood gases regularly. If the PaO_2 decreases during weaning it is likely that you are reducing the MAP too slowly; take a CXR to check for over–distension. Once the MAP is down to 10–12 cm H_2O change back to IPPV. Set the conventional ventilator up to give a similar MAP, adjusting the PIP with a PEEP 3 cm. An alternative is to wean directly from HFOV by reducing the MAP.

Nitric oxide in RDS   Nitric oxide treatment for RDS must be regarded as experimental at the present time. Preliminary results in severe RDS have been disappointing (Subhedar *et al.* 1997). However, in babies who remain persistently hypoxaemic despite all possible endeavour this treatment may be worth trying, after a full explanation has been given to the parents. A UK trial is in progress (INNOVO). ECMO is not an option for babies weighing less than 2.5 kg, and we have not had to resort to ECMO for RDS in more mature babies, although others have. For more detailed advice on using nitric oxide and ECMO, see the section on PPHN (p. 192–194).

OTHER THERAPY

Antibiotics

We put all ventilated babies on antibiotics for three reasons:

1. severe early onset sepsis can masquerade as RDS (p. 239);
2. sepsis can co-exist with surfactant deficient RDS (p. 125);
3. once intubated the lung will be colonized with pathogens which can cause either pneumonia or septicaemia.

We use penicillin and gentamicin (p. 235) until cultures are available at 48 hours. If the initial cultures are negative and the CRP (p. 233) is less than 6 mg/l at 48 hours we stop antibiotics unless the secretions or the CXR suggest that pneumonia is developing.

Analgesia/paralysis (see Chapter 9)

Being on a ventilator is undoubtedly uncomfortable and stressful. High catecholamine levels have been measured in such babies, and there is a relationship between very high levels of stress hormones and adverse outcome. We have found that the combination of a mild sedative such as midazolam with bolus doses of morphine to cover painful procedures and/or a background low dose morphine infusion works well. The aim is to achieve a settled baby who breathes synchronously with the ventilator but in whom a reversal of the sedative effect can be rapidly achieved for weaning. Paralysis with pancuronium is a last resort but is still required from time to time. This drug does have undesirable side effects, but it is clear that it considerably reduces the number of pneumothoraces in babies who are breathing out of phase with the ventilator (Greenough *et al.* 1984). Situations where pancuronium is indicated, apart from severe RDS with asynchrony, include PIE and pneumothorax (pp. 186–187), PPHN (p. 191), meconium aspiration (p. 180), massive pulmonary haemorrhage (pp. 188–189), and diaphragmatic hernia (p. 195). Babies who are given pancuronium because they are fighting the ventilator, are frequently doing a lot of their own "ventilation" and in such cases it will often be necessary to increase the ventilator pressures to achieve adequate blood gases after the pancuronium is given. The other main side effect is that the absence of spontaneous movements causes some peripheral oedema.

Paralysed babies must always be monitored carefully since they are unable to sustain even feeble respiratory efforts if they become disconnected from the ventilator or if their ETT blocks.

Once started, pancuronium should, in general, be continued until the baby requires pressures below 25/5 cm H_2O and below 60% oxygen. It is unwise to stop pancuronium in a baby who is still having problems with air leaks. The effects of pancuronium can usually be allowed to wear off; it is rarely necessary to reverse it with atropine and neostigmine. Infusions should not be used because of the risk of high plasma levels if renal function is inadequate.

SUDDEN DETERIORATION ON IPPV

The steps to be taken when a baby's condition suddenly deteriorates when on IPPV are shown in Fig. 11.12. The important causes of deterioration are:

Blocked endotracheal tube

Check that the chest is moving. This is the key to assessing neonatal ventilation at all times, and a baby whose chest is not moving as well as it was earlier, and whose blood gases are developing increasing hypercarbia, is likely to have a blocked tube. If the problem does not resolve with suction, the endotracheal tube must be changed. If the chest still does not move, the baby has either a blocked trachea, a bilateral pneumothorax or very stiff lungs.

Pneumothorax (pp. 181–187)

The incidence of pneumothorax in ventilated babies is now about 10%. Pneumothorax can cause a catastrophic deterioration with hypoxaemia, hypercarbia and hypotension. If time permits, a CXR should be taken to confirm the diagnosis. In the emergency situation, diagnosis can be confirmed by the clinical signs and by transillumination (p. 184). Any pneumothorax which is associated with a deterioration in blood gases should be drained with a proper chest drain. Occasionally a very small pneumothorax which is found on a routine CXR in an unventilated baby can be observed because the air will absorb. However, if a baby with even a small pneumothorax requires artificial ventilation the air leak is likely to enlarge and become a tension pneumothorax, so a drain should be inserted.

GMH-IVH (pp. 324–326)

A large GMH-IVH may be responsible whenever any baby weighing less than 1.5 kg suddenly deteriorates, whether or not he is receiving IPPV. The baby is difficult to resuscitate, and remains hypoxic and acidaemic with a poor peripheral circulation; there is often also a fall in haematocrit.

Pulmonary haemorrhage

The clue to this diagnosis is a frothy pink endotracheal aspirate. Pulmonary haemorrhage is often associated with haemorrhagic pulmonary oedema because of a patent ductus arteriosus (pp. 355–356). There is usually a coagulopathy. The CXR shows widespread patchy infiltration. Pulmonary haemorrhage is difficult to treat but the best advice is to increase the ventilator settings, paralyze the baby, and replace clotting factors with fresh frozen plasma, cryoprecipitate and platelets as indicated.

GRADUAL DETERIORATION ON IPPV

There are six major diagnoses to consider if a baby's deterioration is more gradual.

1. infection;
2. GMH-IVH;
3. patent ductus arteriosus;
4. partial blockage of the ETT;
5. anaemia/hypotension;
6. slow development of an air leak.

Infection

With the exception of babies who present acutely ill with sepsis (usually GBS) within the first few hours, an infectious cause of deterioration is unusual in the first few days, since antibiotics will have been given to all babies on admission for the reasons given on pp. 166–167, 241. After this period, by far the commonest cause of septicaemia is CONS. CONS is particularly common in babies on long-term IPPV with central lines *in situ* to administer TPN (p. 243). Any other organism can cause septicaemia (pp. 241–242). Pneumonia may also cause problems in the following situations:

1. secondary infection with an organism such as candida or pseudomonas not covered by penicillin and gentamicin;
2. reinfection in a neonate on long-term IPPV some time after an initial course of antibiotics was completed.

Both septicaemia and pneumonia usually present over a period of hours rather than days, with some combination of the following signs:

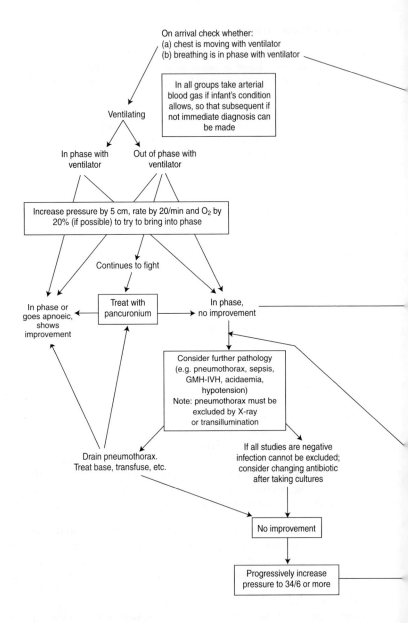

Figure 11.12 Algorithm for action when a baby deteriorates suddenly on a ventilator.

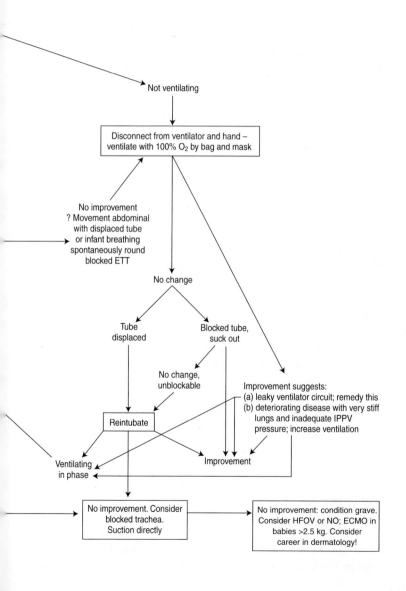

Not ventilating

Disconnect from ventilator and hand –
ventilate with 100% O₂ by bag and mask

No improvement
? Movement abdominal
with displaced tube
or infant breathing
spontaneously round
blocked ETT

No change

Tube
displaced

Blocked tube,
suck out

No change,
unblockable

Improvement suggests:
(a) leaky ventilator circuit; remedy this
(b) deteriorating disease with very stiff
lungs and inadequate IPPV
pressure; increase ventilation

Reintubate

Ventilating
in phase

Improvement

No improvement. Consider
blocked trachea.
Suction directly

No improvement: condition grave.
Consider HFOV or NO; ECMO in
babies >2.5 kg. Consider
career in dermatology!

1. increasing lethargy, decreased peripheral perfusion, pallor;
2. temperature instability;
3. increasing jaundice;
4. nasogastric feeds no longer tolerated, vomiting, abdominal distension;
5. increased thick (purulent) secretions up the ETT and a positive culture of the aspirate;
6. deteriorating lung function – PaO_2 falling, $PaCO_2$ rising;
7. on auscultation, localized or generalized crepitations;
8. CXR changes that are patchy (suggesting pneumonia).

With CONS septicaemia the only clinical features that are usually present are increased lethargy and temperature instability, whereas more clinical features are present in babies with pneumonia. Laboratory confirmation with a raised WBC with a neutrophilia, a raised CRP and a fall in the platelet count is usually obtained.

Most of the above clinical findings are also compatible with deteriorating RDS in a small sick baby, with pulmonary oedema from a PDA or the development of CLD; but since they could also indicate infection, one should start antibiotics or broaden or change the spectrum of cover. If CONS sepsis is a possibility always include flucloxacillin or vancomycin (pp. 233–234). If no organisms grow, this course of antibiotics can be discontinued after 5–10 days.

GMH-IVH (pp. 324–326)

As well as the acute deterioration (*v.s.*), there may be a more stuttering deterioration with the baby becoming pale and unresponsive with deteriorating blood gases. The diagnosis can be confirmed by cerebral ultrasound.

Patent ductus arteriosus (pp. 335–336)

This is a common cause of deterioration towards the end of the first week. The typical clinical and echocardiographic signs will usually be present.

Partial blockage of the ETT

The nurses may suspect this because of difficulties passing the endotracheal suction tube, or there may be conducted sounds audible on chest auscultation. The only way to confirm this diagnosis is to change the ETT.

Anaemia/hypotension

Hypotension may be due to sepsis or GMH-IVH, but can also be due to fluid or blood loss from any cause. Losses due to the blood removed for laboratory analysis must always be replaced by transfusion. (pp. 142–143).

Other causes

Other conditions causing gradual deterioration are:

1. infection in other sites – e.g. meningitis, NEC;
2. development of any type of air leak;
3. electrolyte imbalance, especially marked hyponatraemia, hypocalcaemia, hypo- or hyperkalaemia;
4. hypoglycaemia;
5. development of severe CLD with bronchial hypersecretion.

Weaning off IPPV

Once a baby is stable on the ventilator, off pancuronium, and his gases have been satisfactory for 12 hours or so, and he is no longer dependent on nitric oxide, the weaning process can begin. If, when paralysis is stopped, the blood gases deteriorate and the baby becomes asynchronous with the ventilator then re-paralyse the baby and wait longer before attempting to wean him.

Some babies who were intubated in the labour ward are soon found to have a normal CXR and minimal disease, and in them weaning can be rapid. However, in general, in babies with typical RDS, the temptation to wean them rapidly within the first 48 hours should be resisted; they often deteriorate if this is done, and require vigorous ventilation for resuscitation. Remember that the natural history of RDS is that the disease worsens in the second 24 hour period.

The weaning process using a conventional ventilator is outlined in Table 11.13. This process may take several weeks, or it may be achieved within 24 hours. An alternative method is to use PTV (p. 159), allowing the baby to choose his own rate throughout the process and reducing the pressure until the PIP is virtually the same as PEEP. At this point the baby is effectively on CPAP and can be extubated if he copes on this. Whenever weaning is planned, start caffeine 12–24 hours beforehand, since this reduces the need for reventilation (Henderson-Smart and Davis 1998). PTV can be very

Table 11.13 Weaning from IPPV

Situation	Action
PaO_2 9.0–10.5 kPa (70–80 mmHg) $PaCO_2$ 5–7 kPa (35–50 mmHg) Stable ventilator settings, satisfactory CXR	Start weaning by reducing the PIP and PEEP in 2 cm steps to 12–14 cm PIP and 3 cm PEEP; check blood gases after each step. Reduce F_1O_2. Start caffeine, stop pancuronium
Blood gases satisfactory on F_1O_2 30–40%; PIP/PEEP 12–14/3	Reduce rate in 5 bpm steps to 10/min, watch $PaCO_2$.
Blood gases satisfactory and baby tolerating handling without apnoea at a rate of 20 bpm, low pressures of 12–14/2 and a low F_1O_2 of around 30%	Stop feeds and extubate. Randomized trials show no difference between a head box and CPAP at this point but CPAP should certainly be offered early if the baby develops CO_2 retention or apnoea

useful for weaning but SIMV has not been shown to be better than PTV or conventional ventilation.

Generally speaking, the smaller the baby the slower the process. Certain points in Table 11.13 need expansion.

Following every change in the ventilator setting or F_1O_2 the blood gases should be checked within 1–2 hours to ensure that the PaO_2 and $PaCO_2$ are still satisfactory. If they are not, revert to the previous ventilator settings. In VLBW babies more than 72 hours old who are no longer at high risk of GMH-IVH, it is reasonable to allow the $PaCO_2$ to rise to 7–8 kPa during weaning, as long as the pH is >7.2 (p. 140 and p. 324).

Since more damage is done to the lungs by high pressures than by high oxygen concentrations, try to reduce the pressure first, but always preserve a little PEEP to splint the alveoli open and preserve surfactant. In general, reduce the pressure by 2–3 cm H_2O at a time and the oxygen by 5–10% at a time. Bigger reductions can be made if the PaO_2 is much above 13.3 kPa (100 mmHg) or the CO_2 well below 5.6 kPa (40 mmHg). In general, it is not possible to make more than one such step every four hours.

Once the pressure is in the 12–14/3–4 cm H_2O range, reduce the oxygen to 30–40%, and then reduce the rate to 20/min. If low CO_2 values persist, it means that the lungs are improving rapidly and the pressure and rate can be lowered faster and further. Stop sedation and analgesia as the rate falls below 20 breaths/min.

Extubation Most VLBW babies do not tolerate ETT CPAP at all well when being weaned. Our practice is to extubate small babies from a rate of 10 breaths/min rather than subjecting them to a trial of CPAP, and this routine is supported by the results of a meta-analysis of several small randomized trials (Davis and Henderson-Smart 1998). The extra work of breathing introduced by the resistance of a small bore endotracheal tube exhausts many preterm babies, and the absence of any positive pressure inflations (which act as "sighs") reduces the FRC so that the baby is placed at a disadvantage when the endotracheal tube is removed. Whether it is better to extubate VLBWI directly to nasal CPAP is a question which has been addressed by several studies. The answer appears to be that it makes no difference whether CPAP is offered straight away or only when the baby needs it.

Predicting successful extubation is an imprecise art. In our experience the following precautions make successful extubation more likely:

1. Ensure that, when attempting extubation, the baby is otherwise in optimal condition – his electrolytes and calcium are normal, and his PCV is greater than 40%. Take a CXR to make sure that a small pneumothorax or area of consolidation has not recently appeared, in which case wait until they are corrected before extubation.
2. Ensure that the plasma levels of caffeine or theophylline are in the therapeutic range.
3. Following extubation, ensure adequate humidification of the inspired gases.
4. Be guided by the blood gases. If these rapidly deteriorate after extubation, the time was not right. However, a gradual rise in $PaCO_2$ up to 8.0–8.5 kPa (60–64 mmHg), or a gradual fall in PaO_2, can be allowed so long as the baby is breathing well, looks clinically well and holds his pH above 7.25. These blood gas changes are often transient over the 6–12 hours after extubation, and then improve. Consider nasal prong CPAP in this situation in VLBWI.
5. Stop all oral feeding for 6–12 hours. Feeds decrease the PaO_2. Nasogastric tubes block one nostril, increase the work of breathing, and act as an irritant increasing secretions in the upper respiratory tract.
6. Carefully aspirate the baby's mouth and oropharynx regularly. If secretions were a problem before extubation, the routine used while on IPPV, of regular turning and positioning, plus physiotherapy and suction (if necessary) should be continued every 3–4 hours.

7. Remember the minimal handling rule (Chapter 8). This is difficult when giving physiotherapy and suction, but reduce to the absolute minimum the number of times the baby is interfered with, since any disturbance may cause a fall in PaO_2, an episode of apnoea, and the need for reinsertion of the ETT.

Long-term difficulties with weaning and extubation

Repeated failure to wean a baby off IPPV may be due to any of the following factors:

1. **Persisting problems with secretions.** Leave a nasal ETT *in situ* for 3–5 days, + IMV combined with a vigorous programme of chest physiotherapy, endotracheal tube suction and antibiotic therapy if appropriate before trying again.
2. **Recurrent apnoea once extubated.** The baby should be reintubated and given caffeine. Try again in 1 or 2 days. If apnoea persists off IMV, this may be a sign of a small GMH-IVH, sepsis, or gastro-oesophageal reflux. Image the baby's brain with ultrasound, and consider a pH study or treatment for reflux. Try CPAP but continue IMV if necessary.
3. **PDA and/or pulmonary oedema** (pp. 355–356). Babies in this situation are particularly likely to deteriorate if their PCV is less than 40%. Reintubate, control fluids, give Lasix and indomethacin, and try again. Consider surgery if all else fails.
4. **Chronic lung disease.** If this is severe it may take several months to wean the baby off both IMV or CPAP. Treatment is with patience, minimal ventilator settings, steroids and diuretics (pp. 206–211).
5. **Laryngeal oedema or subglottic stenosis.** In the short term these can usually be circumvented by good humidification and some nasal CPAP. Occasionally, dexamethasone 0.5–1.0 mg IM four times daily for 48 hours before extubation and then discontinued over a further 48 hours may help. If this fails, reinsert a nasal ETT (together with IMV) taking great care to immobilize it. Leave for 48–96 hours before reattempting extubation under dexamethasone cover. In some babies moderate degrees of subglottic stenosis can be controlled with long-term nasal CPAP, until the baby grows and the stenosis resolves. A cricoid split operation can be tried (Seid and Canty 1985) but tracheostomy is a last resort in such babies, since if one is inserted it is very unlikely that decannulation will be possible in under 6 months.

6. **Very small babies** (<1.0–1.20 kg). If after three attempts you have failed to extubate such a baby, restart IMV at 3–5 breaths/min plus 2–3 cm CPAP, and fatten the baby up by the enteral or intravenous route. Ten days and 250 g later, he will probably extubate easily.

7. **Underlying neurological problems.** GMH-IVH was considered above but primary muscle disorders, e.g. dystrophia myotonica may present this way.

TRANSIENT TACHYPNOEA OF THE NEWBORN

This condition affects mainly mature babies, but it does occur in those born prematurely.

AETIOLOGY

TTN is attributed to delayed clearing of the fetal lung liquid after the onset of respiration. It is more common in babies delivered by caesarean section before the onset of labour. In many cases there is a mild abnormality of surfactant.

CLINICAL SIGNS

The baby, who is typically delivered in good condition at 38 weeks gestation by elective caesarean section after an uneventful pregnancy, develops respiratory distress within an hour or two of delivery. He has mild grunting, and little sternal, intercostal or subcostal recession, but the respiratory rate may be 100 breaths/min. On auscultation the chest sounds normal with good air entry and there are no râles. Cyanosis may be present in air but is relieved by putting the baby into 30–40% oxygen.

Another group of babies who probably have the same disease show a different clinical picture. Their body temperatures have often fallen to around 35°C, they breathe quite slowly, and they have varying degrees of recession but grunt loudly. When their body temperature rises to normal, they switch to the more typical clinical pattern of TTN.

The illness usually lasts 24–48 hours, though a form which lasts longer and may need 60–70% oxygen has been described. The differential diagnosis is given in Table 11.5, but in the first few hours of life TTN cannot, with confidence, be distinguished from the early stages of GBS pneumonia or sepsis.

RADIOLOGY

The CXR shows "wet lungs", with prominent vascular markings and fluid in the fissures.

TREATMENT

In mature babies who are not at risk from ROP, peripheral arterial samples and oximetry are adequate for the initial evaluation which usually shows mild hypoxaemia with normal acid–base data. Arterial catheterization is rarely necessary, unless the baby requires more than 40% oxygen, or if there is any doubt at all about the nature or severity of his disease. Because of the risk of GBS sepsis, after taking cultures, we put all tachypnoeic neonates on penicillin until the bacteriology reports are known to be negative. Although the disease is due to delayed clearing of pulmonary fluid, frusemide is of no benefit.

During the first 12–24 hours the baby should be hydrated with IV 10% Dextrose, but oral feeds can often be started by 24 hours of age, if not before. Give 1–2 hourly feeds to start with, and aspirate the nasogastric tube every 4–6 hours to ensure that the stomach is emptying.

As soon as the baby has satisfactory blood gases when he is breathing air, and is tolerating feeds by NG tube if necessary, he should be returned to his mother on the postnatal ward. Respiratory rates of 50–60/min may persist for several days, but this is no reason for keeping the baby on the NNU.

MINIMAL RESPIRATORY DISEASE

This name is given to the condition found in babies who have mild symptoms for 4–6 hours after birth, some grunting or a respiratory rate of 50–60 breaths/min, and then recover. Careful observation, occasionally oxygen and taking care to exclude infection is all that is required.

MECONIUM ASPIRATION

- *MAS is a disease of postmature babies usually born through thick meconium;*
- *vigorous suction of the airway at birth reduces the incidence and severity of MAS;*

• *early treatment with IPPV, paralysis, low levels of PEEP and surfactant can usually prevent progress to severe PPHN requiring NO or even ECMO.*

This condition is confined to mature babies, since premature babies virtually never pass meconium *in utero*. Meconium staining in preterm labour strongly suggests listeria infection (pp. 253–254). Passage of meconium occurs in 10% of all labours at term (15–20% after 41 weeks). Meconium stained liquor is a poor marker of fetal asphyxia unless there are co-existing changes in the CTG or fetal pH.

AETIOLOGY

When meconium is present in the liquor and the upper airway before, during or immediately after delivery, it can be inhaled. Inhalation of meconium causes airway obstruction, air trapping and over-distension of the lungs with a considerable risk of pneumomediastinum and pneumothorax. The irritant properties of meconium also cause a chemical pneumonitis, and the presence of inhaled organic material predisposes to bacterial infection, and denatures surfactant on the alveolar surface.

CLINICAL SIGNS

The baby's skin, nails and umbilical cord are often meconium stained. Respiratory distress appears quickly after birth, and may be very severe. Air trapping causes lung over-distension, anterior bowing of the sternum, and an increased anteroposterior diameter to the chest. On auscultation there are widespread added sounds with rhonchi, and fine or sticky crepitations.

Differential diagnosis is rarely a problem (Table 11.5), but other conditions may coexist, particularly hypoxic ischaemic encephalopathy, pneumothorax and pneumonia. The baby may take 7–10 days to recover.

RADIOLOGY

The lungs appear over-expanded and contain multiple areas of streaky atelectasis. As the disease progresses the lungs become more diffusely opaque due to chemical pneumonitis and/or bacterial superinfection.

TREATMENT

Every effort should be made to prevent this condition by meticulous intrapartum care (pp. 81–82). Three non-randomized studies and one RCT suggest that careful aspiration of the airways at birth reduces the incidence and the severity of MAS. Meconium aspiration syndrome occurs in only 1% of deliveries where the baby is born through meconium stained liquor, and MAS is more likely if the meconium is thick (pea-soup meconium) because this occurs when there is oligohydramnios. Thin, watery pale green liquor, merely tinged with meconium, is not usually followed by MAS. In practice, the difficulty in agreeing definitions of "thick" and "thin" means that paediatricians have to attend all deliveries where the liquor is meconium stained, although their presence at deliveries where the liquor is only faintly stained may be superfluous. As soon as the baby is delivered the upper airway should be cleared under direct vision using a laryngoscope. If meconium is seen at or beyond the vocal cords intubation and tracheal suction should be done. If no meconium is seen at this level more harm than good is done by determined attempts to achieve endotracheal toilet.

The general monitoring and treatment is the same as in severe RDS. However, the following specific points should be noted in babies with meconium aspiration:

1. Blood gas analysis should be carried out with the same regularity as in RDS, and a UAC should be inserted. Although these babies may be profoundly hypoxaemic owing to right to left intrapulmonary shunting, most hyperventilate sufficiently to keep their $PaCO_2$ normal. A progressively rising $PaCO_2$ is an indication of very severe disease with persistent plugging of the airways with meconium. These babies occasionally benefit from bronchial lavage and lavage with surfactant can be tried (*v.i.*).
2. All babies should receive broad-spectrum antibiotic prophylaxis from the moment of birth. Give the usual broad spectrum antibiotic cocktail in use on the unit, often penicillin and gentamicin (p. 235).
3. Surfactant is of value, and should be given to ventilated babies with MAS. Large amounts may be needed.
4. Steroids are of no value.
5. The risk of pneumothorax is very high, and a chest drain set should be readily available.
6. Babies with MAS can be very difficult to ventilate. Pancuronium is virtually always necessary.

7. The ventilator settings are different from those required in RDS, since these babies have gas trapping, an increased airways resistance, and a chemical pneumonitis. Settings should include a long T_E and low levels of PEEP. Suggested early settings are F_IO_2 0.8, rate 60 breaths/min, pressure 20/3, T_I 0.3 s.

8. Many babies with severe MAS have pulmonary hypertension. Dopamine helps to keep the systemic pressure above the pulmonary pressure; nitric oxide may be helpful, as may induction of a metabolic alkalosis and pulmonary vasodilation (p. 192–193).

9. Our experience is that with adequate and vigorous early therapy the need to progress to ECMO is very rare, but as these babies are usually >2 kg and >37 weeks gestation if they remain profoundly hypoxic with an OI of >30, ECMO is an option (pp. 193–194). If babies with MAS are not responding to treatment by 12–24 hours consider ECMO; do not wait for days.

10. The babies have often suffered from hypoxia ischaemia *in utero*, and if they have, they are at risk from HIE and renal problems. Great care is therefore required to avoid fluid overload. Seizures may not be clinically apparent in paralysed babies and consideration should be given to EEG monitoring. Assessment of the CNS is particularly important if ECMO is being considered.

PULMONARY INTERSTITIAL EMPHYSEMA, PNEUMOTHORAX, PNEUMOMEDIASTINUM

- *The incidence of air leaks has been markedly reduced to about 10% of ventilated babies by antenatal steroids, postnatal surfactant and synchronous ventilation.*
- *PIE and pneumothorax can be asymptomatic in preterm babies on IPPV with severe lung disease. To detect air leak, which will alter the type of IPPV applied, a CXR should be done at least daily.*
- *All pneumothoraces should be drained if symptomatic or present in babies requiring IPPV, and the drain should be attached to suction of 10–20 cm H_2O.*
- *Management of PIE is by "gentle" IPPV with permissive hypercapnia using ventilator rates of 80–100 breaths/min. HFOV may be indicated.*

All air leak problems are complications of high pressure ventilation. Air leak increases the mortality rate and the incidence of intracranial haemorrhage. During the last decade the incidence of all air leaks combined has fallen from 30% to 10% of ventilated babies. This is due to increased use of antenatal steroids and postnatal surfactant, and a widespread acceptance of the philosophy of synchronous ventilation with paralysis where necessary. There is a very strong link between air leak of any kind and CLD. Severe PIE such as that shown in Figure 11.13 is now fortunately rare but remains a predictor of severe chronic lung disease.

Pneumopericardium, pneumoperitoneum and subcutaneous emphysema are rare varients of air leak, usually complications of a tension pneumothorax.

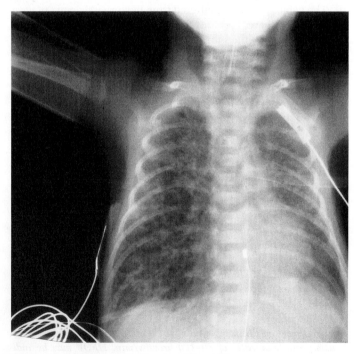

Figure 11.13 Chest X-ray showing severe bilateral PIE.

AETIOLOGY

Air leaks are primarily found in babies on IPPV plus PEEP, but pneumothorax and pneumomediastinum may also occur in the following circumstances:

- following over-vigorous resuscitation at birth, either with a bag and mask or an ETT, especially if a small ETT was inserted, and it slipped down into a lobar bronchus (p. 83);
- in association with any severe lung disease prior to IPPV, especially MAS and RDS;
- spontaneously: healthy neonates may generate inspiratory pressures exceeding 70 cm H_2O, which is well above the pressure at which normal lungs rupture.

When gas leaks out of an alveolus in a neonate it rarely ruptures subpleurally, but tracks along the bronchovascular bundle. If it is trapped within a bronchovascular bundle because there is more interstitial connective tissue in very premature lungs or because of damage caused by IPPV, PIE will develop (Fig. 11.13).

PIE can take two forms. The diffuse form shown in Fig. 11.13 is characteristically seen in ELBW neonates. Another form with more patchy distribution and larger cystic spaces is virtually limited to babies who have required pressures of >30/5 cm H_2O for severe RDS or pulmonary hypoplasia. In both forms of PIE the disease may be unilateral or even affect just one lobe.

If parenchymal gas gets as far as the mediastinum, it will cause a pneumomediastinum. From there it commonly ruptures into the plural cavity, causing a pneumothorax. Occasionally air in the mediastinum ruptures into the pericardium, or tracks down the mediastinal tissues, through the diaphragm and into the retroperitoneal tissues, where it may lodge or rupture out to give a pneumoperitoneum; air may also escape into the subcutaneous tissues.

Terminally air may rupture into the vascular tree causing a fatal air embolus. If babies with air leaks suddenly collapse this diagnosis should be sought by early post-mortem X-ray and at autopsy.

CLINICAL SIGNS

Pneumothorax

A small non-tension pneumothorax may have little effect apart from mild respiratory difficulty or slight deterioration in the condition of a baby who requires IPPV. Radiological surveys of whole neonatal populations have shown an incidence of pneumothorax of 1.0–1.5%; most of these babies are asymptomatic.

Tension pneumothorax is the commonest cause of sudden deterioration in ventilated babies. It presents dramatically because ventilation is severely compromised, with the lung collapsed on the side of the lesion, and mediastinal shift compressing the contralateral lung. The baby becomes increasingly dyspnoeic or apnoeic, and is often pale and/or cyanosed. The mediastinal shift, by distorting the great vessels as they pass through the diaphragm, may impair arterial perfusion to the lower half of the body, or dam back the venous return. This may reduce the cardiac output and can result in the baby being differentially perfused, with striking colour differences above and below the diaphragm.

The affected side will be hyper-resonant on percussion, but on auscultation air entry may sound surprisingly good. The affected side transilluminates brilliantly with an appropriate bright light source.

The abdomen may be distended and appear rigid, due to the tension pneumothorax pushing the diaphragm down and compressing the abdominal contents.

Pulmonary interstitial emphysema

This is often asymptomatic, though when marked (Fig. 11.13) it causes a steady deterioration in the baby's blood gases with hypoxaemia and hypercapnia: it is one of the causes of neonates being impossible to oxygenate (p. 162). The lungs may be very tympanitic, and on auscultation there are often widespread fine crackles. If there are large amounts of trapped intrapulmonary gas, the lungs will transilluminate.

Pneumomediastinum

This is commonly asymptomatic, but there may be anterior bowing of the sternum and the heart sounds may be muffled. Diagnosis can be confirmed with a lateral CXR.

Pneumopericardium

This is often asymptomatic but should be considered in any seriously ill neonate known to be having problems with air leaks who becomes hypotensive (due to tamponade) or in whom the heart sounds become muffled.

Pneumoperitoneum

This also can be an incidental finding on X-ray; if large, the abdomen will become distended and tympanitic. It must be differentiated from perforation of a viscus especially in NEC (*v.i.*).

RADIOLOGY

Diagnosis is made by appropriate X-rays, including a lateral horizontal beam film of the chest and abdomen. This is the only satisfactory way to demonstrate a pneumomediastinum and pneumoperitoneum where, with the baby lying supine, air collects under the sternum or the anterior abdominal wall. A similar view is also valuable for assessing the size of the pneumothorax in RDS where there is always a major degree of lung collapse, even without tension developing.

DIFFERENTIAL DIAGNOSIS

There is rarely any difficulty with the differential diagnosis once an X-ray has been taken. The problem is remembering to exclude air leaks such as pneumothorax and PIE by X-ray in any baby with worsening dyspnoea or hypoxaemia.

The only condition which may pose a problem is pneumoperitoneum which must be differentiated from pneumoperitoneum due to a ruptured bowel (e.g. in necrotising enterocolitis). This can usually be done easily on the basis of the other clinical and X-ray features of NEC. If there is still doubt, a small amount of gas can be aspirated. This will have a low PO_2 in NEC and a high PO_2 in babies with air leaks in high oxygen on IPPV.

TREATMENT

Pneumothorax

Most babies with pneumothoraces already have severe lung disease such as RDS or meconium aspiration, and already have indwelling catheters and monitors attached when the pneumothorax develops. However, in the occasional baby, in whom the pneumothorax is an isolated lesion, the basic routines of respiratory intensive care (p. 137, *et seq.*) should be instituted. However, a baby must never be left severely distressed with a tension pneumothorax while other procedures are carried out.

All tension pneumothoraces, and all pneumothoraces in babies with primary lung disease, should be drained. In an emergency, a 17 or 19 gauge needle can be inserted anteriorly through the second intercostal space in the mid-clavicular line, but must always be followed by an FG10 or FG12 thoracentesis tube (p. 490). Use local anaesthetic and give morphine unless the baby is moribund.

Since air gathers anteriorly, the tip of the drain should also be anterior and not lying in the paravertebral gutter. The tube should be firmly anchored to the chest wall and connected to an underwater seal and attached to suction of 10–20 cm H_2O. Without suction, removal of all the air in babies with severe lung disease is rarely possible. In sick babies the pneumothorax must be almost completely drained. Therefore, always check the CXR after inserting the tube, and if the pneumothorax persists adjust the position of the tube. If this does not work, insert a second chest drain aiming towards the largest residual loculus of air.

After a baby has developed a pneumothorax he is often much more difficult to oxygenate for the next 24–48 hours. Higher pressures, and the manoeuvres outlined on p. 160, *et seq.*, are often required. Most babies are much easier to manage after pneumothorax if they are paralysed or sedated and they must be given adequate analgesia.

Leave the drain *in situ*, with applied suction until the lung has been expanded for at least 24 hours, and longer in babies on IPPV. It is doubtful whether a drain should ever be removed if the baby still requires IPPV with PIP exceeding 25 cm H_2O.

When removing the drain the suction should be stopped, the tube clamped and then removed, checking with an X-ray after each step to ensure that the pneumothorax has not reaccumulated.

In the spontaneously breathing baby with a small non-tension pneumothorax, no underlying lung disease, minimal respiratory distress, and satisfactory blood gases, the pneumothorax can be allowed to resolve spontaneously. If the baby is mature, and beyond the age when ROP is a hazard, the rate of absorption of the pneumothorax can be speeded up by breathing a high inspired oxygen concentration. This washes the slowly absorbed nitrogen out of the pleural space, and replaces it with rapidly absorbed oxygen.

Pneumomediastinum

This commonly coexists with pneumothorax. It cannot be drained, since it consists of multiple small locules of air within the connective tissue matrix of the mediastinum. If it causes symptoms, routine management of respiratory illness should be undertaken, and the rate of absorption of the pneumomediastinum can be accelerated by giving the baby a high oxygen concentration to breathe if he is not at risk from ROP.

Pulmonary interstitial emphysema

In the diffuse generalized form of this disease seen early in the course of RDS, the best initial approach is to paralyse the baby and ventilate him at 80–100 breaths/min using as low a MAP as possible, allowing the $PaCO_2$ to run at 8–9 kPa (60–64 mmHg) if necessary. It is in this situation that HFOV may be valuable if available (Keszler *et al.* 1991) (p. 164). In extreme cases inserting a chest drain into the worst-affected lung and allowing it to deflate may be justified.

If PIE is unilateral the affected lung can be bypassed by selectively intubating the contralateral bronchus. The interstitial bubbles of gas are absorbed within 2–3 days and do not usually reappear when the lung reinflates. Obstructing the bronchus on the affected side with a balloon catheter has also been tried, and also works by deflating the affected lung.

Disappearance of the PIE has also been reported after lying the neonate on the side of the affected lung for several days. Large discrete cysts can be drained using a thoracentesis tube or differential bronchial intubation can be used. Occasionally a lobectomy is necessary.

Pneumopericardium

This is usually an incidental finding on chest X-ray in a baby with other major air leaks (e.g. tension pneumothorax). If it is large it may cause cardiac tamponade.

The pericardium can be drained via the sub-xiphoid route, using a FG 17-19 Medicut which can be left *in situ* if necessary until radiological proof of clearing is obtained (pp. 490–491).

Pneumoperitoneum

If this is under tension and is causing diaphragmatic splintage, it should be drained by paracentesis (pp. 491–492).

Subcutaneous emphysema

This should not, and in fact cannot, be treated.

MASSIVE PULMONARY HAEMORRHAGE

AETIOLOGY

The following factors have been implicated: severe birth asphyxia, hypothermia, rhesus haemolytic disease, left heart failure especially with patent ductus arteriosus or congenital heart disease, fluid overload, oxygen toxicity and haemostatic failure. The unifying concept for all these factors is that they combine left-sided heart failure with pulmonary capillary damage. Initially this will cause pulmonary oedema, but eventually red cells will leak out of the capillaries. The haematocrit of pulmonary haemorrhage fluid is usually less than 10% – i.e. it is a haemorrhagic pulmonary oedema.

In recent years our experience is that this disease occurs most commonly in VLBW neonates who are ventilated for both severe RDS and a large PDA – a situation that is entirely compatible with the heart failure/leaky capillary concept. It has also been reported in babies treated with the synthetic surfactant Exosurf. We have seen one or two catastrophic cases of pulmonary haemorrhage in babies with a coagulopathy secondary to HIE.

CLINICAL SIGNS

The baby, who is usually seriously ill with one of the above conditions, suddenly deteriorates, and becomes pale, cyanosed and limp often over a period of 2–5 minutes. If he is being ventilated, bloody fluid will be found welling up his endotracheal tube. If not, he will usually become apnoeic, and at laryngoscopy bloody fluid is seen welling up the trachea.

RADIOLOGY

In the acute phase the X-ray usually shows homogeneously opaque lungs, with some cardiac enlargement.

TREATMENT

All such babies should be intubated and ventilated, irrespective of whether or not they show any inclination to breathe spontaneously after resuscitation. If they are already on IPPV, the inflating pressure may need to be raised by 5–10 cm H$_2$O. The ventilator settings and the general management are those required for RDS (p. 150 *et seq.*).

Treat the underlying condition, and in addition take the following precautions:

- treat the baby for heart failure with diuretics in the first place;
- arrange an echocardiogram to assess the size of the ductus arteriosus;
- pancuronium is virtually always necessary;
- blood transfusion is usually required to correct the blood loss from the haemorrhage and the ensuing hypotension;
- check the haemostatic state. The baby often has DIC following resuscitation. If DIC is present, treat it accordingly (pp. 449–450);
- control fluid intake very carefully. Fluid overload is often an iatrogenic component in the aetiology of the disease;
- if there is significant flow through the ductus (see above) give indomethacin once the coagulopathy is controlled and the platelet count is more than 100×10^9 /l;
- surfactant – one or two doses depending on response – can be tried.

PERSISTENT PULMONARY HYPERTENSION OF THE NEWBORN

- *Pulmonary hypertension is a common complication in babies with severe lung disease (RDS, MAS). In general, treatment in this group should be aimed at the respiratory problem.*
- *PPHN as a diagnosis should be restricted to those babies in whom pulmonary hypertension is the main (if not the sole) cause of their hypoxaemia, and in these babies treatment should be aimed at lowering the pulmonary artery pressure.*
- *The initial management of PPHN is conservative, keeping all physiological variables within the normal range in a paralysed baby. In particular, it is important to keep the PaCO$_2$ no higher than 5 kPa (37 mmHg) and use strict minimal handling (no physiotherapy).*
- *Babies with PPHN who remain persistently hypoxaemic may respond to induction of a metabolic alkalaemia (pH 7.5), or inhaled nitric oxide.*
- *Weaning NO and IPPV need to be done very slowly and carefully.*

Table 11.14 Conditions in which PPHN can develop

Chronic intrauterine hypoxia resulting in primary PPHN	
Alveolar capillary dysplasia	
Diaphragmatic hernia	p. 195
Congenital heart disease	Chapter 22
Meconium aspiration syndrome	p. 180
GBS septicaemia	p. 239
Pulmonary hypoplasia	p. 194
Hypoxic ischaemic encephalopathy	p. 319
Respiratory distress syndrome	p. 125
Maternal prostaglandin synthetase inhibitor treatment	
Maternal lithium treatment	

This condition is sometimes called persistent fetal circulation. We prefer the term PPHN because the placenta is no longer in the circulation. PPHN has an incidence of one in 1400 live births, and refers to the clinical situation that results when a newborn baby fails to complete the normal cardiorespiratory adaptation necessary for extrauterine life (pp. 344–345). The basic problem in PPHN is a failure of the normal rapid decrease in pulmonary vascular resistance with the accompanying increase in pulmonary blood flow. Pulmonary vasodilation is mediated by prostacyclin, nitric oxide, endothelin 1 and PaO_2. Nitric oxide has recently been shown to be an effective treatment for PPHN (see below). Oxygen is an extremely potent pulmonary vasodilator, and PPHN can occur as a primary entity or accompany many conditions in which hypoxaemia is present (Table 11.14).

PATHOPHYSIOLOGY

Histological examination of the pulmonary arterioles in babies who die from PPHN reveals an excessively muscular media, which extends further down the small arteriolar branches than usual. In animal models, chronic intrauterine hypoxia produces similar medial hypertrophy of the peripheral pulmonary arteries.

CLINICAL SIGNS

PPHN presents with cyanosis in the first 12 hours of life; the babies are blue but the respiratory distress is minimal. P_2 may be loud, and a soft systolic murmur of tricuspid incompetence is occasionally heard. Cardiomegaly and heart failure are not features. The CXR usually shows a normal sized heart with pulmonary vascularity normal to decreased. Characteristically there is a marked variability in the PaO_2 early in the course of the disease. Once PPHN is established there is persistent severe hypoxaemia.

INVESTIGATIONS

There may be a mild decrease in lung markings on the CXR, but unless the PPHN is secondary to hypoxaemia accompanying lung disease (Table 11.14) the CXR is unremarkable. Cross-sectional echocardiography will demonstrate a structurally normal heart. Ventricular function may be reduced, and there may be a patent ductus arteriosus. Indirect assessment of the pulmonary artery pressure is possible with Doppler ultrasound. Colour Doppler may show tricuspid incompetence, in which case the Bernoulli equation (pressure = $4V^2$ where V = peak velocity of the regurgitant jet) can be used to estimate the pulmonary artery pressure. Colour Doppler can also demonstrate right to left shunting across the foramen ovale and at ductal level.

TREATMENT

1. Maintain as many physiological variables within the normal range as possible, paying particular attention to the following:
   - blood gases
   - blood pressure
   - electrolytes and calcium
   - blood glucose
   - PCV.
2. Give antibiotics after taking cultures (risk of GBS).
3. Minimal handling is crucial because slight interference from suction, physiotherapy, or a CXR can cause a dramatic increase in pulmonary artery pressure and clinical deterioration.
4. Monitor all variables as outlined in Chapter 10. Continuous PaO_2 and SpO_2 monitoring is essential, ideally recording from both pre and post ductal sites.
5. Use paralysis, sedation and analgesia liberally.

If the pulmonary artery pressure (and oxygen requirement) does not fall in response to this conservative management, physiological pulmonary artery vasodilatation should be attempted:

1. Increase the pH to 7.5–7.55, preferably by infusing alkali intravenously. Alternatively increasing IPPV to lower the $PaCO_2$ to 3.0–3.4 kPa (25–30 mmHg), or both, can be tried. Hyperventilation can damage the lungs.
2. Use pulmonary vasodilators. Formerly many drugs including tolazoline, prostacyclin, and magnesium sulphate were used, but all have the disadvantages of reducing systemic BP as much as (or more than) they reduce the PAP. The ideal vasodilator would act on only the pulmonary vascular bed, increasing the difference between the systemic and pulmonary pressures. Nitric oxide gas meets this criterion. Inhaled nitric oxide has been shown to be effective in a RCT of term babies with PPHN (NINOS study group 1997). The advantages of nitric oxide include the fact that because it is a gas it is only delivered to ventilated areas of lung. This improves ventilation-perfusion mismatching and avoids systemic side effects.

Using nitric oxide in PPHN

Nitric oxide (NO) is supplied in cylinders with a concentration of up to 1000 ppm, with nitrogen as the balance gas. Cigarette smoke contains 400–1000 ppm of nitric oxide. The gas must be carefully diluted down to a concentration of 10–80 ppm in oxygen/air, and the concentration monitored, before it can be safely administered to babies. Nitric oxide is oxidized to higher oxides of nitrogen (NO_2 to NO_x) in the presence of oxygen. Nitrogen dioxide (NO_2) is a toxic gas, already well studied as a component of car exhaust fumes. Current occupational health guidelines limit exposure of NO_2 to 5 ppm, and histological changes have been seen in lungs exposed to 25 ppm of NO_2. Nitrogen dioxide forms nitric and nitrous acid once it comes into contact with water. For these reasons NO must be added to the baby's inspired gases right at the patient manifold of the circuit, in order to limit contact time between NO and oxygen, and the concentrations of NO_2 to NO_x must be monitored in the expiratory limb. The blender device and any rotameters used must be made of non-ferrous metal to avoid corrosion from acid, and ventilators must be exhaustively purged after use for the same reason. Waste gas must be scavenged in order to avoid contaminating the working environment. Other potential problems with regard to nitric oxide include methaemoglobin formation, increased bleeding time and free radical toxicity. Methaemoglobin reductase activity is lower in the newborn, and a deficiency is common in some ethnic groups, including the Native Americans. This could lead to high concentrations of methaemoglobin if affected babies required treatment with NO. In our practice methaemoglobinaemia has not been a limiting factor in NO treatment.

Starting treatment with nitric oxide

- Use a safe, reliable, specially designed circuit. Add the NO gas to the inspiratory limb of the ventilator circuit as near to the baby as possible and scavenge the waste gas.
- Monitor the concentration of NO and NO_2 in the expiratory limb.
- Set the rotameter to give a concentration of 20 ppm.
- Measure the methaemoglobin concentration after 1 hour of NO administration (reduce the concentration if the levels are >5%).
- Measure the blood gas response after an hour; most babies respond more rapidly than this.
- Try up to 80 ppm if there is no response.

Weaning from nitric oxide

- Once the inspired oxygen concentration is down to 30%, begin weaning NO.
- Wean by 1 ppm every hour whilst the blood gases remain stable (use transcutaneous/continuous monitoring if possible to reduce the number of samples) until 3 ppm is reached.
- Wean the last 3 ppm more slowly, say 1 ppm every three hours. This is because in some babies endogenous manufacture appears to be inhibited during NO therapy.
- Be alert for rebound. Some babies need NO to be restarted.

ECMO

ECMO is a modification of heart-lung bypass technology which has been developed for use in babies with severe pulmonary or cardiopulmonary failure. The main indications for use are MAS and PPHN, and babies with these conditions do best, but RDS, sepsis and CDH are also indications for ECMO in some situations. ECMO candidates must be >2 kg in weight and >34 weeks gestation because of the risk of intracerebral haemorrhage associated with heparin anticoagulation. Infants who are ventilated with an oxygenation index greater than 30–40 (p. 501) should be considered for ECMO because their predicted mortality is very high.

During ECMO, blood is circulated through a membrane oxygenator via a circuit which is primed with blood before connecting it to the baby's vascular system, usually via cannulae in the carotid artery and jugular vein (to the right atrium; Veno-arterial ECMO). Veno-venous ECMO is a possibility if the heart can maintain an adequate blood pressure and this method avoids the need to sacrifice the carotid artery on one side. Roller pumps keep the blood flowing through the circuit, which has access ports and a bridge for emergencies. Blood flows from the atrium under pressure into a bladder, and is then pumped through the oxygenator back into the baby via the arterial catheter. Artificial ventilation is continued at a very low rate, "idling" settings, resting the lungs.

Survival after ECMO in babies with PPHN and MAS is over 90%; mortality in this group was reduced by a half in the UK randomized controlled trial (UK Collaborative ECMO trial group 1996). Outcome remains poor for babies with CDH who require ECMO; these babies usually have irreversible pulmonary hypoplasia. The most feared and common complication of ECMO is bleeding, and platelet consumption is inevitable. Neurological sequelae are quite common, with 16% of this severely ill group having CNS abnormality detectable at a year. Deafness is emerging as a particularly frequent disability in ECMO survivors.

PULMONARY HYPOPLASIA

When it is part of a syndrome such as Potter's (p. 379) or one of the short limbed dwarfs with small chests (p. 309) pulmonary hypoplasia is but one marker of a lethal malformation, should be recognized as such and no intensive care offered. Pulmonary hypoplasia may also occur as an isolated and lethal abnormality which will only be recognized if, at autopsy, lung weights are carefully measured. Two groups of babies with pulmonary hypoplasia are important and should be treated:

- Preterm babies delivered after prolonged preterm rupture of the membranes. In general this type of pulmonary hypoplasia develops only if the membranes rupture before 26 weeks gestation.
- Congenital diaphragmatic hernia.

PULMONARY HYPOPLASIA SECONDARY TO PPROM

These babies can be identified from the history and by the presence of small volume lungs on the initial CXR which may or may not show parenchymal changes, the respiratory failure in some babies being due simply to the small alveolar volume. The management of the (usually) preterm baby in respiratory failure from this variant of pulmonary hypoplasia is the same as that for RDS. The following points should be noted:

- There is a high risk of co-existing infection. Always give antibiotics.
- Surfactant is beneficial in some cases and should be tried.
- High peak pressures (>30 cm H_2O) and longer inspiratory times (up to 1.0 seconds) may be required for 24–48 hours to "open up" the lungs.
- When pressures >25 cm H_2O are being used give pancuronium.
- If despite high pressures, long T_I, a F_IO_2 of 0.95 and surfactant the baby remains hypoxic and hypercarbic a trial of HFOV and nitric oxide is worth attempting. If these measures fail to improve the blood gases and the lungs remain small on a CXR the prognosis is hopeless and intensive care should be withdrawn.

PULMONARY HYPOPLASIA ASSOCIATED WITH CONGENITAL DIAPHRAGMATIC HERNIA

There is usually severe pulmonary hypoplasia on the ipsilateral side and some hypoplasia on the contralateral side, which is squashed *in utero* by the mediastinal shift. The lung hypoplasia causes severe respiratory failure which usually presents within minutes of delivery as a cyanosed dyspneoic baby who may need active resuscitation in the labour ward with IPPV and high concentrations of oxygen.

Up to 50% of babies with CDH, no matter what is tried, never become adequately oxygenated and die within 12–24 hours. We do not currently offer ECMO to this group. Amongst the remainder are some who respond to full intensive care with nitric oxide, paralysis and ventilation *v.s.* and a further subset who are easy to ventilate. This latter group, currently diagnosed antenatally and managed aggressively from birth, are those who would have presented late in former series. We currently spend time stabilizing the baby before carrying out corrective surgery. Several early studies adopting this approach suggested an improved survival rate, although one recent randomized controlled trial showed no benefit (Nio *et al.* 1994).

The surgical management is outlined on pp. 404–405.

PLEURAL EFFUSIONS (CHYLOTHORAX)

These may be part of generalized hydrops (Chapter 29). Isolated neonatal pleural effusions usually become chylous once the baby is feeding. Treatment is recurrent pleural taps, often combined with feeds containing MCT to reduce chyle formation. The prognosis is good.

CONGENITAL MALFORMATIONS AFFECTING THE RESPIRATORY TRACT

CONGENITAL LOBAR EMPHYSEMA

This condition can present at any age in infancy with respiratory distress, cyanosis, and a characteristic CXR showing severe emphysema, usually of an upper lobe, with a mediastinal shift. Differential diagnosis from localized PIE is usually easy on the basis of the history. Cases that present as an emergency should be treated by resection of the affected lobe.

CONGENITAL CYSTIC ADENOMATOID MALFORMATION

CCAMs are now usually recognized during antenatal ultrasound examinations, although the diagnosis is not completely reliable. Antenatally the diagnosis relies on imaging a solid/cystic area within the thorax. An antenatally diagnosed CCAM can disappear during pregnancy. A few enlarge and cause fetal death, hydrops or pulmonary hypoplasia which is fatal after birth.

The majority cause minimal neonatal respiratory illness or are asymptomatic. Those which cause symptoms should certainly be resected. A CXR is insufficient postnatal investigation and can appear normal. CT or MRI of the thorax often reveals the abnormal area of lung. Whether all these cases should be operated to prevent infection or the potential for malignant change remains controversial, but our current practice is to offer resection in infancy. Surgery is much more difficult to perform after infection has occurred.

UPPER AIRWAY OBSTRUCTION

Choanal atresia

In this rare condition the baby can only breathe through his mouth.

Since most neonates are obligate nose breathers, babies with choanal atresia are fine when they are crying, but turn blue and are very breathless when their mouths are closed. This very characteristic clinical picture usually presents immediately after birth and should be instantly recognized despite its rarity (1 in 60 000 live births) – otherwise the baby may die of respiratory obstruction rather than keep his mouth open. The baby should be forced to breathe through his mouth by inserting a Magill airway, or even an endotracheal tube, until appropriate surgery can be carried out on his posterior choanae.

Babies with unilateral atresia, or those who are able to breathe through their mouths, may present much later in infancy with a purulent discharge from the obstructed nostril.

Pierre Robin syndrome (micrognathia, midline cleft palate, and glossoptosis)

This syndrome may cause acute neonatal upper respiratory tract obstruction due to the tongue falling back and obstructing the oropharynx. An airway can usually be sustained in the short term by inserting a Magill airway and lying the baby prone, often with his head extended, allowing the tongue and small mandible to fall forward. If problems persist, a long nasopharyngeal tube connected to a CPAP circuit is often successful. Small laryngeal airways are available and have been used successfully in emergencies in this situation. The laryngeal airway is like a small mask on the end of an endotracheal tube and is designed to sit over the larynx when inserted. There is a soft air filled "Hovercraft" skirt which is blown up when the mask is *in situ*. If none of these approaches work and intubation cannot be achieved (intubation of such babies can be exceptionally difficult owing to the small mandible) emergency tracheostomy should be considered.

In the first week or two of life, using various combinations of palatal obturators, lying the baby prone, nasopharyngeal airways and spoon or tube feeding, it is usually possible to achieve normal growth and often to get the baby home. However, in severe forms of the malformation, tracheostomy and long-term hospital stay may be necessary to allow the baby to breathe, feed and grow before surgical repair is possible. There is a risk of sudden death in Pierre Robin syndrome.

In the long term the mandible grows, and the cleft palate can be repaired. The modern tendency is to close the palate as soon as possible, once the baby is thriving.

Congenital laryngeal stridor/laryngomalacia

Severe forms of this disorder may present in the neonatal period. So long as the baby feeds well and thrives, does not have severe choking episodes, has a normal $PaCO_2$, and does not develop signs of cor pulmonale, a watching brief can be held in the expectation that as his larynx grows the stridor will lessen. In the very small percentage of babies in whom this is not the case, a tracheostomy is necessary in the neonatal period with the recognition that it is likely to remain *in situ* for 6–12 months.

REFERENCES

Ahluwalia, J., White, D.K. and Morley, C.J. (1998) Infant flow driver or single nasal prong continuous positive airway pressure: short-term physiological effects. *Acta Paediatrica* **87**: 325–327.

Ainsworth, S.B., Beresford, M.W., Milligan, D.W.A., Shaw, N.J., Matthews, J.N.S., Fenton, A.C. and Ward Platt, M.P. (2000) Pumactant and poractant alfa for treatment of respiratory distress syndrome in neonates born at 25–29 weeks gestation: a randomized trial. *Lancet* **355**: 1387–1392.

Baumer, J.H. (2000) International randomized controlled clinical trial of patient triggered ventilation in neonatal RDS. *Archives of Disease in Childhood* **82**: F5–F10.

Blayney, M.P. and Logan, D.R. (1994) First thoracic vertebral body as a reference point for endotracheal tube placement. *Archives of Disease in Childhood* **71**: F32–F35.

Bourchier, D. and Weston, P.J. (1997) Randomised trial of dopamine compared with hydrocortisone for the treatment of hypotensive very low birth weight infants. *Archives of Disease in Childhood* **76**: 174–178.

Ceruti, E. (1966) Chemoreceptor reflexes in the newborn *Pediatrics* **37**: 556–564.

Cools, F. and Offringa, M. (1999) Meta-analysis of elective high frequency ventilation in preterm infants with respiratory distress syndrome. *Archives of Disease in Childhood* **80**: F15–F20.

Crowther, C.A. (1997) Antenatal thyrotropin-releasing hormone (TRH) prior to preterm delivery. In: Pregnancy and childbirth module of the Cochrane database of systematic reviews, Neilson, J.P., Crowther, C.A., Hodrett, E.D., Hofmeyr, G.J. and Kierse, M.J.N.C. (eds). Update Software, Oxford.

Crowley, P.A. (1997). Corticosteroids prior to preterm delivery. In: Pregnancy and childbirth module of the Cochrane database of systematic reviews, Neilson, J.P., Crowther, C.A., Hodrett, E.D., Hofmeyr, G.J. and Kierse, M.J.N.C. (eds). *The Cochrane Collaboration*. Issue 3. Update Software, Oxford.

Davis, P.G. and Henderson-Smart, D.J. (1998) Extubation of premature infants from low-rate IPPV vs extubation after a trial of endotracheal CPAP. In: Pregnancy and childbirth module of the Cochrane database of systematic reviews, Neilson, J.P., Crowther, C.A., Hodrett, E.D., Hofmeyr, G.J. and Kierse, M.J.N.C. (eds). Update Software, Oxford

Dawes, G. S. (1966) Pulmonary circulation in the fetus and newborn. *British Medical Bulletin* **22**: 61–65.

Dunn, P. M. (1965) The respiratory distress syndrome of the newborn. Immaturity versus prematurity. *Archives of Disease in Childhood* **40**: 62–65.

Godfrey, S. (1981) Growth and development of the respiratory system: functional developments. In: *Scientific Foundations of Paediatrics*, 2nd edn, Davis, J.A. and Dobbing Wm, J. (eds). Heinemann Medical Books, London, pp. 432–439.

Greenough, A., Milner, A.D. and Dimitriou, G. (1998) Synchronized mechanical ventilation in neonates. In: Neilson, J.P., Crowther, C.A., Hodrett, E.D., Hofmeyr, G.J. and Kierse, M.J.N.C. (eds), Pregnancy and childbirth module of the Cochrane database of systematic reviews. Update Software, Oxford.

Greenough, A., Wood, S., Morley, C.J. and Davis, J.A. (1984) Pancuronium prevents pneumothoraces in ventilated premature babies who actively expire against positive pressure inflation. *Lancet* i: 1–3.

Gribetz, I., Frank, N.R. and Avery, M.E. (1959) Static volume pressure relations of excised lungs of infants with hyaline membrane disease; newborns and stillborn infants. *Journal of Clinical Investigation* **38**: 2168–2175.

Henderson-Smart, D.J. and Davis, P.G. (1998) Prophylactic methylxanthine for extubation in preterm infants. In: Neilson, J.P., Crowther, C.A., Hodrett, E.D., Hofmeyr, G.J. and Kierse, M.J.N.C. (eds), Pregnancy and childbirth module of the Cochrane database of systematic reviews. Update Software, Oxford.

HiFi Study Group (1989) High frequency oscillatory ventilation compared with conventional mechanical ventilation in the treatment of respiratory failure in preterm infants. *New England Journal of Medicine* **320**: 88–93.

HiFo study group (1993) Randomised study of HFOV in infants with severe respiratory distress syndrome. *Journal of Pediatrics* **122**: 609–619.

Jobe, A.H., Mitchell, B.R. and Gankel, J.H. (1993) Beneficial effects of the combined administration of prenatal corticosteroids and postnatal surfactant on preterm infants. *American Journal of Obstetrics and Gynecology* **168**: 508–513.

Keszler, M., Donn, S.M. and Bucciarelli, R.L. (1991) Multicenter controlled trial comparing high frequency jet ventilation and conventional mechanical ventilation in newborn infants with pulmonary interstitial emphysema. *Journal of Pediatrics* **119**: 85–93.

Klaus, M.H. and Fanaroff, A.A. (1979) *Care of the High Risk Neonate.* W. B. Saunders, London, p. 214.

Morley, C.J. (1997) Systematic review of prophylactic versus rescue surfactant. *Archives of Disease in Childhood* **77**: F70–F74.

Neonatal Inhaled Nitric Oxide Study (NINOS) Group (1997) Inhaled nitric oxide in full-term and nearly full-term infants with hypoxic respiratory failure. *New England Journal of Medicine* **336**: 597–604.

Nio, M., Haase, G., Kennaugh, J. *et al.* (1994) A prospective randomised trial of delayed versus immediate repair of congenital diaphragmatic hernia. *Journal of Pediatric Surgery* **29**: 618–621.

Robertson, P.A., Sniderman, S.H., Laros, R.K. *et al.* (1992) Neonatal morbidity according to gestational age and birth weight from five tertiary care centres in the United States 1983–1986. *American Journal of Obstetrics and Gynecology* **166**: 1629–1645.

Seid, A.B. and Canty, T.G. (1985) The anterior cricoid split procedure for the management of subglottic stenosis in infants and children. *Journal of Pediatric Surgery* **20**: 388–396.

Sinha, S.K. and Donn, S.M. (1996) Advances in neonatal conventional ventilation. *Archives of Disease in Childhood* **75**: F135–F140.

Subhedar, N.V., Ryan, S.W. and Shaw, N.J (1997) Open randomised controlled trial of inhaled nitric oxide and early dexamethasone in high risk infants. *Archives of Disease in Childhood* **77**: F185–F190.

UK Collaborative ECMO Trial Group (1996) UK collaborative trial of neonatal ECMO *Lancet* **348**: 75–82.

Vain, N.E., Prudent, L.M., Stevens, D.P., Weeter, M.M. and Maisels, M.J. (1989) Regulation of oxygen concentration delivered to infants via nasal cannulas. *American Journal of Diseases of Children* **143**: 1458–1460.

Whyte, S., Birrell, G. and Wyllie, J. (2000) Premedication before intubation in UK neonatal units. *Archives of Disease in Childhood* **82**: F38–F41.

Ziegler, J.W., Ivy, D.D., Kinsella, J.P. and Abman, S.H. (1995) The role of nitric oxide, endothelin and prostaglandins in the transition of the pulmonary circulation. *Clinics in Perinatology* **22**: 387–403.

FURTHER READING

Greenough, A. (1999) Respiratory physiology. In: Rennie, J.M. and Roberton, N.R.C. (eds). *Textbook of Neonatology*, 3rd edn. Churchill Livingstone, Edinburgh, p. 455–481.

Greenough, A. and Roberton, N.R.C. (1999) Acute Respiratory Disease. In: Rennie, J.M. and Roberton, N.R.C. (eds). *Textbook of Neonatology*, 3rd edn. Churchill Livingstone, Edinburgh, p. 481–607.

Greenough, A., Roberton, N.R.C. and Milner, A.D. (1996) *Neonatal Respiratory Disorders*. Edward Arnold, London.

12

CHRONIC LUNG DISEASE

- *CLD develops in up to 30% of VLBW and 50% of ELBW babies.*
- *Prevention is difficult; steroids and/or surfactant do not prevent CLD but "gentle" ventilation, careful fluid balance and avoidance of infection probably do.*
- *Treatment at 7–10 days with systemic steroids is currently the most effective therapy, but may increase the risk of cerebral palsy.*
- *Long term treatment with diuretics, inhaled steroids or bronchodilators or theophylline are not of proven benefit.*
- *Babies who are still ventilator dependent at 50 days often have a poor prognosis, with a high chance of death or disability.*

Chronic lung disease is now the preferred term to describe the persisting pulmonary disorder that is frequently seen in VLBW survivors of neonatal intensive care. The term bronchopulmonary dysplasia, if used at all, should be limited to describing the small number of babies with the severe cystic end stage lung disease first described 30 years ago. CLD is one of the most serious problems in neonatal medicine. Every neonatologist is all too familiar with the very preterm infant who initially does well, but who then spends many months in the NNU because of oxygen dependence.

CLD is very rare in babies born at more than 31 weeks of gestation, although the occasional case is seen in term infants who require ventilation. About 30% of ventilated babies develop CLD (Shaw *et al.* 1993, Bohin and Field 1994, Manktelow *et al.* 2001). Amongst the UK cohort of babies born at less than 26 weeks gestation in 1994 50% were still oxygen-dependent on their expected date of delivery, and of these children 16% remained in oxygen at a year. Improved survival and surfactant treatment have not led to a consistent reduction in the incidence of CLD. Many centres have reported an increase (Shaw *et al.* 1993, Fenton *et al.* 1996), although others have described a decrease (Corcoran *et al.* 1993, Todd *et al.* 1997).

Two criteria are widely used for the diagnosis of CLD (Bancalari *et al.* 1979):

(a) Babies who remain oxygen dependent for more than 28 days after requiring mechanical ventilation in the first week, with persistent X-ray changes.

(b) The same clinical criteria applied at 36 weeks postconceptional age.

AETIOLOGY

The typical infant who develops CLD is an extremely premature baby who initially requires only gentle ventilation with air at low pressures, more for poor respiratory effort than for severe RDS. As the weeks go by the baby cannot be weaned off IPPV. Often, in the presence of heart failure from a PDA or infection, his lung disease gets worse, both in terms of gas exchange and radiologically, and he develops severe CLD.

We still see, occasionally, more mature babies who develop CLD as a sequel to severe lung disease requiring high pressure IPPV with high oxygen concentrations. Their primary disease may be RDS, meconium aspiration, PPHN, diaphragmatic hernia, pulmonary hypoplasia or GBS sepsis; in fact any condition which causes severe neonatal respiratory failure. To the classic description of the aetiology of CLD "oxygen plus pressure plus time" can now be added immature lung structure, infection, and PDA. Mechanical ventilation is clearly important, because of either pressure (barotrauma) or volume (volutrauma) damage to the lungs. The effects of oxygen, positive pressure ventilation, and inflammation combine to damage the lung during a critical period of active growth. Infection, by releasing cytokines and preventing normal alveolar growth, is of crucial importance (Jobe and Ikegami 2001). Acquired CMV may worsen the lung disease (p. 257). Sadly, neither antenatal steroids nor postnatal surfactant have dramatically reduced the incidence of CLD.

The factors implicated in CLD are summarized in Table 12.1.

NATURAL HISTORY

The fact that a ventilated neonate is developing CLD is usually apparent by 7–10 days of age. He either stops improving or actually deteriorates both clinically and radiologically. The CXR shows increasing haziness with or without cysts. At this stage marked bronchorrhea may occur, the aspirate consisting of dysplastic and metaplastic epithelial cells, macrophages and polymorphs. Infection

Table 12.1 Aetiological factors in CLD

1. high pressure, long inspiratory time ventilation with or without air leak (PIE)
2. ventilation with variable volume delivery, perhaps because of insufficient PEEP
3. pulmonary oxygen toxicity
4. persisting immaturity of the surfactant system
5. very immature lungs (easily damaged by 1 and 2 and 3)
6. PDA and fluid overload
7. infection, including maternal and via inflammatory cytokine release
8. disturbance of the elastase/protease system in the lung destroying the parenchyma
9. gastro-oesophageal reflux and inhalation of gastric contents
10. intralipid damage to the lungs
11. male sex

probably contributes to increased bronchoconstriction via inflammatory mediators, and raised neutrophil counts and elevated levels of leukotrienes and/or platelet activating factor have all been found in the tracheal aspirate of babies developing CLD.

CLINICAL FEATURES

If still ventilated, the baby has a falling PaO_2 and rising $PaCO_2$. If he is not ventilated he is permanently dyspnoeic, often with an over-inflated chest. Crackles and wheezes are frequently heard throughout both lung fields even in the absence of heart failure. If heart failure does develop there will be tachycardia, a triple rhythm, hepatosplenomegaly and peripheral oedema. Cor pulmonale should be suspected when there is a pronounced RV heave, a loud P_2 and sometimes the murmur of tricuspid regurgitation. Feeding is hard work for these babies, and is often accompanied by episodes of desaturation, vomiting, and increased breathing difficulties.

INVESTIGATIONS

The ECG will show RV overload, and echocardiography can be used to measure the size of the right ventricle and to estimate the degree of pulmonary hypertension(p. 191). Pulmonary function tests show increased airways resistance, increased airway reactivity and reduced compliance.

DIFFERENTIAL DIAGNOSIS

The definition of CLD is given above. On this basis there is effectively no differential diagnosis. The radiological changes of Wilson-Mikity syndrome (p. 213) are not dissimilar from the cystic changes of milder CLD, but the antecedent history clearly differentiates the two conditions.

HISTOLOGY

In established disease alveolarisation is markedly reduced and there is widespread destruction of the pulmonary tissue which is replaced by areas of collapse and emphysema, surrounded by organizing fibrous tissue. There is peribronchial fibrosis, and the bronchial walls are thickened with muscular hypertrophy. There is often necrosis proceeding to mucosal hyperplasia and squamous metaplasia of the bronchial lining. Smaller bronchi may be obliterated. There are changes of pulmonary hypertension in the arteries.

RADIOLOGY

The radiological changes of the original disease often with superimposed PIE gradually merge into one of the two types of change which Hyde *et al.* (1989) found to be prognostically valuable at 28 days. These are type I disease, in which there is homogenous opacification without coarse reticulation and type II, in which there is coarse reticulation and streaky density with small cystic translucencies. The prognosis of type I disease is better than that of type II. The trachea often becomes enlarged.

By 4–5 months the changes may still be severe with a characteristic broad chest and high diaphragm (Fig. 12.1). Cardiomegaly is a terminal event, but osteoporosis, rickets and even rib fractures may be seen in these babies, whose calcium and phosphate intakes have not been sufficient to prevent osteopenia of prematurity (pp. 309–310).

PREVENTION

Much effort has gone into trying to prevent or minimize CLD, but with little success. Neither antenatal steroids, antenatal TRH nor surfactant have any effect.

Minimizing barotrauma/volutrauma using modern techniques of CPAP and IPPV is important, but the role of HFOV in preventing CLD remains controversial (Bhuta and Henderson-Smart 1998, Cools and Offringa 1999).

Meticulous control of fluid balance and early treatment of a PDA may also reduce the incidence of CLD. Prophylactic measures such

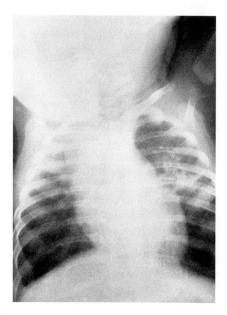

Figure 12.1 Chest X-ray of severe CLD.

as vitamins A and E, and superoxide dismutase have not proved to be successful either.

There is considerable variation in the incidence of CLD in different units and there is a widely held belief that this is related to careful fluid balance and/or "gentler" ventilation techniques in ELBW babies. Some Scandinavian units have remarkable success with very early CPAP and a "minitouch" technique, which has yet to be replicated elsewhere.

MONITORING

Babies with CLD should have electrolytes and a blood count measured two or three times a week. Regular monitoring of CRP may provide early warning of infection, and surveillance cultures should be obtained weekly in ventilated babies. Acid–base status in these babies can be monitored effectively by capillary samples, and pulse oximetry comes into its own as the ideal way of monitoring oxygenation in this group. Occasional arterial blood gas measurements can be taken but these often make the baby very distressed, and the results are impossible to interpret if he was howling at the time the stab was done. X-rays should be taken once or twice a month until it is clear that the disease is improving.

INFECTION

In the fluctuating clinical course that is characteristic of CLD it can be formidably difficult to decide whether an episode of deterioration is due to infection. Changes in the temperature, WBC, CRP, CXR and the nature of any aspirate from the airway can be very helpful.

Because one cannot afford to ignore the possibility of infection in babies with CLD who deteriorate, these babies inevitably receive many courses of broad spectrum antibiotics. Fungal infection can emerge. Antibiotics should be stopped after 2–3 days if there is no laboratory confirmation of infection.

Intercurrent viral infections, especially RSV bronchiolitis, are a major threat. Care should be taken to protect babies with CLD from contact with staff or relatives who have respiratory infections. If they develop RSV positive bronchiolitis they should be treated with Ribavirin. Influenza vaccine should be given to babies with CLD in the winter months in addition to the usual vaccines including pertussis. The AAP now recommend prophylactic RSVIG for infants under 2 years of age with CLD, but this therapy has not been adopted worldwide. Our current practice is to give RSV immunoglobulin (Palivizumab, Abbott) to protect only those babies who are in home oxygen (*v.i.*) during the winter months.

MANAGEMENT

There is no specific treatment other than to keep the baby alive without further damage to his lungs, in the hope that the restrictive changes in his airways will resolve or can be controlled pharmacologically, pulmonary hypertension and cor pulmonale (and other complications, see Table 12.2) can be prevented and that the normal growth of alveoli from approximately 30×10^6 at 28/52 to 250×10^6 at 8 years will steadily progress. The chief aspects of management are discussed below and include the following:

- Management of oxygen therapy and respiratory support, preventing pulmonary hypertension

Table 12.2 Complications associated with CLD

Poor growth
Airway hyper-reactivity
Airway problems – tracheomalacia, subglottic stenosis from prolonged intubation
Neurodevelopmental delay
Respiratory tract infection
Pulmonary hypertension
Systemic hypertension
Metabolic bone disease
Gastrointestinal reflux, vomiting
Steroid side effects (see Table 12.3)
Nephrocalcinosis from diuretic therapy

- Management of nutrition and fluid balance
- Prevention and treatment of infection
- Steroid therapy
- Other measures, e.g. bronchodilators.

Respiratory support

The most important single factor in getting the baby with CLD off the ventilator is being prepared to accept $PaCO_2$ values in the range 8.0–9.5 kPa (60–70 mmHg) or even higher so long as PaO_2, pH and vital signs are stable. The process of weaning should progress exactly as outlined on pp. 173–177, albeit slowly. Use the lowest possible PIP, but high levels of PEEP may help to maintain alveoli at a constant volume. Caffeine, and other drugs (see next section) may help.

In general, if the baby can be kept off IPPV for a sustained period of say 2–3 weeks, he will survive unless he develops some other complication. An intercurrent viral respiratory infection can be devastating and fatal in these babies. Reventilation is usually required after inguinal hernia surgery and this apparently simple operation can end in disaster in a baby with CLD.

Oxygen

One of the causes of death in CLD is cor pulmonale secondary to pulmonary hypertension. To minimize the degree of hypoxic pulmonary vasoconstriction, although $PaCO_2$ can be allowed to rise to 9.5 kPa (70 mmHg), PaO_2 should be kept in the range 8–12 kPa (60–90 mmHg) (SpO_2 90–95%). These babies are virtually always too mature to develop ROP so there is no risk from hyperoxaemia, and unusually for neonatal intensive care it is better to be liberal with oxygen than to restrict it. The exact level of oxygen saturation which is adequate to prevent pulmonary hypertension is unknown, but a consensus view is that saturation levels should be kept above 92%. The oxygen carrying capacity of the blood should be maintained by transfusion, and we aim to keep the PCV above 35% when the baby requires more than 35% oxygen.

Once the baby is no longer CPAP dependent and the oxygen requirements have diminished oxygen can be given very effectively by nasal cannula (p. 147, Fig 11.8). This system enables the baby to be picked up, played with and to be fed orally by breast or bottle.

Fluids/nutrition

These need to be carefully supervised, balancing the risks of over-hydration and heart failure against the increased caloric requirements of these babies. Most babies with CLD tolerate enteral feeds, which should be given at 150–180 ml/kg/24 h, and of sufficient caloric density to ensure a weight gain of approximately 30 g/day in those weighing more than 2.0 kg.

Every effort should be made to encourage bottle feeding (within reason) once it is possible to nurse a baby with CLD in nasal cannula oxygen. Experience has taught us that unless this is done early these babies can become phobic of any stimuli round their mouths, and consequently become extremely difficult to feed orally in the weeks and months ahead.

In some babies, vomiting and GOR is a problem; if this cannot be controlled easily by lying the baby prone or thickening his feeds, fundoplication will have to be considered.

Diuretics

These improve lung compliance and airways resistance in the short term in CLD. Frusemide 1–2 mg/kg is useful as an interim measure when babies are breathless, with increased oxygen requirements and excessive weight gain. An alternative regimen, with chlorthiazide and spironolactone, can also be helpful in the short term. Using diuretics long term can have serious consequences and there is no evidence that they shorten the course of CLD. Frusemide may cause hypercalciuria, nephrocalcinosis and haematuria, although these usually resolve when the drug is stopped.

Hyponatraemia, hypocalaemia and hypochloraemia are also common with any diuretic regimen. Hypochloraemia with the resultant metabolic alkalaemia can be a particular problem, and is an adverse prognostic finding. Hypochloraemic alkalaemia may depress ventilation and increase the $PaCO_2$ – thus diuretics can worsen the very problem for which they were prescribed. Vigorous chloride replacement giving 10–20 mmol/kg/24 h may be necessary.

Steroids

Since they were first introduced 20 years ago the use of steroids in CLD has generated controversy. The initial wave of enthusiasm is currently waning as full appreciation of their side-effects dawns.

Clinical experience shows that in some babies the response to 0.5 mg/kg/24 h of dexamethasone is a dramatic decrease in respiratory support and oxygen requirement, often accompanied by marked weight loss and diuresis (Gladstone et al. 1989, Halliday and Ehrenkrantz 1999). At the other extreme some babies, particularly those who earlier had severe PIE, show virtually no response. Bhuta and Ohlsson (1998) used meta-analysis to show that steroids given between 7 and 14 days reduced the incidence of CLD and mortality. Halliday, analysing similar trials, agrees (Halliday 1999). Strictly speaking, a meta-analysis of these trials is not valid because of the vast differences in the enrolled populations and the steroid dose used. Although there are acute improvements with a reduction in ventilatory requirements, a reduction in tracheal inflammatory markers, and better pulmonary mechanics these improvements are not necessarily sustained nor do they translate into a better long term outcome.

Steroids are clearly of some value in CLD, and we consider treatment at 7–10 days in babies who are still ventilated in more than 50% oxygen, are free of infection and have radiological features of CLD. We discuss the potential risks and benefits of treatment with the baby's parents. We now use a lower dose than previously (v.s.), of 0.1 mg/kg/24h of dexamethasone. If there is no response within 72 hours then steroids are stopped; there is no evidence that a short course affects adrenal reserve. If the baby responds, and it is possible to reduce the inspired oxygen concentration by more than 20% or wean the ventilation completely, then steroids are continued for 7–10 days. Very short courses of steroids do not appear to work; Bhuta and Ohlsson (1998) suggested that more than 14 days of steroids were of no additional benefit although one trial (Cummings et al. 1989) did show some benefit from a long course.

Table 12.3 Side effects of steroids in CLD

Reduced growth, including lung growth
Increased protein catabolism (raised urea)
Hypertension*
Hyperglycaemia[+]
Cardiomyopathy
Sepsis (especially fungal)
Possible later neuromotor effects, including cerebral palsy
Osteomalacia
Cataract
Gastrointestinal haemorrhage[~]
Adrenal supression[^]
Reduced immunological response to immunizations

(* treatment p. 370, [+] treatment p. 294, [~] treament p. 392, [^] treatment p. 280).

A second course of 7–10 days is considered if the baby relapses or does not respond the first time, but we do not offer steroid treatment to unventilated babies. Attempts to use inhaled steroids have met with no success, even when delivered carefully into the pharynx (Cole *et al.* 1999).

Whenever starting parenteral steroids there is always anxiety about sepsis. Baseline cultures should be taken and a WBC and CRP measured. We do not use antibiotics routinely when starting steroids, but would choose to be cautious in the case of a baby who was already on an antibiotic cocktail, and in such babies we would continue antibiotic treatment. Prophylactic oral nystatin should be given to babies on antibiotics and steroids in view of the risk of fungal sepsis.

Steroid treatment of CLD has accumulated a formidable list of side effects (Table 12.3). Most of these are reversible by drug withdrawal. Yeh*et al.* (1998) found an excess of neuromotor dysfunction and poor growth (boys) in steroid treated babies compared to controls, and this worrying finding has now been confirmed. So far five studies have reported on neurodevelopmental outcome 1–3 years after steroid treatment, with a relative risk of late morbidity of 1.6 (95% confidence intervals from 1.0 to 2.6) (Tarnow-Mordi and Mitra 1999, Doyle and Davis 2000).

Bronchodilators

Giving β-mimetics and occasionally ipratropium by inhalation may improve these babies. In some babies the bronchial musculature is playing an active role in maintaining airway patency, and giving bronchodilators including theophylline (in effect muscle relaxants) makes the disease much worse. In the wheezing non-ventilated baby with CLD the response to a trial of these agents is worth considering. If they help, use them – if they do not, desist.

Airway intervention

Some babies with CLD have tracheomegaly and/or peripheral airway collapse; tracheobronchomalacia. This can only be diagnosed by bronchoscopy or tracheobronchography. Nevertheless, the possibility should be borne in mind because treatment can be offered in the form of balloon dilatation of the stenosed airway, or aortopexy.

Baby stimulation and parental support

Babies with CLD spend many months in the nursery, and thought needs to be given to the provision of an appropriate environment for them and their parents.

"SPELLS"

Babies with severe CLD have characteristic episodes in which they become agitated, are cyanosed, pale and sweaty, become bradycardic and may go into heart failure with rapid deterioration of their blood gases. Precisely what causes these spells is not known, but some are probably due to airways collapse where bronchomalacia or tracheomalacia has been caused by damage to the cartilage after long-term intubation or infection. The spells can be treated by increasing the inspired oxygen concentration, giving diuretics and using CPAP or ventilation as indicated.

DISCHARGE

Some babies make a full recovery within 3–4 months, while others are still oxygen dependent at this stage. Babies who require less than 30% inspired oxygen, are stable, off steroids and diuretics, and feeding orally can be discharged home receiving nasal cannula oxygen. We give RSV humanized monoclonal antibody, palivizumab (Synagis, Abbott Laboratories) 15 mg/kg IM once a month for the five months of the RSV season to babies at home in oxygen. This is obviously a major exercise involving the family, the NNU, the GP and the community services and the management is beyond the remit of this book.

PROGNOSIS

The longer the baby stays on the ventilator the less likely he is to survive. Babies who are still ventilator dependent at 3 months or in more than 50% oxygen at 6 months have a very poor prognosis. We reported virtually no intact survivors amongst babies ventilated for more than 50 days in the late 1980's, although the situation has improved since then (Wheater and Rennie 1994, Galliard *et al.* 2001). The mortality in the first year is about 11%, and of those babies with severe cystic BPD as many as 40% die. Among those who do go home, growth is poor, and most have multiple severe lower respiratory tract infections requiring readmission and often reventilation during the first 24 months. Severe restrictive airways disease may persist throughout childhood, and growth is poor.

Neurologically these children fare badly, with many long-term survivors having a DQ <85 and others showing an odd encephalopathic illness affecting the basal ganglia (Perlman and Volpe 1989). A dysmature EEG, which changes more slowly or not at all with increasing postconceptional age, has been described.

WILSON-MIKITY SYNDROME

This is a disease of very low birth weight babies who, characteristically, have not had any serious respiratory disease in the first week or two of life.

AETIOLOGY

This is not known, but it has been suggested that it is due to air trapping behind the highly compliant, and collapsible airways in VLBW babies. Trapped air causes alveolar distension, rupture and fibrosis. Pulmonary function studies confirm an increased TGV and airways resistance. Another theory is that Wilson-Mikity syndrome is due to chronic aspiration of milk into the upper lobes of the lung.

CLINICAL SIGNS

A previously healthy low birth weight baby becomes progressively dyspnoeic during the second and third weeks of life, and requires supplementary oxygen. There may be a few fine crepitations in his lungs. His blood gases initially show hypoxaemia and mild CO_2 retention.

In most babies the disease spontaneously begins to recover by the sixth to eighth week of life, and the babies are asymptomatic by the age of 3 months. A small percentage has progressive disease culminating in death from respiratory failure and cor pulmonale at 3–4 months.

RADIOLOGY

The CXR shows a honeycomb appearance, with coarse interstitial fibrosis outlining areas of hyperaeration. These changes are most prominent in the upper lobes, and may take over 12 months to clear.

HISTOLOGY

This shows areas of emphysema, septal thickening and fibrosis corresponding to the honeycomb appearance of the chest X-ray. The bronchial tree is histologically normal.

TREATMENT

There is no specific treatment other than supplementary oxygen, and treating heart failure if it develops. Babies who require IPPV rarely survive. Most cases of the disease occur at a gestation where ROP is still a major hazard, but they are too old for umbilical artery catheterization. SpO_2 measurements are valuable in monitoring these babies, and if the baby is in more than 40% O_2, peripheral arterial samples must also be taken regularly for blood gas analysis.

CHRONIC PULMONARY INSUFFICIENCY OF PREMATURITY (CPIP)

Some low birth weight babies, who may or may not have had RDS, become mildly dyspnoeic around the second to fifth week of life, with an increased frequency of apnoeic attacks. Clinically they are indistinguishable from those with Wilson-Mikity syndrome. Radiologically, however, they have a diffusely hazy CXR. Pulmonary function studies show a decreased FRC and TGV, and normal airways resistance. Krauss *et al.* (1975) ascribe the condition to transient postnatal surfactant deficiency.

The condition has a benign course: extra oxygen should be given but monitored very carefully in order to prevent ROP.

Theophylline, and occasionally CPAP, is required to prevent the apnoeic attacks.

REFERENCES

Bancalari, E., Abdenour, G.E., Feller, R. and Gannon, J. (1979) Bronchopulmonary dysplasia: the clinical presentation. *Journal of Pediatrics* **95**: 819–823.

Bhuta, T. and Henderson-Smart, D.J. (1998) Rescue high frequency oscillatory ventilation vs conventional ventilation in preterm infants with pulmonary dysfunction (Cochrane Review) In: *The Cochrane Library*, 4th Edition, Update Software, Oxford.

Bhuta, T. and Ohlsson, A. (1998) Systematic review and meta-analysis of early postnatal dexamethasone for prevention of chronic lung disease. *Archives of Disease in Childhood* **79**: F26–F33.

Bohin, S. and Field, D.J. (1994) The epidemiology of neonatal respiratory disease. *Early Human Development* **37**: 73–90.

Cole, C.H., Colton, T., Shah, B.L. *et al.* (1999) Early inhaled glucocorticoid therapy to prevent bronchopulmonary dysplasia. *New England Journal of Medicine* **40**: 1005–1010.

Cools, F. and Offringa, M. (1999) Meta-analysis of high frequency ventilation in preterm infants with respiratory distress syndrome. *Archives of Disease in Childhood* **80**: F15–F20.

Corcoran, J.D., Patterson, C.C., Thomas, P.S. and Halliday, H.L. (1993) Reduction in the risk of bronchopulmonary dysplasia from 1980–1990: results of a multivariate logistic regression analysis. *European Journal of Pediatrics* **152**: 677–681.

Cummings, J.J., D'Eugenio, D.B. and Gross, S.J. (1989) A controlled trial of dexamethasone in premature infants at high risk for bronchopulmonary dysplasia. *New England Journal of Medicine* **320**: 1505–1510.

Doyle, L.W. and Davis, P.G. (2000) Postnatal corticosteroids in preterm infants: systematic review of effects on mortality and motor function. *Journal of Paediatrics and Child Health* **36**: 101–107.

Fenton, A.C., Mason, E., Clarke, M. and Field, D.J. (1996) Chronic lung disease following neonatal ventilation. II. Changing incidence in a geographically defined population. *Pediatric Pulmonology* **21**: 24–27.

Galliard, E.A., Cooke, R.W.I. and Shaw, N.J. (2001) Improved survival and neurodevelopmental outcome after prolonged ventilation in preterm neonates who have received antenatal steriods and surfactant. *Archives of Disease in Childhood* **84**: F194–F196.

Gladstone, I.M., Ehrenkranz, R.A. and Jacobs, H.C. (1989) Pulmonary function tests and fluid balance in neonates with chronic lung disease during dexamethasone treatment. *Pediatrics* **84**: 1072–1076.

Halliday, H.L. (1999) Clinical trials of postnatal corticosteroids: inhaled and systemic. *Biology of the Neonate* (suppl) **76**: 29–40 (http://BioMedNet.com/karger).

Halliday, H . and Ehrenkranz, R.A. (1999) Early postnatal corticosteroids for preventing chronic lung disease in preterm infants (Cochrane Review), and Delayed (>3 weeks) treatment for preventing chronic lung disease in preterm infants (Cochrane Review). In: *The Cochrane Library* Issue 2, 1999. Update Software, Oxford.

Hyde, I., English, R.E. and Williams, J.E. (1989). The changing pattern of chronic lung disease of prematurity. *Archives of Disease in Childhood* **64**: 448–451.

Jobe, A.H. and Ikegami, M. (2001) Prevention of bronchopulmonary dysplasia. *Current Opinion in Pediatrics* **13**: 124–129.

Krauss, A.N., Klein, D.B. and Auld, P.A.M. (1975). Chronic pulmonary insufficiency of prematurity (CPIP). *Pediatrics* **55**: 55–58.

Manktelow, B.N., Draper, E.S., Annemelei, S. and Field, D. (2001). Factors affecting the incidence of chronic lung disease of prematurity in 1987, 1992 and 1997. *Archives of Disease in Childhood* **85**: F33–F35.

Perlman, J.M. and Volpe, J.J. (1989). Movement disorder of premature infants with severe bronchopulmonary dysplasia: a new syndrome. *Pediatrics* **84**: 215–218.

Shaw, N., Gill, B., Weindling, M. and Cooke R.W.I. (1993) The changing incidence of chronic lung disease. *Health Trends* **25**: 50–53.

Tarnow-Mordi W. and Mitra, A. (1999) Postnatal dexamethasone in preterm infants. *British Medical Journal* **319**: 1385–1386.

Todd, D.A., Jana, A. and John, E. (1997) Chronic oxygen dependency in infants born at 24–32 weeks' gestation: the role of antenatal and neonatal factors. *Journal of Paediatrics and Child Health* **33**: 402–405.

Wheater, M. and Rennie, J.M. (1994) Poor prognosis after prolonged ventilation for bronchopulmonary dysplasia. *Archives of Disease in Childhood* **71**: F210–F211.

Yeh, T.F., Lin, Y.J. and Huang, C.C. (1998) Early dexamethasone therapy in preterm infants: a follow up study. *Pediatrics* **101**: E7.

13

APNOEIC ATTACKS

- *The definition of a clinically significant apnoea is a pause in breathing for more than 20 seconds, or any apnoea associated with a bradycardia or colour change.*
- *Apnoea must be distinguished from periodic breathing which is very common in newborn babies.*
- *Ideopathic apnoea is a diagnosis of exclusion; any baby who develops symptomatic apneoic attacks must be carefully assessed to exclude the causes of secondary apnoea, including sepsis.*
- *Apnoea of prematurity may be obstructive, central or mixed and usually stops by 34 weeks gestational age.*
- *Babies with apneoic attacks have normal lungs and ROP is a significant risk if oxygen is administered indiscriminately.*
- *Most premature babies with apneoic attacks respond to oral methyl-xanthines.*

DEFINITION OF APNOEA AND PERIODIC BREATHING

Most entirely normal babies, both term and preterm, have periodic breathing in which periods of regular breathing are separated by short episodes of apnoea (3–15 seconds). Clinically significant apnoea is associated with swallowing movements (never seen in periodic breathing), and with bradycardia and desaturation. In some babies desaturation occurs after very short apnoeas, leading to one proposed definition of apnoea as "that non-breathing interval which a given infant cannot tolerate without bradycardia and cyanosis". The bradycardia usually starts after a time lag and is probably caused by the reduced oxygenation, although there may be a common brain stem pathway which gives rise to the apnoea and bradycardia together. Apnoea is more common in active sleep, and may be associated with episodes of gastro-oesophageal reflux. Feeding hypoxia is also a common problem in preterm babies who are learning to swallow, and can cause apnoea. Monitoring for apnoea is described on p. 96–97.

SYMPTOMATIC APNOEA

Apnoeic attacks in a baby who is already unwell are a sign of deterioration. In a previously asymptomatic baby the onset of apnoea may be the first indication of serious disease. Whenever a baby develops apnoeic attacks the following causes should be considered, and if necessary excluded by investigation:

1. Infection (p. 231).
2. Metabolic disorders e.g. hypoglycaemia (p. 286), hypocalcaemia (p. 29); inborn errors of metabolism (Chapter 18).
3. Upper airways obstruction; obstruction of the neck by flexion.
4. CNS disorders; GMH–IVH (pp. 324–326); seizures (p. 312); Arnold-Chiari malformation; very occasionally congenital central hypoventilation syndrome (Ondine's curse).
5. Respiratory depression from drugs.
6. Gastro-oesophageal reflux (p. 389–390); aspiration of feed; feeding hypoxia.
7. Wrong environmental temperature setting (p. 11–12).
8. Anaemia of prematurity (p. 169, 437).
9. RDS can present with apnoea but should have been diagnosed much earlier by the usual criteria (p. 133).
10. Other lung disease; remember apnoea can recur with viral infections especially RSV (p. 257).
11. Post-operative; all preterm babies must be monitored for apnoea post-operatively (p. 409).
12. Heart failure – especially pulmonary oedema with a PDA (p. 356).

RECURRENT APNOEA OF PREMATURITY

When all the problems outlined above have been excluded, one is left with a group of otherwise entirely healthy preterm babies who develop apnoeic attacks. Characteristically the attacks develop on the fifth or sixth day of life, and irrespective of the gestation at birth usually disappear by 34–36 weeks gestational age (Fig. 13.1).

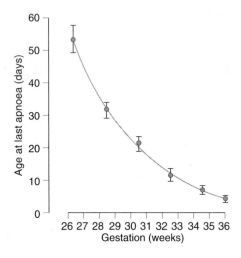

Figure 13.1 Mean postnatal age (±SE) when last apnoea was detected versus gestational age (from Henderson-Smart 1981).

PATHOPHYSIOLOGY

In babies who are otherwise well and who have recurrent apnoea of prematurity there are three types of apnoeic attack, namely obstructive, central and mixed (Fig. 13.2). In obstructive apnoea the upper airway becomes occluded by laryngeal adduction while the baby continues to make (ineffective) respiratory movements. About 10% of neonatal apnoeic attacks are of this type, which is more common in babies with a neurological problem. The neurological problem may be either congenital (e.g. Down syndrome, neural tube defect) or acquired (post GMH-IVH). In the common central apnoea the baby just stops breathing at end expiration with his larynx open, but in a proportion of these the larynx adducts during the attack converting it into a mixed attack (Upton *et al.* 1992). About 10% of short attacks are mixed, but the proportion is greater in the more prolonged attacks.

The exact aetiology of apnoea of prematurity is unknown and is probably multifactorial. The potential factors are:

Neurological immaturity: This is undoubtedly important, and the incidence of apnoeic attacks can be shown to decline in association with

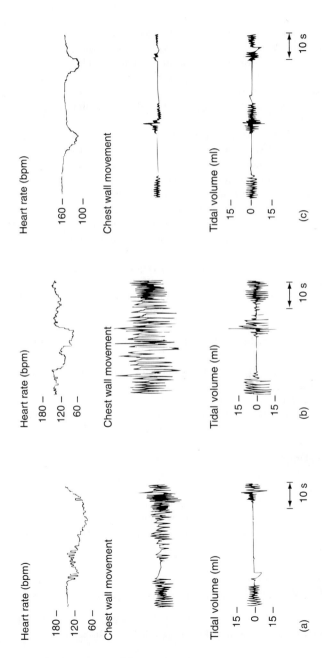

Figure 13.2 (a) Mixed apnoea. Obstructed breaths precede and follow a central respiratory pause. (b) Obstructive apnoea. Breathing efforts continue, although no nasal airflow occurs. (c) Cenral apnoea. Both nasal airflow and breathing efforts cease simultaneously. (From Miller, 1986.)

maturation of various brain stem functions. Brain stem compression, as in the Arnold-Chiari malformation, can cause apnoea.

Hypoxia: This depresses respiration in neonates (p. 119).

Abnormal CO_2 response: Preterm babies have a flattened CO_2 response curve (p. 120).

Anaemia: Once the PCV is below 40% the frequency of attacks increases.

Reflexes from the upper airway: It can be shown that liquids other than liquor amnii, saline or species-specific milk applied to the upper airway induce reflex apnoea. This may be the mechanism of gastroesophageal reflux induced apnoea.

Airway obstruction: Curiously this may actually perpetuate the apnoea – the baby just gives up when his airway is occluded. Examination of the upper airway with an ultra-thin fibreoptic scope has shown that the aryepiglottic folds are large and obstructing the airway in some babies.

Sleep state: Respiration is much more irregular and apnoeic attacks are much more common in active sleep. In part this is a manifestation of the inherent tendency for respiratory rate to cycle in active sleep, but an additional reason is that with the marked hypotonicity of active sleep, the rib cage may be distorted sufficiently during inspiration for the chest wall mechanoreceptors to inhibit the inspiratory drive (p. 120).

Temperature change: It is an old observation that if the incubator gets too hot the frequency of apnoeic attacks increases (p. 11–12).

Feeding: A common observation is that the number of apnoeic attacks increases in the 20–30 minutes after a bolus nasogastric feed.

Handling: One of the reasons for the minimal handling rule is the recognition that disturbing the baby for any reason – changing his nappy, taking blood – may precipitate a run of apnoeic attacks.

Post-operative: Any surgical procedure/anaesthetic no matter how trivial may be followed by an increase in the number of apnoeic attacks.

Immunizations/viral infections: Surviving ex-preterm babies who are given their routine immunizations while still on the NNU (particularly those with CLD) can experience frequent apnoeic attacks in the 24–48 hours after immunization.

RADIOLOGY

The CXR in babies with recurrent apnoea is usually normal, but should always be taken in order to exclude other diseases.

TREATMENT

As many as possible of the triggering factors for apnoea which are present should be corrected, including changing to continuous pump feeding, but not resorting to intravenous feeding in the first place.

Anaemia should be corrected, and the incubator temperature must be controlled. The baby should lie with his head well supported, and his neck comfortably extended by putting a small folded nappy under his neck and shoulders. Check the blood gases, and if these show a mild hypoxaemia – say PaO_2 of 6.6–8.0 kPa (50–60 mmHg); the inspired oxygen concentration can be very cautiously increased, 2% at a time.

Great care must be taken with oxygen therapy. These very premature babies usually have normal lungs, and once they are breathing normally in an oxygen-enriched atmosphere may achieve PaO_2 values well in the ROP-inducing range.

Recurrent apnoea should be treated with a methylxanthine administered intravenously (aminophylline) or orally (theophylline and caffeine). After a loading dose, therapy should be continued, guided by a plasma level measurement (Table 13.1). Doxapram (1.5 mg/kg/h) can be tried intravenously in difficult cases.

For the few babies in whom recurrent apnoea persists despite theophylline, low-pressure (3–4 cm H_2O) nasal CPAP will usually control the attacks. CPAP works by slightly increasing the FRC and reducing the distortion of the rib cage during inspiration, and partly by keeping the upper airways open. It is rarely necessary to ventilate a baby with apnoea. However, if this is necessary, since the lungs are normal and very compliant, the initial ventilator settings should be as follows: 25% O_2, rate 25/min, inspiratory time 0.3 s, pressures 13/2 cm H_2O. Once the baby is intubated and attached to the ventilator at these settings, the blood gases can be checked, and

Table 13.1 Methylxanthines for recurrent apnoea

Drug	Loading dose	Maintenance dose/24 h	Plasma level therapeutic range	Dose frequency
Theophylline	5.0 mg/kg	6–8 mg/kg	5–15 mg/l = 27–81 μmol/l	3–4 /day
Caffeine	10 mg/kg	2.5 mg/kg	5–20 mg/l = 25–100 μmol/l	daily

it is then usually possible to drop back to IMV at 5–10 breaths/min in most cases.

It is often very difficult to wean a baby with recurrent apnoea off IMV, and this may take 10–14 days in some cases. The methylxanthines should always be used to help the process.

TREATMENT OF AN APNOEIC ATTACK

As soon as an apnoeic attack is detected, the baby's head should be gently extended, and if he has aspirated a feed his upper airways should be *carefully* sucked out. All this may provide enough stimulus to start him breathing, but if not, the soles of his feet should be flicked while checking his heart rate. Most babies will respond to these simple remedies. If they do not, and their heart rate is falling, they should be ventilated, using a bag and mask, with the gas mixture they are normally breathing. *At no time should they be given 100% oxygen by face mask since this is a sure recipe for ROP.* Oxygen should only be given if there is a progressive bradycardia despite adequate lung inflation with the bag and mask, and then only under medical supervision, with careful monitoring of SpO_2 during the resuscitation and rapid reduction of the F_IO_2 after resuscitation. It is rare for such a baby to need intubation, provided that the attack is detected early and bag and mask ventilation is properly administered.

REFERENCES

Henderson-Smart, D. J. (1981) The effect of gestational age on the incidence of recurrent apnoea. *Australian Pediatric Journal* **17**: 273–276.

Miller, M.J. (1986) Diagnostic methods and clinical disorders in children. In: Edelman, N. and Santiago, T. (eds) *Breathing disorders of sleep.* Churchill Livingstone, New York.

Upton, C.J., Milner, A.D. and Stokes, G.M. (1992) Upper airway patency during apnoea of prematurity. *Archives of Disease in Childhood* **67**: 419–424.

FURTHER READING

Milner, A.D. (1999) Apnoea and bradycardia. In: Rennie, J.M. and Roberton, N.R.C. (eds), *Textbook of Neonatology,* 3rd edn. Churchill Livingstone, Edinburgh, pp. 630–637.

14

INFECTION

- *Meticulous hand washing is the best way to prevent cross-infection in a NNU.*
- *Infection remains an important cause of morbidity and mortality at all birth weights and gestations.*
- *The organisms that most commonly infect babies are GBS and E. coli, with CONS a frequent cause of late onset sepsis in VLBWI.*
- *Any baby suspected of sepsis must have investigations including a blood culture carried out immediately.*
- *Initial treatment with penicillin and an aminoglycoside should be started unless a senior paediatrician assesses the risk of infection as being very low.*
- *Neonatal bacterial meningitis still has a poor prognosis. All cases should be managed in large centres with appropriate neuroradiological and neurosurgical expertise.*

INFECTION CONTROL IN NEONATAL UNITS

Babies usually emerge from a sterile intrauterine environment, and it follows from this that most infections in babies admitted to neonatal units are hospital-acquired, or nosocomial, infections. The risk of nosocomial infection is directly proportional to the number and crowding of babies in the unit, the number of infections in those babies, shortages of staff, and the number of people (visitors and staff) going in and out of the unit. Clearly, therefore, units should be spacious and designed so that only those who need to enter them pass through, babies should only be admitted to the NNU if absolutely necessary, and staffing levels should be maintained (p. 1–5).

Scrupulous attention to hand washing is the single most important factor in the prevention of cross-infection. Hands and forearms should always be washed in an antiseptic soap (Betadine or chlorhexidine), before and after handling a baby. Watches and jewellery must be removed. To minimize skin irritation, after initial washing, a hand wash consisting of 2.5% chlorhexidine in 70% alcohol (Hibisol) can be used on a repeated basis over the next few hours unless the hands become dirty, or contaminated with urine, faeces or blood, in which case thorough washing must be repeated.

There is no evidence that the use of gowns, masks and overshoes by staff or parents makes any difference to the level of cross-infection in a NNU. Gowns and masks should only be used when it is necessary to protect the staff during outbreaks of serious infection.

Staff with a current infectious disease such as a respiratory illness, boils, gastroenteritis or weeping dermatitis should be excluded from the unit. Staff with cold sores should cover them, and those with herpetic hand infections must not work. Parents with these problems, and mothers with wound infections, vaginal discharge or known pathogens on their HVS should be allowed in, but any exposed lesions should be covered and their hand washing should be supervised and particularly fastidious.

Communal equipment such as stethoscopes and thermometers are a major source of cross-infection. Individual pieces of equipment should therefore be provided. Disposable equipment should be used where possible, for example blood pressure cuffs.

Neonates with infections which could be a hazard to other babies should be nursed in separate rooms if possible. An incubator provides a moderately secure microenvironment for most infected neonates if the hand washing technique is rigorous, and is adequate for asymptomatic carriers of pathogenic organisms.

When confronted by epidemic infectious disease (e.g. recurrent Serratia septicaemia or enterovirus infections), there is no alternative but to close the unit to new admissions.

With the current trend to early discharge, babies can be readmitted to the NNU from the community. However, babies who require readmission and who have symptoms of viral infections such as RSV must not be readmitted to neonatal units unless they can be isolated, as epidemics can follow. Viral infections can be life-threatening to babies with CLD.

HOST DEFENCES IN THE NEWBORN

The body defends itself against infection in three ways – physical, cellular and humoral. Neonates, especially premature ones, are deficient in all three of these defences.

PHYSICAL DEFENCES

The neonatal skin is very thin, easily damaged and infected. The umbilical stump becomes necrotic after birth and acts as a locus for infections which can then disseminate. The passage of an endotracheal tube, a nasogastric tube or an intravascular catheter provides a route for pathogenic organisms to enter the body.

The newborn baby is virtually germ-free at birth, apart from organisms that become smeared over him as he passes through the vagina. He therefore lacks the protection afforded by having a resident flora of non-pathogenic organisms. A normal neonate is colonized by generally non-pathogenic organisms acquired from his mother, including those in her vagina and rectum to which he was exposed during delivery. However, particularly if he is in an NNU, he may also be colonized by, and subsequently infected with, potentially pathogenic organisms acquired from the hospital environment.

CELLULAR IMMUNITY

Lymphocyte function is well developed even in the 28-week fetus. The absolute number of T-cells present is similar to adult values. T-cell function seems to be adequate with some decrease in cytotoxic T-cell function and in the ability to respond to sensitizing agents such as dinitrochlorobenzene.

A full complement of B-lymphocyte types is present by the end of the second trimester, and these cells can respond by synthesizing antibodies although their function is still sub optimal (De Vries *et al.* 1999). A swift antibody synthetic response by the neonatal lymphocyte is dependent on the presence of some IgG in the plasma to help process the antigen. The response of the neonate will be improved if he has an adequate level of transplacental maternal IgG, or if he has received an infusion of intravenous immunoglobulin postnatally (*v.i.*).

PHAGOCYTE FUNCTION

Polymorphonuclear leucocytes from healthy preterm and full-term babies when suspended in normal adult serum show normal phagocytosis and bactericidal activity, but some reduction in chemotaxis and adherence. However, when suspended in neonatal serum which is deficient in the opsonic activities of immunoglobulins and complement, their phagocytic activity is seriously reduced. The bactericidal capacity of neonatal polymorphs *in vivo* is also reduced in the presence of severe concurrent illness such as RDS or meconium aspiration pneumonitis (Wright *et al.*, 1975).

HUMORAL IMMUNITY

The normal neonate, irrespective of gestation, has virtually no circulating IgA, IgD, IgE or IgM. If any of these are present in cord blood or the early neonatal period they have been manufactured by the fetus and imply fetal infection. IgG, on the other hand, is both actively and passively transported across the placenta from about the twentieth week of gestation, and by full term the baby's IgG level is higher than that of his mother. Following delivery, the level of IgG in the baby's plasma falls with a half-life of about three weeks, and until he produces adequate amounts of IgG, IgM and IgA there is a transient postnatal hypogammaglobulinaemia. This is rarely clinically important in a term baby; but a premature baby is born before much IgG has crossed the placenta and is therefore at increased risk of infection from the time of birth for several weeks until after the postnatal hypogammaglobulinaemia has been corrected. At the trough, about 3–4 weeks after delivery, the preterm baby may have IgG levels less than 0.2 g/l.

Since the neonate acquires his IgG from his mother, he is immune to the infections to which she is immune, except for those conditions in which immunity is IgM mediated or cell mediated (*E. coli*, TB).

The levels of the components of the complement cascade, and the alternative complement pathway in the neonate, are 50–80% of adult values, and even lower in premature babies.

The neonate is immunodeficient because he lacks these defence mechanisms. However, it is important to recognize that he is immunocompetent since he can, and does, respond to the antigenic challenges he receives postnatally, particularly if he has adequate levels of IgG. The normal baby has a "good enough" immune system for his needs, which are usually limited.

BACTERIAL INFECTION IN THE NEWBORN

The major bacterial pathogens now encountered are *E. coli*, the group B β-haemolytic streptococcus (GBS; *Step. agalactiae*), and

Staphylococcus epidermidis (coagulase negative staphylococcus; CONS) which are responsible for 80–85% of severe neonatal infections. Other bacteria which are commonly responsible for serious infection are:

1. *Pseudomonas aeruginosa*;
2. other Gram-negative bacilli (*Klebsiella, Proteus, Enterobacter, Haemophilus*);
3. *Staphylococcus aureus*;
4. *Pneumococcus* and other streptococci (Groups A, D, G and viridans);
5. *Listeria monocytogenes.*

However, a wide spectrum of both Gram-negative and Gram-positive organisms, as well as fungi and viruses can cause early and late onset neonatal infection.

SUPERFICIAL INFECTIONS

Bacterial infection of the umbilicus and skin

The umbilical cord should be treated at birth with a broad-spectrum antibiotic powder. If this is done properly, even local infection around the umbilicus will be rare. If infection does occur, with periumbilical redness and local discharge, it is usually due to staphylococci or *E. Coli*, and, after taking a swab, it usually responds to topical antibiotics. Occasionally systemic antibiotics (p. 235) will be indicated if the discharge is copious or oedema and inflammation are spreading up the falciform ligament.

Effective umbilical cord care is important, not only to prevent ascending infection with portal pyaemia, but also to keep the umbilical stump sterile in case catheterization of the umbilical vessels is required. It also reduces the incidence of other superficial infections including those of the baby's skin and eye, and the mother's breast.

Staphylococcal skin infection is now rarely seen other than as very minor superficial blisters which respond to 5 days treatment with oral flucloxacillin. Occasionally toxic epidermal necrolysis (Ritter's disease) develops. This responds to adequate parenteral fluid replacement and intravenous flucloxacillin.

Thrush

This is usually a trivial oral or perianal infection in otherwise healthy term babies. It presents as white plaques on the buccal mucosa and tongue which cannot be wiped off, or as the typical bright erythematous perianal rash with discrete lesions looking like the base of thin roofed blisters, lying peripheral to the confluent rash. This usually responds promptly to treatment with topical miconazole gel or nystatin suspension.

Thrush is more common in VLBW babies who are on broad spectrum antibiotics for a prolonged period of time, especially if they are also receiving steroids for CLD (p. 209–210). In such babies systemic candidiasis may occur. For these babies prophylactic oral nystatin should be considered, although there is no convincing evidence that it is effective.

Conjunctivitis

The diagnosis and management of this condition is outlined in Table 14.1.

Table 14.1 Management of neonatal conjunctivitis

Organism	Age at presentation	Diagnosis	Treatment
Gonococcus	1 day (some recognized in 1st week)	Maternal history Profuse conjunctival discharge Urgent Gram stain on pus shows Gram-negative intracellular diplococci. Culture of swab sent in transport medium	Intravenous penicillin 75 000 units/kg/24 h given in two divided doses for a week. Also penicillin eye drops hourly for 24 hours, then 4 hourly for a week. Notifiable disease. Remember to organize treatment for mother and contact tracing
Chlamydia trachomatis	5 days or more	No distinguishing clinical features. May be maternal history. Conventional cultures can be sterile. Antigen detected in eye swab by immunofluorescence	Systemic erythromycin (45 mg/kg/24 h in three divided doses) for at least 2 weeks to prevent pneumonia. Well absorbed orally. Also use 1% chlortetracycline eye ointment
Others; commonest are Staph aureus, E coli, Haemophilus, Strep pneumoniae	3–5 days peak, but may be at any time including day 1	Culture of swab	If mild; sterile saline cleaning. If severe, use 0.5% chloramphenicol eye drops

SUPERFICIAL ABSCESSES

These develop at the site of IV infusions, heel sticks or any other place where the skin is damaged. The local lesion is obvious, but care should be taken to ensure that the underlying bone is not affected. If fluctuant, the abscess should be aspirated and the pus sent for Gram stain and culture. The other routine investigations for infection should also be carried out (pp. 232–234). Treatment with IV flucloxacillin and gentamicin should be given initially for 7 days or until the lesion is healed.

SYSTEMIC BACTERIAL INFECTION

The comparative immunodeficiency of the neonate not only predisposes him to infection, but also means that when infection occurs it may disseminate very rapidly, with septicaemic shock and death occurring within 12 hours of the first signs of illness. This dissemination – which is particularly rapid in the most immature – has two major implications:

1. Early diagnosis is essential. Even very trivial clinical findings that suggest infection demand full laboratory evaluation.
2. Initial therapy must be started on the basis of clinical suspicion. There is not time to wait for the laboratory results to come back 24–48 hours later.

Shrewd and vigilant observation by the nurses who are with the babies all the time is the cornerstone of early diagnosis. Woe-betide the neonatal resident who ignores such observations made by an experienced nurse.

History

Apart from verifying the presenting history, the following points should always be checked:

1. Is the baby compromised in any way that would predispose him to infection (eg very premature, indwelling catheter, endotracheal tube)?
2. Was there anything in the perinatal history suggesting an infectious risk (e.g. maternal illness or pyrexia, prolonged rupture of membranes, pathogens known in the mother's HVS)?
3. Is there a risk of nosocomial infection from relatives, staff, or other sick babies on the unit?

Early symptoms and signs

Temperature change Hypothermia and hyperthermia are often due to deficiencies in the control of the environmental temperature (Chapter 2). These can usually be excluded rapidly by taking a history, and noting the environmental temperature! A body temperature below 36°C or above 37.5°C sustained for more than an hour or two in an appropriate environmental temperature is due to infection until proved otherwise. The higher or lower the temperature the more significant it is. A core-peripheral temperature difference of 73°C (p. 11, 106) can be an early marker of sepsis.

Anorexia When a previously healthy baby refuses to feed from breast or bottle, infection should be suspected.

Poor weight gain This, without any other symptoms, can indicate occult infection, though it is obviously not a feature of rapidly progressing sepsis.

Listlessness, lethargy, hypotonia, pallor, mottled skin These are often the first, mild, non-specific signs that a baby is unwell. The baby just does not seem "right".

Irritability A baby who is irritable and will not stop crying or whimpering, even for a feed, may be developing septicaemia or meningitis.

Jaundice If this develops rapidly in a baby without haemolytic disease, sepsis is present until proved otherwise, although the yield of infection screens when jaundice is the *only* presenting sign is very low.

Vomiting If persistent, this is suggestive of infection (as well as intestinal obstruction). Diarrhoea and vomiting are not necessarily signs of gastroenteritis in neonates, and are much more commonly non-specific features of early infection.

Ileus/intestinal obstruction Sepsis may present as vomiting, abdominal distension and constipation due to an ileus, particularly when there is intra-abdominal infection (e.g. necrotising enterocolitis, pp. 383–388).

Pseudoparalysis The lack of movement owing to limb pain may alert the clinician to the presence of arthritis or osteomyelitis before local or generalized signs develop.

Apnoea Commonly the first sign of infection in premature babies.

Tachypnoea Tachypnoea accompanying any of the above signs is often the first sign of pneumonia or septicaemia.

Cardiovascular signs Tachycardia is common in any infection, and marked in cardiac infections. Delayed capillary filling is a useful early sign; skin blanched by pressure should return to normal colour within 1–2 seconds.

Late signs and symptoms

These are usually specific to one organ system. If infection presents in this way it suggests that the diagnosis could have been made earlier if the baby had been more carefully and expertly observed.

Respiratory Cyanosis, grunting, respiratory distress, cough.

Abdominal Bilious or faeculent vomiting, gross abdominal distension, livid flanks, indurated abdominal skin and periumbilical staining, absent bowel sounds.

CNS High pitched cry, retracted head, bulging fontanelle, convulsion.

Haemorrhagic diathesis Petechiae, bleeding from puncture sites.

Sclerema This is a late feature of any serious illness, especially in preterm neonates. It has no specific significance nor specific therapy.

Clinical examination

The baby should be completely undressed and carefully examined, paying particular attention to the following points:

1. Confirm the presenting signs (e.g. fever, jaundice, pallor, grunting).
2. Are there any lesions on the skin, subcutaneous tissues or scalp?
3. Is there periodic breathing or tachypnoea at rest?
4. Is there tachycardia or murmurs suggesting cardiac disease?
5. Are there added sounds on auscultation of the chest?
6. Is there hepatosplenomegaly which accompanies generalized infection as well as hepatitis?

7. Is there kidney enlargement? Cortical swelling of the kidneys may be present in early septicaemia as well as UTI.

8. Is the umbilicus red and tender with a thickened cord of inflamed umbilical vein extending up the falciform ligament?

9. Can osteomyelitis and arthritis be excluded by the presence of full and painless limb movements?

10. Are bowel sounds present? Does the baby cry during palpation of his abdomen, suggesting peritonitis?

11. Do not forget otitis media in the neonate.

12. Meningism is rare in neonatal meningitis, but check the spinal cord, column and skull for pits or other skin defects that might be the entry site for spinal infection.

13. Assess the baby's overall neurological state (p. 311) – is he in coma?

14. Babies do not have dysuria or frequency, but with pyelonephritis they may have loin tenderness which can be detected by gentle pressure on the renal angle.

15. Is the baby dehydrated? Has he lost more than 10% of his birth weight, suggesting major gut fluid loss?

Investigations

Whenever there is any suspicion of infection on the above features, the following tests should *always* be carried out:

1. Take swabs. There is little if any benefit from taking swabs from any site other than the ear and throat when assessing babies in the first 6–12 hours (Dobson *et al.*, 1992). Gram stains of gastric aspirate are more often confusing than helpful. Large numbers of gastric aspirate specimens have organisms and white cells present, but very few of these babies develop symptoms. Gastric aspirate reflects the liquor and the contents of the birth canal.

2. In the presence of early onset sepsis a maternal HVS should always be cultured.

3. In late onset sepsis or NEC, stool culture or effective rectal swabs are helpful.

4. Endotracheal tube aspirate (if applicable).

5. Bag urine in investigation after 24 hours of age. The vulva or penis should be cleaned as carefully as possible, and any infection noted, to assist interpretation of the result. The urine should be decanted from the bag into a sterile container as soon as possible after voiding. Results from bag specimens of urine

collected from neonates should always be viewed with grave suspicion unless pus cells or bacteria were seen immediately on examination of the sample. If any doubt exists, urine must be obtained by suprapubic bladder puncture.

6. Blood culture. Great care should be taken in interpreting positive results when more than one organism is grown or the organisms grown are also skin commensals. Unless these grow in pure culture within 24–48 hours, they are probably contaminants and the blood culture should be repeated, particularly if antibiotics have not already been started.

7. WBC and differential. Polymorph counts above $7.5–8.0 \times 10^9/l$ ($7500–8000/mm^3$) or below $2 \times 10^9/l$ ($2000/mm^3$), more than 0.8×10^9 myelocytes/l ($800/mm^3$) an I:T ratio of >0.2 (the ratio of immature to total neutrophils) and a left shift or toxic granulation of the white cells are all suggestive of neonatal bacterial infection after the third day of life. On the first day of life a polymorphonuclear leucocytosis is not a sign of infection, but neutropenia, an I:T ratio of >0.2 and the presence of immature cells, and toxic granulation are. Thrombocytopenia (<100 $\times 10^9/l$) is common in infected babies.

8. C-reactive protein. A CRP above 6 mg/l suggests infection, but the levels take 12 hours to rise. CRP is more helpful for monitoring progress than for establishing the diagnosis. The levels of other acute phase proteins such as haptoglobin also rise, but measuring them adds nothing to the measurement of CRP. Measuring cytokine response to infection (e.g. IL6) is promising but not yet readily available.

The following investigations should also be carried out in most situations:

1. Lumbar puncture. This should be carried out in all babies with suspected sepsis with the exception of babies with RDS in whom antibiotics are started at birth (p. 241) or those with CLD on IPPV who develop lung infection (p. 206).

2. CXR. This often gets forgotten – unwisely! CXR should be done unless there is an obvious extrapulmonary focus of infection.

3. Abdominal X-ray. If the symptoms suggest intra-abdominal pathology, if there is any abdominal distension, or if there is blood in the stool.

4. Blood gases. A metabolic acidaemia is often present in severe infections, and if the base deficit is above 8 mmol/l, not only does it suggest sepsis, but it should be corrected. Hypoxia,

hypercapnia or apnoeic attacks are indications for ventilation in sepsis.

5. The plasma electrolytes, urea, glucose, calcium and albumin should also be checked; not only may they be abnormal when sepsis presents, but also a base line measurement is important when planning fluid and electrolyte balance in the next few days.

Interpretation of results

When the baby first presents a quick decision has to be made about whether or not to treat with antibiotics. Of the tests initially carried out, those which give the definitive answer – the cultures – take 24–48 hours to come back, and so the clinician has to rely on tests with a turn-round time of an hour or two to help him make that decision. Results that would mandate to the early use of antibiotics include the following:

1. significant changes in the neutrophil count, especially neutropenia $<2 \times 10^9/l$;
2. platelets $<100 \times 10^9/l$;
3. a raised CRP;
4. pneumonic changes on the CXR;
5. leucocyturia;
6. CSF changes – an increase in white cells, or organisms seen on microscopy.

The more of the above results that are positive, the more likely it is that infection is present. However, there is no test which effectively *excludes* infection within the first 12–24 hours, and because of the neonate's great susceptibility to infection, the decision to start antibiotics has to be a clinical one.

If in doubt, treat.

Treatment of systemic bacterial infection

Antibiotics (Isaacs and Moxon 1999; Dear 1999)   Any baby in whom it is remotely possible that an infection is responsible for the abnormal clinical and laboratory findings should be given antibiotics. These can be stopped in 5 days or less if the baby's condition rapidly improves and cultures are negative. Proven infections should be treated for at least 10 days, rising to 14 days in most babies with septicaemia (except CONS – p. 243) and at least 21 days in meningitis (*v.i.*). In virtually all cases the antibiotic should be given intravenously; intramuscular antibiotics in a neonate may cause nerve and muscle damage. Oral antibiotics have no place other than in the treatment of UTI (*v.i.*), chlamydial conjunctivitis (Table 14.1.) or trivial superficial skin infection in babies who are systemically well.

The choice of antibiotics in the neonatal period is becoming increasingly difficult, with the availability of the third generation cephalosporins, the rising incidence of CONS sepsis and the emergence of multiply antibiotic resistant organisms such as MRSA. However, we know of no evidence that cephalosporins are preferable to the well-tried combination of a penicillin plus aminoglycosides for routine use in the neonatal period. We keep cephalosporins as second line alternatives for this reason.

Two antibiotics should be given to babies with suspected systemic infection. One of these should be an aminoglycoside to deal with the coliform group of organisms. We use gentamicin, although tobramycin, amikacin or netilmicin can be used.

Depending on which of the following organisms are common in the unit, select the second or third antibiotic to be given intravenously with the aminoglycoside:

- Group B β-haemolytic streptococcus – penicillin G.
- *Staphylococcus aureus or epidermidis* (CONS) – flucloxacillin, vancomycin.
- *Pseudomonas aeruginosa* – ceftazidime, piperacillin.
- *Listeria monocytogenes* – ampicillin.
- Anaerobes – metronidazole.

Our current practice is to give penicillin and gentamicin to babies less than 48 hours old in whom streptococci (particularly GBS) and pneumococci are a problem. Beyond 48 hours we use flucloxacillin plus gentamicin to cover staphylococcal disease. We add ceftazidime or piperacillin if there is clinical suspicion or microbiological proof of pseudomonas infection, and use cefotaxime and vancomycin in babies in whom CONS is likely and who are very ill, or who are not responding to flucloxacillin and gentamicin. In babies with intra-abdominal sepsis and NEC, we add metronidazole to the other two antibiotics to deal with anaerobic infections. Where flucloxacillin resistant CONS is becoming a problem in VLBW babies vancomycin may be used instead of flucloxacillin as second line.

Third-generation cephalosporins are very effective against most Gram-negative bacilli, and they penetrate the CSF well. However, they are not effective against *Streptococcus fecalis, Listeria, Enterobacter* species and (with the exception of ceftazidime) *Pseudomonas,* and there is anxiety about their efficacy against Gram-positive cocci (Goldberg 1987). Furthermore, their routine use may result in alterations in the resident flora in the unit, selecting for multiple antibiotic resistant Gram-negative organisms and anaerobes, such as *Bacteroides.*

Once the culture and antibiotic sensitivity results are available, changes in the antibiotics can be made. For example, in babies with proven coliform septicaemia we would give both a cephalosporin (cefotaxime) and gentamicin, and for *Strep. faecalis* we would give ampicillin plus gentamicin. The antibiotic therapy in meningitis is outlined on pp. 246–248. Whenever an aminoglycoside is being given plasma levels should be checked several times a week. The trough level should be taken just before a dose is due, and a peak level 1 hour later. Acceptable levels are given in Table 14.2. If the trough level is too high the dose frequency needs to be decreased to 24 hourly or even 36 hourly (and vice versa). The peak levels assess dose, if too high reduce the dose, if too low increase it. Plasma levels do not need to be measured when giving cephalosporins or penicillins.

Whichever antibiotic policy is decided upon, a close watch must be kept on which organisms are actually responsible for the serious infections in the unit, and whether their antibiotic resistance pattern is changing. The routine antibiotic cocktail can then be continuously adapted and updated. However our own brew of penicillin/flucloxacillin plus gentamicin has remained satisfactory for two decades.

Table 14.2 Drug levels of some commonly used antibiotics

Drug	Sampling time	Target range
Amikacin	1 hour post dose	15–20 microg/ml
	pre-dose	<4 microg/ml
Gentamicin	1 hour post dose	6–10 microg/ml
	pre-dose	<2 microg/ml
Netilmicin	1 hour post dose	10–12 microg/ml
	pre-dose	<2 microg/ml
Tobramycin	1 hour post dose	4–8 microg/ml
	pre-dose	<2 microg/ml

Immunotherapy

The use of intravenous immunoglobulin has been intensively investigated in neonatology in two situations:

1. prophylactically in VLBW neonates who are likely to develop postnatal hypogammaglobulinaemia;
2. therapeutically in all neonates with probable septicaemia.

Prophylaxis Even meta-analyses disagree! The most recent one (Jensen and Pollock 1997) suggests benefit from regimens that usually involve giving 0.5g/kg of IVIG weekly for the first 4–6 weeks. If there is benefit from prophylaxis it is primarily in preventing late onset nosocomial infection with CONS. Our current practice is not to use prophylactic immunoglobulin. Prophylaxis may be of greater benefit in those parts of the world where early and late onset sepsis are more common than in the UK, Europe and the USA (Haque *et al.* 1986, Dear 1999).

Therapy A Cochrane review of four trials that enrolled a total of 208 babies with suspected infection showed a 50% reduction in mortality which was not significant when the results of one German quasi-randomized trial were excluded or when only cases with proven infection were considered (Ohlsson and Lacy 1999). Further randomized trials are planned. In the meanwhile it may be worth giving IVIG 0.5 g/kg daily for four days to babies with septicaemia, except for those with CONS sepsis who do well with conventional treatment. According to Jensen and Pollock (1997) this improves the likelihood of survival six fold.

Exchange transfusion This is a complex way of infusing immunoglobulins and white blood cells, and its use in severe sepsis has to some extent been superseded by the availability of immunoglobulin and cytokines. However, exchange transfusion gives many other opsonins, as well as coagulation factors, and washes out assorted toxic metabolites, so a single volume exchange using blood which is as fresh as possible still has a place in the management of the occasional baby with fulminating sepsis.

WBC transfusion, G-CSF and GM-CSF Severely septic neonates of all gestations may have a marked neutropenia. Granulocyte transfusions were used in the past with varying degrees of success, but their use has now been superseded by G-CSF and GM-CSF. Both these agents raise the neutrophil leucocyte count in septicaemic neutropenic babies and preliminary results suggest they are safe. These agents should not be used except as part of a prospective randomized controlled trial.

Other management

Fluid and electrolyte balance All babies being treated with antibiotics will have an intravenous line *in situ* for administration of the drugs. In babies in whom the infection is mild, or in whom the antibiotics are being given on suspicion of infection only, it may be possible to continue oral feeding by nasogastric tube. However, in the seriously ill baby with septicaemia or meningitis, an ileus lasting several days may develop, so that feeding should be stopped and fluid balance will need to be maintained intravenously taking great care to avoid fluid overload (Chapter 3). Plasma biochemistry should be checked at least daily during the acute illness.

Acidaemia/blood gases Septicaemic babies are often acidaemic and hypoxic, and require frequent blood gas analyses. Umbilical arterial catheters should probably be removed from babies with blood stream infection, but peripheral arterial cannulae are essential in this situation. The implications for, and management of, intravenous base, supplementary oxygen and IPPV are identical to those in RDS. CPAP is rarely helpful.

Cardiovascular therapy Hypotension is common in septicaemic babies, and the mean blood pressure must be kept above 30 mmHg and ideally above 35 mmHg. Hypotension should be treated initially with plasma expanders or blood giving 15 ml/kg, but intravenous dopamine 5–10 microg/kg/min or dobutamine are often required. In severe sepsis PPHN may develop (pp. 189–194).

Haematology The full blood count should be checked daily and the baby transfused if the haemoglobin is less than 12 g%. Haemolysis after blood transfusion due to the agglutination of neonatal red cells by normal adult serum (T-activation) can occur in neonatal sepsis and NEC. DIC may also occur in severe septicaemia, and clotting studies and a platelet count should always be done. If DIC is confirmed, it should be treated with infusions of fresh frozen plasma, platelets, or blood (pp. 449–450).

RAPID-ONSET NEONATAL SEPTICAEMIA

The most dramatic form of neonatal septicaemia is the fulminating pneumonic/septicaemic illness which can develop in babies of all gestations. Characteristically this is caused by GBS, but many organisms may be responsible.

Group B streptococcal septicaemia

It is convenient to divide neonatal GBS infections into the following three categories:

1. Acute postpartum disease presenting at birth or within 2–4 hours of delivery; septicaemic and pneumonic; all GBS serotypes.
2. Early-onset disease: average age of onset 20 hours; all serotypes of GBS; equal numbers of cases with meningitis, pneumonia and septicaemia; all serotypes.
3. Late-onset disease: usually greater than 7 days old, predominantly GBS serotype III; 85% of cases are meningitis.

The group 1 babies who have been infected *in utero* are often in poor condition at birth and difficult to resuscitate. More typically, with intrapartum infection the baby presents at age 1–2 hours with mild grunting and recession, but then rapidly deteriorates if not promptly and vigorously treated, soon becoming apnoeic, hypotensive and oliguric, and dying during the first 24–48 hours. The treatment for groups 1 and 2 is identical and is outlined below.

Differential diagnosis

This early onset form of GBS sepsis can sometimes be differentiated from RDS by the following:

1. known positive culture of GBS from the maternal vagina, perineum or urine;
2. early onset of apnoea and hypotension (particularly in mature babies);
3. comparatively easy to control $PaCO_2$, but very difficult to oxygenate i.e. PPHN (pp. 189–194);
4. laboratory tests – WBC may be very low in GBS sepsis (p. 233)
   (a) Gram stain – Gram-positive cocci in deep ear swab in GBS sepsis;
   (b) L:S ratio – less than 1.5:1 suggests RDS;
   (c) Latex tests (if available) – positive for GBS.

In some patients, however, early onset GBS disease and surfactant deficient RDS coexist.

Prevention of early onset GBS

The alternative strategies recommended by the AAP are summarized in Fig 14.1. One is based on giving intrapartum prophylaxis based on the results of surveillance cultures taken at 35–37 weeks of pregnancy, and the second strategy is to offer treatment on the basis of risk factors without culture. It is estimated that the first approach would prevent 90% of early onset GBS, and the second 69% (AAP 1997).

Current minimum best practice should include a protocol to treat the following high risk groups:

• previous child with GBS disease;
• pregnant woman known to carry GBS;
• raised temperature in labour >37.8°C;
• GBS bacteriuria in pregnancy.

Other groups which should be considered for treatment include:

• preterm labours;
• prolonged rupture of membranes – these women should have a swab taken so that their GBS status is known; if GBS is grown then intrapartum antibiotic prophylaxis should be given once labour commences.

Neonatal treatment

1. Babies of under 37 weeks gestation born to carrier mothers who received any prophylaxis, and more mature babies whose mothers received an incomplete course of treatment (antibiotics less than 6 hours before delivery) should have a full blood count, including a differential white count, and a blood culture performed. They should be treated with intravenous penicillin and gentamicin until the cultures are known to be negative, and if they are symptomatic an LP should be done. This also applies to babies born to mothers who should have received treatment, but did not.

2. Babies of ≥37 weeks gestation whose mothers received prophylaxis more than 6 hours before delivery do not need to be investigated. Opinions differ on whether these babies can be offered early discharge from the hospital; our own practice is to observe them for 48 hours.

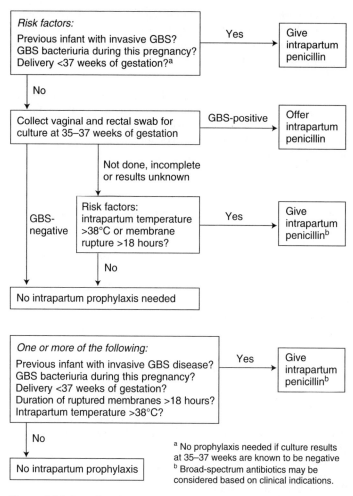

Figure 14.1 Prevention of early onset GBS (American Academy of Pediatrics 1997).

3. All babies with respiratory illness, including those with RDS (p. 125) and TTN (p. 178), should have cultures taken at presentation and receive penicillin and gentamicin until the cultures are known to be sterile.

4. If GBS sepsis seems likely on the basis of history, clinical course, presence of maternal infection, or the presence of Gram-positive

cocci in the ear swab taken immediately after birth, plus appropriate WBC changes or latex studies, then penicillin 100 mg (150 000 units)/kg/24 h should be given in two divided doses, with gentamicin in conventional doses added for its synergistic effect against the organism.

If the cultures are negative antibiotics can be discontinued in 48 hours, but if they are positive they should be continued for 14 days. Correct use of a selective intrapartum antibiotic policy has proved very effective in a number of centres, including our own, over the last few years.

Supportive treatment

Babies with severe early onset GBS are critically ill. They need the full panoply of neonatal intensive care outlined on pp. 137–143. IPPV is virtually always necessary, as is correction of metabolic acidaemia (p. 139) and support for the blood pressure with transfusion plus dopamine and/or dobutamine.

Severe cases develop PPHN probably due to the release of vasoactive agents such as thromboxane A from the pulmonary vascular epithelium in response to the infection. These babies are sometimes helped by nitric oxide and ECMO.

OTHER CAUSES OF RAPID-ONSET SEPTICAEMIA

Many other organisms acquired from the maternal birth canal have been isolated from babies with an identical clinical picture to that seen with the Group B streptococcus. Organisms responsible for this type of illness include the following (Stoll *et al.* 1996b, Dear 1999):

1. pneumococci;
2. groups A, D and G streptococci;
3. *Enterococcus faecalis*;
4. *Haemophilus* species (*H. influenzae*, *H. parainfluenzae*, *H. aphrophilus*);
5. anaerobes;
6. coliforms, including *E. coli*.

These are all adequately treated by the initial penicillin and gentamicin cocktail; for optimal treatment these will need to be changed once the culture and sensitivity results become available.

In particular, ampicillin should be given for *Streptococcus faecalis* and ampicillin or a cephalosporin for *Haemophilus* species.

COAGULASE NEGATIVE STAPHYLOCOCCAL (CONS) SEPTICAEMIA

In most neonatal units this has become the single most important cause of late onset neonatal septicaemia (Stoll *et al.* 1996a). In part this is due to the large number of ELBW neonates surviving with intravenous cannulae left *in situ* for a long time, and also receiving intralipid which seems to predispose to this infection (Freeman *et al.* 1990). The bowel acts a reservoir for CONS in the newborn. There are more than 20 species of CONS, although in clinical practice 80% of infections are caused by *Staphylococcus epidermidis* or *Staphylococcus haemolyticus*. Slime producing strains cause particular problems with line and shunt infections because the slime enables the organism to migrate along the catheter. The risk of line infection is a function of time and the number of times the catheter is used for injections. For this reason long lines should only be used for TPN or very high concentrations of dextrose.

Clinical features

These organisms do not cause fulminating illness, although CONS may be grown from blood cultures in babies with NEC. CONS may cause meningitis especially in babies with shunts. Characteristically it presents after the first week in ELBW neonates with indwelling lines for TPN or arterial access. The signs are the more subtle ones listed on pp. 230–231, with just a gradual decline in the baby's condition, pallor, worsening blood gases and decreasing tolerance of feeds. Often there are no signs initially, and the infection is detected because of changes in routinely collected blood tests.

Investigation

As well as growing the organism from the blood culture, there will often be a rise in the WBC and CRP, and a fall in the platelet count. Acid base, electrolyte or radiological changes are rare.

Treatment

Give flucloxacillin and gentamicin intravenously for 10 days. In some units a large number of CONS are flucloxacillin resistant, in which case vancomycin should be used intially; otherwise vancomycin should be reserved for resistant strains. Vancomycin has to be given slowly intravenously and may be associated with an intense transient erythema of the skin. Teicoplanin is another option, although the clinical experience with this agent in the newborn is limited. Urokinase infusion may also help (p. 60). Central lines should preferably be removed, but if vascular access is a problem the line can be left *in situ* and vancomycin given through it. This will be effective in 50–60% of cases, and in virtually all cases will transiently eliminate the infection.

Outcome

CONS is usually a mild infection and few babies should die as a result of it.

PNEUMONIA

The organisms responsible for pneumonia are those responsible for neonatal septicaemia (pp. 239, 241–242). Viral pneumonia also occurs in the neonate.

Neonatal pneumonia presenting within 2–4 hours of delivery, and caused by one of the many organisms that are resident in the maternal birth canal, is discussed in the preceding section. Pneumonia that develops in babies on IPPV is discussed on pp. 169–172. Pneumonia, often viral, is a major problem for the long-term patient with severe CLD (p. 206).

Respiratory distress developing after 4 hours of age in any neonate who does not have some other diagnosis readily made on clinical examination or CXR – such as pneumothorax, some lung malformation or heart failure – is due to pneumonia until proved otherwise.

Cultures should be taken (p. 232–233) and the baby started on the antibiotic cocktail appropriate for his age and the known bacterial flora in the NNU. These should be continued for 7–10 days.

Irrespective of the organisms responsible, the other aspects of management are those for any severe respiratory illness described on p. 137 *et seq.*

ENDOCARDITIS

This has been recognized with increasing frequency in critically ill VLBW neonates with central lines. Vegetations form on the valves or the endocardium. The organisms responsible are usually *Staphylococci aureus* and CONS, and candida. In addition to the standard features of infection (pp. 230–231) these babies characteristically have murmurs, haematuria, and thrombocytopenia. The vegetations can be demonstrated echocardiographically, and the other investigations are those listed on pp. 232–234. Treatment is with a 6-week course of an appropriate antibiotic. Occasionally valve damage requires surgery. The prognosis is poor.

OSTEOMYELITIS/ARTHRITIS

These conditions frequently co-exist. Multiple bone involvement may occur in babies with central lines, the usual organism being *Staphylococcus aureus*. If a single site is involved GBS is more common. The condition presents with the usual signs of infection together with pseudo-paralysis, or accidentally when the affected bone is X-rayed. Ultrasound examination can be helpful in establishing the diagnosis. The usual work-up for infection is indicated, and the appropriate antibiotics should be given for 4–6 weeks. Survival is the rule, but early advice from a paediatric orthopaedic surgeon must be sought if the diagnosis is confirmed. The infection often ruptures into a joint (e.g. the hip) or into soft tissue in which case drainage is important. Permanent damage to the growth plate of the bone or the joint is common, and the effects of these serious complications can be reduced by correct early orthopaedic management.

NEONATAL MENINGITIS

Clinical signs

The traditional signs of this disease, namely a bulging fontanelle, head retraction and a high-pitched cry, are the signs of established meningitis which may have progressed to a cerebritis with cortical thrombophlebitis. The mortality and long-term neurological morbidity of such babies is high, and every effort should be made to detect neonatal meningitis on the basis of the early and non-specific signs of infection listed on pp. 230–231. For this reason it is important always to have a low threshold for carrying out an LP in sick babies. Basically, there has to be a very good reason *not* to perform an LP when sepsis is suspected.

Organisms

About 40% of neonatal meningitis is due to *E. Coli* and a further 40% to GBS. *Listeria monocytogenes* causes about 10%, but the remaining 10% can be caused by any organism including (rarely) the three bacteria causing meningitis in older children – *Haemophilus, Pneumococcus* and *Meningococcus*. Gram-negative bacillary meningitis is usually complicated by ventriculitis.

Diagnosis

The normal neonatal CSF may contain up to 30 white cells/mm^3, although these are usually predominantly lymphocytes. A WBC count greater than this usually indicates meningitis. However, following an intracranial haemorrhage, especially a GMH-IVH, the polymorph count may exceed 100/mm^3, and the picture is further confused by the CSF glucose level, which in these babies is often less than 1.0 mmol/l (18 mg%). In the presence of a traumatic tap, the RBC:WBC ratio should be approximately 500:1, but wide variations occur, particularly if there is concomitant erythroblastosis when nucleated cells may be nucleated *red* cells.

The normal CSF protein concentration is 0.6 g/l (range 0.4–1.0 g/l) in term and preterm babies, with an upper limit of 1.5–2.0 g/l. Values up to 3.0 g/l (300 mg%) may be seen in premature babies. CSF sugar levels must always be estimated on a sample collected into fluoride. In the neonate, *always* measure simultaneous blood sugar and CSF sugar levels (collect the blood sample first to avoid an elevated glucose level from the stress of the LP). Many cases of neonatal hypoglycaemia have been diagnosed in this way! However, a CSF glucose less than 1 mmol/l usually indicates meningitis. The CSF should be expertly Gram-stained and cultured. If a traumatic tap makes diagnosis impossible, and meningitis remains a distinct clinical possibility, it is safest to treat the baby and repeat the LP next day. If the findings suggest meningitis but no organisms are seen think of viral meningitis and consider acyclovir. A base line brain ultrasound examination should be performed looking for cerebral oedema, ventricular size and ventriculitis (p. 248).

Antibiotic treatment (Table 14.3)

It cannot be emphasized too strongly that neonatal meningitis is a major neonatal emergency, with a high complication rate, and such babies must be transferred to a centre with all the microbiological,

Table 14.3 Antibiotics for neonatal meningitis

Organism	Antibiotic	Total daily dose IV	Number of doses per 24 hours	Intrathecal dose
Group B streptococcus or	Penicillin	100 mg/kg (150 000 units/kg)	3	1000 units
pneumococcus	+ gentamicin	7.5 mg/kg	2–3	1–2 mg
Listeria monocytogenes	Ampicillin	150 mg/kg <7 days, 200–300 mg/kg >7 days old	2 3	5 mg
	+ gentamicin	7.5 mg/kg	2–3	
E coli and other coliforms	Gentamicin	7.5 mg/kg	2–3	1–2 mg
	+ cefotaxime	150 mg/kg	2–3	
Staph aureus	Flucloxacillin	100 mg/kg	4	
Strep faecalis	Ampicillin and gentamicin	As above		
Haemophilus	Cefotaxime	As above		
Pseudomonas	Gentamicin Piperacillin or Ceftazidime	As above 300–400 mg/kg 150 mg/kg	3–4 3	5 mg
Blind therapy if no organisms identified	Ampicillin + cefotaxime + gentamicin	i.v. as above		

neurosurgical and neuroradiological facilities required to carry out the therapy described below.

The baby usually has a concomitant septicaemia, and his basic treatment should follow the routine described on p. 234 *et seq.* for severe infection. Certain additions to the treatment are required if meningitis is present.

In no other infectious disease are opinions more bitterly divided about the appropriate antibiotics to give, and by what route, as in neonatal meningitis. Cases are comparatively rare, and no one unit sees a sufficient number of cases to carry out trials. Multicentre trials have been bedevilled by hetrogeneous patient populations which render the results virtually uninterpretable (McCracken *et al.* 1980). However, the ease with which the third generation cephalosporins penetrate the CSF has helped the therapeutic problems, and survival after neonatal meningitis has improved in the UK (Holt *et al.* 2001).

GBS meningitis For this, give benzyl penicillin 100 mg/kg/24 h combined with a standard dose of IV gentamicin, as the two drugs have a synergistic effect on the organism. Most babies respond clinically to antibiotic therapy within 48 hours, but it is wise to check the CSF at this stage, with repeat LP even earlier (24–36 hours) if there is no clinical improvement. If the CSF has failed to sterilize, intraventricular penicillin is indicated. The speed of sterilization of the CSF is a prognostic indicator.

Listeria meningitis This will respond to large doses of intravenous ampicillin 200–300 mg/kg/24 h given in two or three divided doses; as with GBS meningitis it is probably worth adding IV gentamicin in conventional doses.

E. coli and other Gram-negative enteric organisms An appropriate initial therapy is cefotaxime 150 mg/kg/24 h in three divided doses, plus gentamicin in conventional doses. A repeat LP at 24–48 hours is mandatory in Gram-negative meningitis because there is a significant failure rate after systemic treatment. If the CSF fails to sterilize and the white cell count remains high, the alternatives are to add another CSF-penetrating antibiotic to which the organism is sensitive, to instil appropriate antibiotics into the ventricles, or both. Whichever is chosen, what matters most is that daily assessments continue, to ensure that therapy is being effective. Given the poor outlook if a rapid response is not achieved an aggressive approach, including intraventricular treatment, is warranted.

Blind therapy If no organism is seen on the original CSF and the antigen detection tests are negative we would give ampicillin, gentamicin and cefotaxime in large doses until culture results were available. If these were negative but the clinical signs and CSF findings suggested meningitis we would continue all three for 21 days (*v.i.*). Remember viral meningitis can give a confusing picture.

Intraventricular therapy There is no point in putting antibiotics into the lumbar theca, since they rarely penetrate beyond the basal cisterns.

Intraventricular therapy is the most contentious area in the treatment of neonatal meningitis. However, if meningitis is not responding to systemic therapy after 24–48 hours, as assessed by changes in the CSF, ventriculitis should be considered, especially in coliform meningitis and ventricular puncture should be considered unless the ventricles are tiny and squashed when visualized with cranial ultrasound.

The ventricular puncture should be performed under ultrasound guidance. If the ventricular CSF is clear then all is well, and the baby's poor condition is presumably due to overwhelming sepsis. If ventriculitis is present, then an antibiotic to which the organism is sensitive (e.g. 1 mg gentamicin) should be instilled. The ventricular puncture should then be repeated next day. A decision to stop should be guided by the response to treatment, but most cases of coliform neonatal meningitis treated in the way described show a rapid response within 24–48 hours.

When ventricular punctures are performed, porencephalic cysts may form along the line of the needle track. Therefore, if the second ventricular puncture is not sterile, neurosurgical help should be sought, and a Rickham or Ommaya device inserted. Intraventricular antibiotics can then be safely and easily administered until the infection is controlled.

Assessment of progress

Babies must have a lumbar puncture daily for the first few days, unless the infecting organism is GBS or *Listeria* and there is rapid clinical improvement. Every sample of CSF must be subjected to cytology, chemistry and culture. A lumbar puncture should always be done 2–3 days after cessation of therapy to confirm that the infection has been eradicated.

If aminoglycosides are being used they must be monitored by measuring serum levels. It is particularly important to check ventricular aminoglycoside levels if these drugs are being given directly into the CSF.

A careful neurological examination of the baby should be carried out daily – including head circumference measurements – so that hydrocephalus in particular can be rapidly detected and dealt with. Regular cranial ultrasound imaging will also help to detect complications.

Duration of treatment

Intravenous antibiotics should always be given for 21 days. The only exceptions to this rule are GBS and Listeria meningitis with a rapid clinical and microbiological response and a normal cranial ultrasound scan, in which two weeks of treatment may be adequate. If there is any suggestion of ventriculitis in GBS meningitis, with strands seen within the ventricular cavity on cranial ultrasound images, we treat for three weeks.

Supportive treatment

Many babies with meningitis have fits and cerebral oedema. Fits should be treated with anticonvulsants, beginning with phenobarbitone (p. 314). Cerebral oedema can be treated with mannitol if the intracranial pressure elevation appears to be life-threatening, but the effect of mannitol is short-lived. If raised ICP is clinically apparent, then the blood pressure should be supported in order to maintain cerebral perfusion rather than attempting to reduce ICP. Consideration should be given to an intraventricular tap or insertion of an intraventricular reservoir to measure the pressure and drain CSF. At present there is insufficient evidence to justify steroid treatment in neonatal meningitis.

Fluid and electrolyte balance should be monitored carefully, since these babies are particularly susceptible to inappropriate ADH secretion (pp. 22–23). Fluid intake should be reduced to 40–60 ml/kg/24 h for the first few days of the illness.

Problems in the treatment of neonatal meningitis

Treatment failure If antibiotic therapy is given as outlined above, this will be rare, although it may be necessary to continue treatment for four or occasionally six weeks with unusual Gram-negative organisms. If the lumbar CSF is slow to clear, careful assessment of the baby initially by ultrasound, but then using CT or MR scans is indicated.

Abscess Intracerebral abscesses are particularly common with *Citrobacter* and *Proteus* meningitis. If these organisms are grown, serial ultrasound assessments and other neuroimaging should be performed, either CT or MR. Most abscesses respond to prolonged (6–8 weeks) intravenous antibiotics but often require operative drainage.

Hydrocephalus This will be detected using OFC measurements and ultrasound. If infection is present in the ventricles an intraventricular device must be inserted to give antibiotics and control the ventriculomegaly. If hydrocephalus persists after bacteriological cure, a shunt will need to be inserted.

Outcome

Despite the improvements in care and imaging, the results have remained depressingly poor over the last decade, with 10% dying and 25% being seriously handicapped (Holt *et al.* 2001). The results are worse in preterm babies, and for Gram-negative infections.

URINARY TRACT INFECTION

This commonly presents with mild symptoms such as vomiting, poor weight gain, persisting anaemia, or mild jaundice, although sometimes all the signs of severe sepsis are present. The danger of diagnosing UTI purely on the basis of results of bag urine has already been emphasized (pp. 232–233). If culture of a bag urine is sterile then the baby does not have a urinary tract infection. Bag urine samples with no more than 50 cells/mm^3 without bacterial growth, or significant bacterial growth (>10^5 organisms/ml) without sufficient pus cells, should not be treated as a UTI without confirmation from urine obtained by suprapubic bladder puncture. However, a bag urine with a pure growth of more than 10^5 organisms/ml, with a WBC of more than 100–200/mm^3, is adequate proof of urinary tract infection, provided that there was no local infection of the perineum or foreskin when the bag sample was collected. In urine obtained by a suprapubic stab, anything grown in pure culture, irrespective of the numbers of organisms present, indicates a UTI.

Whenever a UTI is diagnosed, the baby should be carefully examined to exclude renal, bladder or genital abnormalities, and in particular posterior urethral valves should be considered in male babies (pp. 405–406).

In babies with few or no symptoms, treat with oral antibiotics such as trimethoprim; but if the baby is more seriously ill a parenteral aminoglycoside should be used. The antibiotic can be altered appropriately once sensitivities are available, and should be given for 7–10 days.

Once a UTI has been diagnosed, all neonates should have their blood pressure measured and their urea and electrolytes checked, and these tests should be repeated following completion of therapy. The renal tract must be investigated because 30–50% of these babies will have abnormalities, mainly reflux. All cases of neonatal UTI should be investigated with a renal ultrasound scan, a DTPA scan and a micturating cystogram. Whilst awaiting the results of the MCU give prophylactic trimethoprim in case the baby has reflux.

GASTROENTERITIS

Severe nursery epidemics of gastroenteritis due to Salmonella, Shigellae, enteropathogenic *E. coli* and viruses still occasionally occur, although most of the cases of gastroenteritis that are now seen in the neonatal period are sporadic. Infection with rotavirus is endemic in some neonatal units without the babies becoming symptomatic.

Diagnosis

Stool cultures should be sent from all babies with diarrhoea, although the yield of positive cultures is low.

Treatment

Whenever any neonate develops mild gastroenteritis he should be fed with one of the standard oral glucose electrolyte solutions such as Dextrolyte. In most cases his symptoms will settle within 24 hours, and he can restart milk feeding. If the diarrhoea and vomiting do not settle, or if dehydration develops, intravenous therapy will be required for 24–48 hours before restarting oral fluids. Gastroenteritis in preterm babies usually requires a 24–48 hours period of IV therapy before symptoms subside.

Antibiotics should not be given for sporadic cases of neonatal gastroenteritis unless there is systemic spread of the illness. During nursery epidemics, consider using oral non-absorbable antibiotics such as colomycin or neomycin which minimize the amount of cross-infection, but may prolong the carrier state.

If a term baby develops gastroenteritis on the postnatal ward, he should not be admitted to the NNU. If he can be managed with oral treatment, transfer him with his mother to the isolation unit in the maternity hospital; but if the baby requires intravenous therapy he should be transferred to the unit that manages infectious gastroenteritis in older babies. If the baby is already on the NNU he should be kept there, but full barrier nursing routines must be used.

Babies who have recovered, but who are still shedding pathogens in their stools, can go home if they are feeding and gaining weight well. If, however, they have to stay in the NNU they should be isolated.

Two other points to note about gastroenteritis in the newborn:

1. Severe diarrhoea without vomiting which responds to clear fluids but relapses when milk is reintroduced suggests congenital lactose (or other sugar) intolerance.
2. Many completely asymptomatic babies carry enteropathogenic *E. coli* (usually derived from their mothers) in their stools. No action is required.

PROLONGED RUPTURE OF MEMBRANES

In the absence of maternal GBS carriage, if a term baby is asymptomatic, no matter how long the period for which the membranes were ruptured, no cultures need to be done nor therapy given.

If a baby, who is born after prolonged (>24 hours) rupture of the membranes, develops any symptoms in the first 24 hours of life, these should be attributed to infection until proved otherwise. Cultures should be taken from the mother and the baby, and antibiotic treatment started.

Preterm babies (< 37 weeks) born after PPROM should be investigated for infection and treated until culture results are available.

LISTERIOSIS

Neonatal listeriosis has become very rare in the UK since advice about not eating unpasteurized cheese in pregnancy became widespread, and the food industry developed better techniques for sterilizing cook-chill foods and paté. The PHLS have recorded only about 20 cases per year since 1989, when the Government advice regarding these foods was released. Maternal listeriosis can result in fetal infection and premature labour (with meconium stained liquor), severe early onset sepsis, or neonatal meningitis.

In the severe early onset disease, the features are those of generalized sepsis and pneumonia together with, in some cases, characteristic 2–3 mm pinkish grey granulomas in the skin. These granulomata are widespread throughout all tissues hence the name granulomatosis infantisepticum for this form of the disease.

Later onset sepsis with meningitis is indistinguishable from similar illness caused by other organisms.

The investigations are those conventionally carried out, and there are no findings specific to *Listeria*. The diagnosis is made by culturing the Gram-positive coccobacillus from blood or CSF. Treatment is with ampicillin and gentamicin for at least two weeks.

VIRUS INFECTIONS

Viruses are now being identified in many severe neonatal infections. The signs and symptoms are identical to those seen in bacterial infections and the management is exactly the same, including the use of exchange transfusion. Antibiotics are given to such babies, since the clinical signs are identical to those seen in bacterial sepsis. They can be stopped once a viral aetiology is established.

Any baby who shows the signs and symptoms of serious infection but in whom no bacteria are found after 48 hours of culture should be suspected of a viral infection. Samples of stool, CSF and nasopharyngeal aspirate in appropriate virus transport medium should be examined. This should also be done at postmortem in all unexplained "septicaemic" neonatal deaths.

COXSACKIE GROUP B MYOCARDITIS

This condition presents in full-term babies towards the end of the first week with fever, listlessness, tachycardia, tachypnoea, cyanosis, mottling and poor peripheral circulation. The baby is in heart failure with a triple rhythm, hepatosplenomegaly and a soft systolic murmur. He is usually hypotensive and oedematous. Chest X-ray shows cardiomegaly and the ECG shows changes of cardiomyopathy. There may be a coexisting aseptic meningitis. In such a baby samples of stool and CSF should be sent for viral cultures.

Differential diagnosis from other forms of septicaemia is usually easy, because of the primarily myocardial impact of the disease and the coexistence of an aseptic meningitis. Differentiation from other cardiac diseases, including congenital heart disease, can usually be made on the basis of the associated clinical signs of infection, the ECG changes, and echocardiography.

Treatment

The baby should receive all possible intensive care support, taking particular care to avoid fluid overload. Specialized advice is essential in these cases, and may involve the use of digoxin (with great care), diuretics, dopamine or captopril. Some babies will recover and their long-term prognosis is good, although digitalization and captopril may be needed for several months or years. The majority, despite all forms of therapy, die in low-output heart failure.

NEONATAL HERPES

If a baby is born through a birth canal which is infected with herpes virus hominis, he may develop severe postnatal herpes. About 75% of cases are due to the type II (genital) strain, with 25% caused by the type I (oro-pharyngeal) strain. The risk is greatest in the babies of women who are suffering their first herpetic infection and who have overt disease in labour, because these women will not have protected their infants with transplacental immunoglobulin. The majority of cases of neonatal herpes occurs in babies born to women who were asymptomatic in pregnancy, never knowingly having suffered from herpes. A small number of cases are acquired nosocomially from oral or cutaneous herpes.

Clinical features

There are several forms of neonatal herpes which show some overlap. Localized disease presents during the second week with lesions in the skin, eyes and mucous membranes. Systemic upset is rare. Disseminated disease presents earlier by the end of the first week with severe multi-system disease. CNS disease presents at about 10 days with features that are not materially different to those of bacterial meningitis. Finally, disease can be isolated to the lung with pneumonitis.

Investigation

The usual tests for infection should be done (pp. 232–234). Fluid from superficial lesions should be examined by electron microscopy and culture. The diagnosis will only be made in the CNS, pulmonary and disseminated forms of the disease if viral cultures are obtained.

Treatment

There is little that can be done to prevent the disease other than to deliver all women with overt genital herpes within a few hours of membrane rupture, by caesarean section.

In any baby in whom herpes is a possibility, including the asymptomatic baby born through an overtly infected birth canal, intravenous acylovir should be given (30 mg/kg/24 h) for at least 14 days, or until the possibility of herpes has been excluded. Skin or mucous membrane lesions can progress to involve the CNS or other organs so all herpetic lesions should be aggressively treated. In addition, all the usual intensive therapy for the hypotensive seriously ill neonate with a coagulopathy may be required (pp. 137–143, 449–450).

Outcome

Babies with localized disease usually survive intact, but with disseminated and CNS disease the mortality is 20–30% with 50% being handicapped. The outlook is better for those with type I herpes. Even after two weeks of intravenous acyclovir relapses are not uncommon, and require a further two-week course of therapy.

VIRAL MENINGITIS

In the neonate the CSF findings are identical to those for viral meningitis in older children, with a normal CSF sugar level, and a CSF cell count of less than $1000/mm^3$. This may be partly polymorphonuclear in the early stages, but is usually lymphocytic. Appropriate viral cultures should be sent in the presence of these findings. The disease is rarely severe, no specific treatment is required, and neurologically intact recovery is the rule.

ENTEROVIRUS INFECTIONS

Echoviruses of serotypes 6, 7, 12, 14, 17 and especially 11 have been responsible for several epidemics of severe and often fatal neonatal disease in recent years. The babies often present with the non-specific signs of severe sepsis, but characteristically have some abdominal distension and tenderness. In severe cases the course is rapidly downhill with apnoea, hypotension, jaundice and DIC unresponsive to all therapy. Milder cases have just an aseptic meningitis. If the illness is recognized early enough, injections of pooled immunoglobulin may be helpful, and such injections seem to be of major benefit in preventing epidemics within a nursery (Nagington et al., 1983).

RESPIRATORY VIRAL INFECTIONS

Neonates, particularly VLBW survivors who require long-term IPPV and have CLD, may be in the NNU for 3–4 months, and during this time they may well develop a viral respiratory infection contracted from their parents or the staff.

The treatment of these babies is no different to that of any other baby with a viral URTI or bronchiolitis.

Respiratory syncytial virus

Infections with RSV in babies with CLD can be devastating. The severe bronchiolitis often precipitates apnoea, and the neonates once more need IPPV and high oxygen concentrations – often for a further 1–2 weeks – before they can be weaned off. In other babies it provokes terminal respiratory failure from which the baby cannot be retrieved by long-term IPPV, antibiotics and further courses of steroids or diuretics. We currently use immunoglobulin prophylaxis for babies at home in oxygen (p. 211).

If a neonate with CLD does develop RSV bronchiolitis he should be treated with Ribavirin.

Cytomegalovirus

Many babies acquire asymptomatic CMV in the neonatal period, and a small number who are preterm and have been transfused with blood from a CMV-positive donor may develop CMV hepatitis or pneumonitis, the latter making the prognosis in CLD very much worse.

The disease is untreatable and occasionally fatal in CLD. Attempts at prevention must include transfusing neonates only with blood from CMV negative donors, but occasionally babies with CLD acquire CMV from a nursery visitor.

HEPATITIS

The various forms of hepatitis can all be transmitted to the neonate at the time of birth, but because of their long incubation period they rarely present in the neonatal period. Babies born to mothers carrying hepatitis B must be immunized (Table 14.4). Immunization effectively prevents the babies becoming chronic carriers with the attendant risk of hepatocellular carcinoma in later life.

The current shortage of specific immunoglobulin in the UK means that only babies of mothers with high infectivity are offered this treatment. Mothers with high infectivity (more commonly Asian women) are defined as those who are e antigen positive, e antibody negative OR both e antigen and e antibody negative. Their babies must be given 2 ml of immunoglobulin as well as vaccine, ideally within the first 12 hours of life. Vaccine is not always effective in babies, so that four doses are recommended at birth, one, two and twelve months with a blood sample at 14 months to check antibody levels. There are two vaccines available in the UK; Engerix B (SmithKline Beecham) and H-B-VaxII (Pasteur Merieux MSD). The dose is contained in 0.5 ml of vaccine for both preparations; the dose of Enerix B is 10 microg, and that of H-B-VaxII is 5 microg.

SYSTEMIC FUNGAL INFECTION

The baby may be colonized initially by maternal vaginal candidiasis, and fungal infection of the skin and lungs is more common in babies born to mothers with an IUCD *in situ* which has failed to prevent pregnancy. Fungal septicaemia and/or meningitis is a particular problem in ill preterm babies who have received multiple courses of antibiotics.

The presenting features are those of any severe neonatal infection, though endophthalmitis and endocarditis are specific manifestations. Skin lesions are common – many babies have a patchy erythematous skin rash on their trunk.

The usual investigations for sepsis should be carried out (pp. 232–234). In addition appropriate samples – ETT aspirates, urine, can be examined microscopically for budding yeasts and hyphae, and the blood should be cultured in a special media. Microscopic examination of the buffy coat of blood can also help.

Treatment should begin with liposomal amphotericin B 1.0 mg/kg/day to a total dose of 20–30 mg/kg. Liposomal amphotericin (ambisone) is well tolerated and effective (Friedlich *et al.* 1997). If the infection does not respond, consider adding flucytosine 100 mg/kg/day. Image the renal tract and the brain as well as performing ophthalmoscopy and an echocardiogram to look for organ infection with fungus.

MYCOPLASMA/UREAPLASMA

Both these organisms may rarely cause serious illness in the neonate (Dear 1999). The jury is still out on whether ureaplasmas are important in the pathogenesis of CLD. The balance of evidence is at present against such an association.

CONGENITAL INFECTIONS

CONGENITAL RUBELLA, CYTOMEGALOVIRUS, TOXOPLASMOSIS

In their severe form these three conditions have relatively similar clinical findings:

1. low birth weight for gestational age;
2. jaundice;
3. hepatosplenomegaly;
4. thrombocytopenia and purpura;
5. cataract;
6. chorioretinitis;
7. abnormalities of head growth/intracranial calcification;
8. osteitis;
9. congenital heart disease.

If combinations of these abnormalities are present, appropriate cultures and serology should be carried out. A congenitally infected neonate will have the same high titre of IgG in his plasma as his mother, but the diagnostic test is the titre of specific IgM in his plasma against the micro-organism in question. In addition, throat swabs and samples of urine or swabs from any lesions should be sent for culture.

CONGENITAL RUBELLA

This disease should now become even rarer with MMR vaccine being offered to all children in the UK. The babies should be treated symptomatically, in particular a PDA should be closed, cataracts extracted and hearing tests done early to identify and treat those who are deaf. There is no other treatment.

CONGENITAL CMV

Most cases of congenital CMV are asymptomatic in the neonatal period. Such babies are at increased risk of deafness in later life, and, if congenital CMV is diagnosed hearing testing must be offered. There is no treatment for any form of the disease, although some have tried ganciclovir there is as yet no convincing evidence that this can reverse existing damage. We do not at present attempt to treat congenital CMV unless there is active eye disease.

CONGENITAL TOXOPLASMOSIS

This may present with many of the features listed above or just with chorioretinitis. Many countries screen pregnant women for this infection. If congenital infection of any form is found, the baby should be given spiramycin 100 mg/kg/day for 4–6 weeks alternating with pyrimethamine (1 mg/kg/day) plus sulphadiazine (50 mg/kg/day) for 3 weeks for a whole year. This will reduce the likelihood of long-term sequelae, particularly chorioretinitis.

CONGENITAL HERPES

Transplacental passage of herpes is much rarer than perinatally acquired herpes and it causes widespread CNS damage. It is untreatable and virtually always fatal. Babies are usually profoundly damaged with microcephaly or hydranencephaly and skin lesions.

CONGENITAL VARICELLA

This is a rare complication of maternal varicella in the first 20 weeks of pregnancy and affects mainly female fetuses. It causes widespread damage to the CNS, eyes, limb atrophy and cutaneous scars. Most cases die in early infancy.

CONGENITAL PARVOVIRUS B19 INFECTION

This is the virus of erythema infectiosum (fifth disease) and it also causes aplastic crisis in patients with haemolytic anaemias such as spherocytosis and sickle cell anaemia. Most maternal infections cause no problems, but a small number will abort, and about 1% of their fetuses will develop hydrops. If such a baby is born he has a treatable condition and his management is outlined on pp. 457–459.

CONGENITAL HTLV I INFECTION

This virus, common in patients from Japan or the Caribbean, causes T-cell lymphoma and leukaemia in adults. It is transmitted in breast milk. Sero-positive women from these communities should therefore be advised not to breast feed their babies.

CONGENITAL SYPHILIS

This disease is still rare in the UK, though increasing in other parts of the world. In clinical practice the commonest problem occurs with positive serology in mothers who had yaws in childhood. If the mother's serology is consistent with this, and she gives an accurate history, our practice is to monitor the baby for falling antibody titres as an outpatient but not to treat the baby.

Diagnosis in the neonatal period is difficult due to the poor specificity and sensitivity of all the antitreponemal tests (e.g. IgM FTA) when used in the neonate.

All babies with symptoms and positive tests, who are born to mothers not treated adequately during pregnancy should receive benzyl penicillin IV for ten days. This also treats congenital neurosyphilis. However because of residual uncertainty asymptomatic babies, even of fully treated mothers, should receive a single dose of benzathine penicillin 30 mg/kg (Risser and Hwang 1996). Do not forget to check the treatment status of the mother – and her consorts!

CONGENITAL LYMPHOCYTIC CHORIOMENINGITIS

This viral infection spreads from animals, usually rodents, to humans. Mice and hamsters can shed the virus in their urine for months without developing symptoms. LCV infection during pregnancy can result in abortion or a congenital infection with hydrocephalus and chorioretinitis. Neonatal meningitis has been described following maternal infection just before delivery.

AIDS

Fortunately congenital HIV infection is still a relatively rare disease in the UK, with less than 600 HIV positive babies reported to the British Paediatric Surveillance Unit by January 1999, half of whom have developed AIDS. Most of the HIV infected children in the UK are of black African origin and live in London. Nevertheless, the numbers are increasing steadily, and due to an increased uptake of pregnancy screening the neonatal resident may be faced with immediate management of the baby born to an HIV positive mother. Many of these women have already been extensively counselled and offered several options for reducing the chance of transmission of the virus to their fetus, including the option of an elective caesarean section delivery.

In perinatal HIV:

1. All babies born to HIV infected mothers have transplacentally acquired antibody. If they do not become infected, the antibodies disappear by 18 months of age. This means that other tests, including estimation of HIV RNA viral load and PCR for HIV proviral DNA are required to make the diagnosis.

2. Perinatal transmission can be reduced by caesarean section delivery combined with antiviral drugs (see next point).

3. Perinatal transmission can be reduced by two thirds by giving zidovudine (2mg/kg four times a day orally) to HIV positive mothers antenatally and continuing this treatment to the baby for six weeks (Connor *et al.* 1994) (www.hivatis.org). The first dose needs to be given within 4 hours of delivery.

4. Additional antiviral drugs are indicated in some cases, where the mother is already on combination treatment. These include nevirapine 2 mg/kg as a single dose after birth at 48–72 hours and DDI 20 mg twice a day. Lamivudine (3TC) has caused neonatal death as a result of mitochondrial toxicity and its use in the newborn is currently under review. Check www.hivatis.org.

5. At the time of writing antenatal detection of HIV positive women in the UK is woefully incomplete (Mercey 1998). Unlinked anonymous screening has shown that only about 25% of cases are detected by the current system of voluntary screening. This means that many babies are denied the benefits of intervention. Without intervention, about 15–20% will become infected.

6. Cross infection routines on the labour ward, especially in high risk areas (London, Glasgow), must be designed to assume that all women are HIV positive. Gloves should be worn for resuscitation procedures and for testing the suck reflex during the newborn examination.

7. For babies of women known to be HIV positive, hospital guidelines must be followed. The baby should stay with his mother who should not breast feed him.

8. Babies of HIV positive women are at risk from other problems including other sexually transmitted diseases and drug withdrawal syndromes.

9. Confidentiality is an important issue. The mother's HIV status may not be known by her partner, or her immediate family.

Tests to be performed on the baby's blood (not cord blood which may be contaminated) after birth include a full blood count, liver function tests, immunoglobulins and T-cells, HIV viral load, P24 antigen, PCR for proviral DNA.

Table 14.4 Effect of perinatal maternal infections and their effect on breast feeding

Illness	Access to baby and desirability of breast feeding	Treatment to baby
Acute enteric infections (cholera, typhoid)	Nil during acute phase, mother too ill	Nil, encourage breast feeding if possible; immunize baby if appropriate
*Acute respiratory infection (RSV, flu)	Access with masking and hand washing; breast feeding allowed no restrictions	Nil
Chlamydia	No restrictions	Nil if baby is asymptomatic, but see p.228
CMV	No restrictions on access or breast feeding	Nil
*Gastroenteritis	Access with meticulous hand washing	Nil
Hepatitis A	No restrictions but meticulous hand washing	250 mg of immunoglobulin to baby
Hepatitis B	No restriction, breast feeding not contraindicated if full immunization given	Give first dose of vaccine within 12 hours. In addition give 200 i.u. (2ml) of hepatitis B immunoglobulin stat to high infectivity groups (pp. 259–260)
Hepatitis C	No restriction	Nil recommended, but 250 mg standard immunoglobulin may reduce the risk of transmission
Herpes simplex (genital)	No restriction, but meticulous hand washing and gloves	Acyclovir orally to mother (see also pp. 255–256 – treat symptomatic babies aggressively)
*Herpes simplex (labial, whitlow, etc)	No restriction, but mother to wear face mask and treat lesions with acyclovir	None unless symptomatic, when herpes must be excluded
HIV (see pp. 261–262)	Free access, no breast feeding	Start antiretroviral therapy if mother agrees (p.262)
Leprosy	No restrictions	Continue maternal treatment
Malaria	No restrictions on access or breast feeding if mother's general health acceptable	Test baby's blood for parasites especially if mother has falciparum malaria or the baby develops symptoms; treat congenital infection with chloroquine or quinine

Table 14.4 contd

Condition	Restrictions	Action
*Measles	No restrictions	Give 250 mg normal immunoglobulin to the baby (hyperimmune if available)
*Mumps	No restrictions	Nil
Rubella	No restrictions	No problem to neonate, but keep mother away from other antenatal patients
Sexually transmitted diseases (gonorrhoea, syphilis)	Access with meticulous hand washing; no restrictions on breast feeding if mother being treated	Assess baby carefully to check that he is not infected, especially with maternal syphilis (p. 261) and give eye prophylaxis for *Gonococcus* (Dear 1999)
*Skin infections (boils, impetigo)	Access; meticulous hand washing; antibiotics to mother	Nil
*Streptococcal illness or carriage	No restrictions. Meticulous hand washing and masking especially for group A strep respiratory infections	Nil
Toxoplasmosis	No restrictions	Treat the baby (p. 260)
Tropical diseases (trypanosomiasis, schistosomiasis, filariasis)	Usually no restrictions	Nil, but consult local tropical diseases hospital
*TB — open	No restriction if mother's general health satisfactory; drugs do not pass in sufficient quantity into breast milk to contraindicate breast feeding	INAH to baby; BCG at 6 months if baby PPD negative or give INAH resistant BCG at once
TB — closed	As above	As above; normal BCG routine to baby
Ureaplasma colonization	No restrictions	Nil
*Varicella	Access restricted until lesions crusted; mother gowned, masked and gloved	Give 250 mg (one vial) ZIG to baby if maternal disease develops between 7 days before and 14 days after delivery; give acyclovir if vesicles appear
Zoster	Access	Nil; baby immune from transplacental IgG

* conditions where mother may have access to her own term baby, but not allowed into the NNU or have access to other babies.

EFFECT OF PERINATAL MATERNAL INFECTIONS

In most situations a maternal infectious illness, such as urinary tract infection or respiratory infections, poses no risk to the baby. In other situations (e.g. meningitis) the mother will be too ill to keep her baby.

If the mother is suffering from one of the illnesses listed in Table 14.4, appropriate precautions should be taken while allowing access to a normal baby. If, however, the baby is on an NNU, mothers with conditions marked by an asterisk in Table 14.4 should not be allowed to visit the unit because of the risk to other babies.

REFERENCES

American Academy of Pediatrics (1997) Revised guidelines for prevention of early onset streptococcal (GBS) infection. *Pediatrics* **99**: 489–496.

Connor, E.M., Sperling, R.S. and Gilbert, R. (1994) Reduction of maternal infant transmission of human immunodeficiency virus type 1 with zidovudine treatment. *New England Journal of Medicine* **331**: 1173–1180.

De Vries, E., de Groot, R., de Bruin-Versteeg, S., Comans-Bitter, W.M. and van Dongen, J.J.M. (1999) Analysing the developing lymphocyte system of neonates and infants. *European Journal of Pediatrics* **158**: 611–617.

Dobson, S.R.M., Isaacs, D., Wilkinson, A.R. and Hope, P.L. (1992) Reduced use of surface cultures for suspected neonatal sepsis and surveillance. *Archives of Disease in Childhood* **67**: 44–47.

Freeman, J., Goldman, D.A., Smith, N.E., Sidebottom, D.E., Epstein, M.F. and Platt, R. (1990) Association of intravenous lipid emulsion and coagulase negative staphylococcal bacteremia in neonatal intensive care units. *New England Journal of Medicine* **323**: 301–308.

Friedlich, P.S., Steinberg, I., Fujitani, A. and de Lemos, R. (1997) Renal tolerance with the use of Intralipid-Amphotericin B in low birth weight neonates. *American Journal of Perinatology* **14**: 377–383.

Goldberg, D. M. (1987) The cephalosporins. *Medical Clinics of North America* **71**: 1113–1133.

Haque, K.N., Zaidi, M.H., Haque, S.K. *et al.* (1986) Intravenous immunolgobulin for prevention of sepsis in preterm and low birthweight infants. *Pediatric Infectious Disease Journal* **5**: 622–625.

Holt, D.E., Halket, S., de Louvois, J. and Harvey, D. (2001) Neonatal meningitis in England and Wales: 10 years on. *Archives of Disease in Childhood* **84**: F85–F89.

Isaacs, D. and Moxon, E.R. (1999) *Handbook of Neonatal Infections: a practical guide.* Saunders, London.

Jensen, H.B. and Pollock, B.H. (1997) Meta-analyses of the effectiveness of intravenous immune globulin for prevention and treatment of neonatal sepsis. *Pediatrics* **99**: 246.

McCracken, G.H., Mize, S.G. and Threlkeld N. (1980). Intraventricular gentamicin therapy in Gram-negative bacillary meningitis of infancy. *Lancet* i: 787–791.

Mercey, D. (1998) Antenatal HIV testing. *British Medical Journal* **316**: 241–242. This editorial is followed by a series of articles: *BMJ* **316**: 253–307.

Nagington, J., Gandy, G., Walker, J. and Gray, J.J. (1983) Use of normal immunoglobulin in an Echorvirus 11 outbreak in a special care baby unit. *Lancet* ii: 443–446.

Ohlsson, A. and Lacy, J.B. (1999) Intravenous immunoglobulin for suspected or subsequently proven neonatal infection (Cochrane Review). In: *The Cochrane Library*, Issue 2. Update Software, Oxford.

Risser, W.L., Hwang, L-Y. (1996) Problems with the current case definitions of congenital syphilis. *Journal of Pediatrics* **129**: 499–505.

Stoll, B.J., Gordon, J., Korones, S.B. *et al.* (1996a) Late onset sepsis in very low birthweight neonates: A report from the National Institute of Child Health and Human Development Neonatal Research Network. *Journal of Pediatrics* **129**: 63–71.

Stoll, B.J., Gordon, J., Korones, S.B. *et al.* (1996b) Early onset sepsis in very low birthweight neonates: A report from the National Institute of Child Health and Human Development Neonatal Research Network. *Journal of Pediatrics* **129**: 72–80.

Wright, W.C., Ank, B.J., Herbert, J. and Steihm, E.R. (1975) Decreased bactericidal activity of leucocytes of stressed newborn infants. *Pediatrics* **56**: 579–584.

FURTHER READING

Dear, P.R.F. (1999) Neonatal infections. In: *Textbook of Neonatology*, 3rd edn. Rennie, J.M and Roberton, N.R.C. (eds), Churchill Livingstone, Edinburgh, pp.1109–1202.

Isaacs, D. and Moxon, R.E. (1999) *Handbook of neonatal infections: a practical guide*. Saunders, London.

Remington, J.S. and Klein, J.O. (eds) (2001) *Infectious Diseases of the Fetus and Newborn Infant*, 5th edn. W. B. Saunders, Philadelphia.

15

EYE DISORDERS

- *The incidence of ROP can be minimized by meticulous attention to oxygen therapy, always keeping the PaO_2 less than 10 kPa and avoiding wide swings.*
- *ROP develops over a relatively narrow range of maturity, with 75% of the cases developing between 30 and 36 weeks of gestation.*
- *ROP developing after 36 weeks of gestation is unlikely to need treatment.*
- *All babies <32 weeks gestation and <1.5 kg must have regular (1–2 weekly) ophthalmological assessment beginning at 32 weeks postconceptional age or 6 weeks actual age whichever is the sooner, in order to identify those with threshold ROP who require treatment.*
- *Cryotherapy or laser therapy is painful and must be performed using full general anaesthesia.*
- *Vision is impaired in 30% of babies who require treatment for ROP.*
- *Not all visual loss in ex-preterm survivors is due to ROP; some is due to cortical damage.*

RETINOPATHY OF PREMATURITY

This disorder, formerly known as retrolental fibroplasia, is unique to the neonate and is one reason why oxygen therapy is so difficult in babies with lung disease. It is a disease of prematurity (Tables 15.1 and 15.2) with a very low incidence in babies over 32 weeks gestation and 1500 g birth weight. The mildest stages of ROP, which do not progress to permanent damage, are best regarded as a normal variant in babies <28 weeks gestation. As more and more ELBW babies survive, this type of ROP is more commonly seen. There is a new epidemic of ROP in countries where neonatal intensive care has been introduced without adequate resource for ophthalmic screening.

A baby is at risk from ROP until he passes the post-menstrual age of about 32–34 weeks. Thus a baby of 24 weeks gestation is at risk for

Table 15.1 Incidence of ROP

Gestation (weeks)	Percentage developing ROP	Birth weight (g)	Percentage developing ROP
24/25	83	500–699	50
26/27	44	700–899	53
28/29	17	900–1099	32
30/31	8	1100–1299	11
32	5	1300–1499	6
33+	0		

Source: Darlow 1988

Table 15.2 Incidence of cicatricial ROP

Birth weight	All cicatricial ROP (%)	Blind (%)
<1000 g	30	8
1001–1500	2.2	0.5

Source: Phelps 1981

8–10 weeks after birth, whereas a baby of 32 weeks is probably only at risk for a few days.

CLASSIFICATION OF ROP

This is done in three ways (Committee for the Classification of ROP 1987)

1. A classification of the acute stage. This is based on the fact that ROP is a disease of abnormal vascularization of the retina (Table 15.3). The eye is said to show plus disease if there is dilatation and/or tortuosity of the retinal vessels.
2. A description of the region of the retina affected (Fig. 15.1). Zone 1 is twice the distance from the disc to the macula. Zone 2 extends beyond this to the equator of the eye, and Zone 3 beyond the equator on the temporal side of the disc. The area involved can then be described by both Zone and "clock hour". "Threshold" disease, an indication for therapy (v.i.) occurs if there are stage 3 changes in zone 1 or 2 involving five contiguous or eight cumulative clock hours with evidence of plus disease. The risk of blindness in such cases, if left untreated, is 50%.
3. A description of the regressed or cicatricial stage of the disease.

Table 15.3 Classification of acute ROP

Stage	Description
Stage 1	Demarcation line: a simple border or line see at the edge of vessels dividing vascular from avascular retina.
Stage 2	Ridge: the line structure of the previous stage has now acquired a volume and risen above the surface of the retina to become a ridge.
Stage 3	Ridge with extraretinal fibrovascular proliferation: from the surface of the ridge, this extraretinal tissue may extend into the vitreous.
Stage 4	Subtotal retinal detachment: forces developed from proliferating tissue in the vitreous or retina result in a traction type of retinal detachment. This is subdivided into: a) detachment not involving the macula; b) subtotal retinal detachment involving the macula – resulting in poor vision.
Stage 5	Total retinal detachment: a total funnel-shaped retinal detachment with very poor visual prognosis.

Documentation of the zone reached by the normal wave of vascularization – stage 0 – is useful in order to avoid stopping screening too soon.

AETIOLOGY

The fundamental problem is a combination of prematurity plus hyperoxaemia affecting the retinal vasculature. Although it is clear that the longer the baby is in oxygen and the higher his PaO_2 the more likely he is to develop ROP, there is no figure for the shortest exposure to hyperoxaemia that may prove damaging. Furthermore, babies in the "at risk" gestations may be exposed to high PaO_2 levels for many hours without developing ROP. It is doubtful whether ROP ever develops without added oxygen except in ELBW babies for whom the PaO_2 achieved when breathing room air may damage the retina. ROP in mature babies may be due to a different disease, familial exudative vitreoretinopathy (Moore 1999).

However, it was established between 1950 and 1960 that preterm babies were much more likely to develop ROP if they were breathing more than 40% oxygen. At that stage of maturity this level of inspired oxygen when breathed by a baby with normal lungs gives a pre-ductal PaO_2 of about 20–21.3 kPa (150–160 mmHg). If sampling is carried out post-ductally (e.g. from a UAC), to keep the

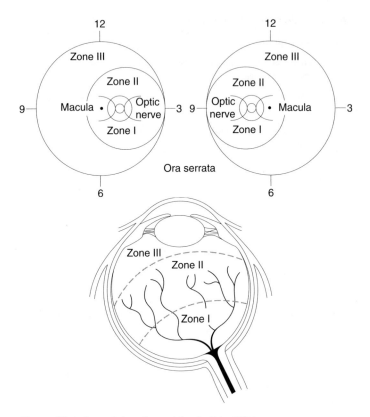

Figure 15.1 Zones of the retina used for classifying ROP in neonates.
Source: Committee for the Classification of ROP 1987 and Phelps 1998.

pre-ductal levels below this value, the post-ductal PaO_2 must be kept below 12–13.3 kPa (90–100 mmHg). During the last decade, with the resurgence of ROP in ELBW babies, even tighter controls have been recommended aiming to keep the post-ductal PaO_2 below 10 kPa (75 mmHg). The BAPM recommend an upper limit of 10 kPa (BAPM 1999), and the AAP (AAP 1997) recommend that the PaO_2 be kept in the range 6.7–10.7 kPa (50–80 mmHg).

Since ROP was first recognized half a century ago many factors have been suggested which increase the baby's susceptibility (Table 15.4). None of these (apart from low gestational age) have as yet

Table 15.4 Factors which may predispose to ROP

Low gestational age and birth weight (see Table 15.1)
Sepsis
GMH-IVH
Hypercapnia and hypocapnia
Light
Recurrent apnoea
Exchange and top up transfusion
Hypoxaemia
Fluctuating PaO_2
Vitamin E deficiency
Prolonged oxygen therapy
Surfactant
Intralipid
Indomethacin
Hyperviscosity
Jaundice

withstood the test of time or been evaluated in prospective trials. Currently fashionable are hypoxaemia (again!) vitamin E (again!), light exposure and PaO_2 lability.

What has also emerged is that so long as the PaO_2 is kept below12 kPa (10 kPa in ELBW) throughout the time a baby is at risk from ROP, cicatricial ROP causing blindness is exceptionally rare.

PREVENTION

By far and away the most important component of prevention is strict monitoring of PaO_2. Transcutaneous PO_2 monitoring and oximetry are not adequate unless backed up by intermittent (4 hourly) arterial sampling (pp. 97–104).

DIAGNOSIS AND SCREENING

Guidelines for screening have been published and should be adhered to (RCOpth and BAPM 1995). All babies delivered at 31 weeks or less and/or <1501 g birth weight should be screened at 6–7 weeks postnatal age or at 35 weeks post menstrual age, whichever is the sooner (Fig. 15.2). For 23 week gestation babies this means screening when they reach 30 weeks even if they are still critically ill on IPPV. Do not forget 31 week 1800 g babies!

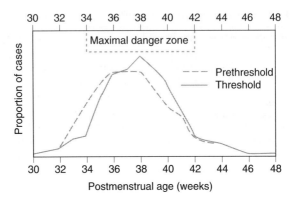

Figure 15.2 Relationship of likelihood of developing ROP related to postmenstrual age.
Source: Phelps 1998

Babies who qualify for screening must be re-examined fortnightly until vascularization has progressed to zone 3, but more frequent checks may be indicated in those with early onset progressive disease.

The eyes should be examined by an experienced ophthalmologist (not the neonatal SHO!) using indirect ophthalmoscopy and after dilating the pupils with 0.5% cyclopentolate and 2.5% phenylephrine eye drops. An alternative is a combination preparation of tropicamide 0.2% and phenylephrine 1%.

MANAGEMENT

In most babies with acute stage 1 and 2 ROP, and stage 3 limited to zone 3, the disease regresses. For babies with this type of disease a watching brief is indicated, but in any baby whose disease progresses to threshold disease (*v.s.*) cryotherapy is indicated. The hope is that by damaging the peripheral avascular retina the release of angiogenic factors, which promote the progression of the disease, will be halted. Unfortunately treatment is not a guarantee of success and 20% of treated eyes still have little or no vision. Myopia appears to be more common when cryotherapy is used, rather than laser treatment. The reason for this may be that cryotherapy induces more scleral damage, affecting the long term growth of the eye.

PROGNOSIS

With meticulous control of oxygen therapy and effective screening and treatment, blindness from ROP should now steadily decline in incidence. However, survivors of both regressed and treated ROP have an increased incidence of myopia and squint and should be carefully followed up. Not all visual problems at follow up are due to ophthalmic problems; there is a significant incidence of cortical visual problems too (p. 466). In the recent Epicure study of all births less than 26 weeks gestation in the UK in 1995, 17% of survivors had visual impairment at 2.5 years and 1.8% were blind (Wood and Marlow 1999). Almost 20% of the whole cohort had required treatment for ROP.

BUPHTHALMOS (NEONATAL GLAUCOMA)

The baby presents with irritability (due to pain), photophobia and tearing from the eye, which has an acute increase in intraocular pressure. The eye has an enlarged corneal diameter (>11 mm) and is injected. This is an ophthalmic emergency if blindness is to be avoided.

CATARACT

If a cataract is seen in the neonatal period urgent ophthalmic referral is indicated, particularly for bilateral disease to prevent amblyopia developing. Cataract is the commonest cause of preventable childhood blindness. Many cases are genetic and further investigation is indicated.

CONJUNCTIVITIS (p. 228)

STRABISMUS

All babies have a tendency to transient alternating convergent strabismus. This is of no significance, and the eyes gradually straighten by 3–6 months of age. Unless the eye position is constantly abnormal observation is appropriate until the baby is 4 months old. A fixed strabismus may occur following birth trauma (usually a transient VI th nerve paralysis), or it may be associated with retinoblastoma (p. 411). In the latter case early diagnosis can be life saving.

REFERENCES

American Academy of Pediatrics and American College of Obstetrics and Gynaecology (1997) *Guidelines for Perinatal Care*, 4th edn. Library of Congress, pp. 188–192.

BAPM (1999) Guidelines for the management of neonatal RDS. Full text available from www.bapm-London.org

CCRP (Committee for the Classification of Retinopathy of Prematurity) (1987) The classification of retinal detachment. *Archives of Ophthalmology* **105**: 906–916.

Darlow, B.A. (1988) Incidence of retinopathy of prematurity in New Zealand. *Archives of Disease in Childhood* **63**: 1083–1086.

Moore, A.T. (1999) Neonatal ophthalmology. In: Rennie, J.M. and Roberton, N.R.C. (eds), *Textbook of Neonatology*, 3rd edn. Churchill Livingstone, Edinburgh and London, pp.903–916.

Phelps, D. (1981) Vision loss due to retinopathy of prematurity. *Lancet* i: 606.

Phelps, D. (1998) Using new information in retinopathy of prematurity. In: *Current Topics in Neonatology 3*. Hansen, T.N. and McIntosh, N. (eds), W B Saunders, London, pp. 174–190.

Wood, N. and Marlow, N. (1999) Developmental and neurological disability in extremely preterm children at two and a half years. Proceedings of the Royal College of Paediatrics and Child Health Spring Meeting. *Archives of Disease in Childhood* Suppl 1, v.

FURTHER READING

Moore, A.T. (1999) Neonatal ophthalmology. In *Textbook of Neonatology*, 3rd edn. Rennie, J.M. and Roberton, N.R.C. (eds), Churchill Livingstone, Edinburgh, pp. 903–916.

Royal College of Ophthalmologists, British Association of Perinatal Medicine (1995) *Retinopathy of Prematurity, Guidelines for screening and treatment*. Available from the BAPM, 55 Hallam Street, London or via the BAPM website at www.bapm-London.org

USEFUL WEBSITE

http://www.konnections.com/eyedoc/icrop.html

16

ENDOCRINE DISORDERS

- *The commonest cause of ambiguous genitalia is CAH causing masculinization of baby girls (female pseudohermaphroditism).*
- *All cases of ambiguous genitalia require urgent investigation so that gender identity can be confirmed as soon as possible and any necessary treatment begun.*
- *Consider Addisonian collapse due to CAH in any baby who presents in shock at 7–14 days with hyponatraemia, hypoglycaemia and hypotension.*
- *Neonatal thyrotoxicosis can cause serious illness which requires urgent treatment if it is not to be fatal.*

INTRODUCTION

Endocrine disease is rare in the neonatal period. Pituitary disease may occasionally cause hypoglycaemia and diabetes mellitus can present in the first weeks of life. Think of pituitary disease in babies with midline facial defects. Inappropriate (and appropriate) ADH secretion is common and is dealt with on pp. 22–23. Diabetes insipidus is occasionally seen, sometimes in association with a massive intracranial haemorrhage.

Parathyroid disorders are exceptionally rare in the neonatal period but the diagnosis should be considered if the other, much commoner, causes of hyper- or hypocalcaemia have been excluded.

THE NEONATE WITH AMBIGUOUS GENITALIA

Do not ask the parents to choose, and never, ever guess! Admit that you are in doubt, and reassure the parents that the cause can be determined and the appropriate sex assigned with little delay in nearly all cases.

Ambiguous genitalia may be due to:

Table 16.1 Causes of pseudohermaphroditism (From Cheetham and Barnes 1999)

Male pseudohermaphroditism
    Anti Mullerian Hormone deficiency
    Testosterone deficiency
        Deficient – 20,22 desmolase
                 – 3β-hydroxysteroid dehydrogenase
                 – 17α-hydroxylase
                 – 17,20 desmolase
                 – 17 ketosteroid reductase
        Leydig cell hypoplasia
        Gonadotrophin deficiency or resistance
    Impaired peripheral androgen responsiveness
        5α-reductase deficiency
        androgen insensitity, partial or complete
    Dysmorphic syndromes
    Idiopathic

Female pseudohermaphroditism
    Virilizing congenital adrenal hyperplasia
        Deficient
                 – 21α-hydroxylase
                 – 11β-hydroxylase
                 – 3β-hydroxysteroid dehydrogenase
    Aromatase deficiency
    Maternal androgen excess
        Endogenous
        Exogenous
    Dysmorphic syndromes

1. male pseudohermaphroditism; incomplete virilization in a genetic male (Table 16.1);
2. female pseudohermaphroditism: virilization in genetic females (Table 16.1);
3. disorders of gonadal development
   (a) chromosomal abnormalities, e.g. Turner's syndrome;
   (b) true hermaphroditism;
   (c) other.

MANAGEMENT OF THE NEONATE WITH AMBIGUOUS GENITALIA

Explain the situation carefully to the parents. Take a detailed family history, and also note any history of maternal drug exposure during pregnancy.

Carefully examine the baby. Measure the size of any phallus, and note the position of the urethral orifice. The following features are vitally important in helping to establish the diagnosis, planning the investigations, and guiding the initial discussions with the parents, but it is important to follow the advice given above (Table 16.1) and wait for an expert:

1. Are testes palpable outside the abdominal cavity? The baby is then a *male* pseudohermaphrodite.
2. Can a uterus be demonstrated with ultrasound or on an X-ray "genitogram"? The baby is then a *female* pseudohermaphrodite.
3. Could the external genitalia ever be fashioned into a sexually functional penis? If not, it should be considered whether or not to rear the baby as a female. This is a contentious area.
4. Is the baby hypertensive? This localizes the abnormality in the adrenal.

Send blood samples for urgent chromosome analysis and also send blood and urine samples for urgent analysis to establish the diag-

Table 16.2 Steps in establishing the diagnosis in an infant of uncertain sex

Clinical feature

Palpable gonads	+	+	+
Uterus present*	+	−	−
Increased skin pigmentation	−	−	±
Sick baby	−	−	±
Clinical diagnosis	Gonadal dysgenesis with Y chromosome	Partial androgen insensitivity	Block in testosterone synthesis

Investigation

Serum 17-OHP	Normal	Normal	Normal
Electrolytes	Normal	Normal	Normal
Karyotype	45, X/46, XY or other pattern	46, XY	46, XY
Testosterone response to HCG	Definite response	Good response (both testosterone and DHT)	Blunted or absent response
Gonadal biopsy	Dysgenetic gonad, +/− tumour	Normal testis, (+/− Leydig cell hyperplasia)	Normal testis
Other	−	Genital skin fibroblast culture	Measure testosterone precursors

* use ultrasound

nosis of CAH (*u.i.*). This is the commonest cause of ambiguous genitalia and can cause fatal Addisonian collapse within the first 10–14 days so diagnosis is urgent.

If CAH is not confirmed, on the basis of a clinical examination and the other investigations further radiological and biochemical investigations can be carried out in a more leisurely manner to detect the conditions listed in Table 16.2.

CONGENITAL ADRENAL HYPERPLASIA

The incidence is 1 in 10 000. There are two main enzyme defects: absent 21α-hydroxylase (>90%) and absent 11β-hydroxylase (<10%).

Other rare enzyme deficiencies exist (Fig. 16.1, Table 16.1). All are autosomal recessive and antenatal detection and treatment are now possible. Population screening, measuring 17-hydroxyprogesterone on the "Guthrie" blood spots has been carried out, but there are no plans to introduce it into the UK.

21α-hydroxylase deficiency usually presents with virilization and/or a salt-losing state, depending on the severity of the defect.

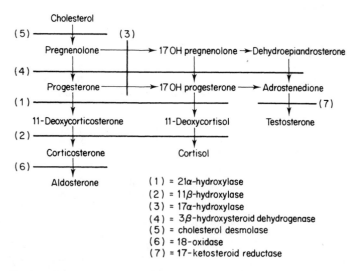

Figure 16.1 Synthetic pathway for adrenal steroids showing the site of block in different inherited enzyme deficiency states.

11β-hydroxylase deficiency usually presents with virilization and/or hypertension (since the block is distal to the salt-retaining deoxycorticosterone). Identifying the virilized female is easy. Male babies may have increased pigmentation but often present either in Addisonian crisis or, if they are not salt losers, with precocious puberty later in life.

The genetics of this condition have been extensively studied and the gene is located on chromosome 6. Prenatal diagnosis is possible, and administration of dexamethasone to the mother of a female baby with CAH can reduce the virilization and the need for extensive surgery.

INVESTIGATION OF THE CHILD WITH AMBIGUOUS GENITALIA TO ESTABLISH CAH

1. Measure serum 17-hydroxyprogesterone and/or 11-deoxycortisol (cortisol precursors). These are raised in CAH and differentiate 21α-hydroxylase deficiency from 11β hydroxylase deficiency (Fig. 16.1).
2. Measure ACTH. This is a non-specific indicator of cortisol deficiency and is raised in CAH.
3. Measure plasma and urinary electrolytes daily to check for salt loss.
4. Monitor the blood glucose carefully.
5. Measure blood pressure daily. Salt losers may become hypotensive, but hypertension rarely presents in the newborn.
6. If CAH is confirmed, or if there are symptoms such as vomiting and weight loss, or the electrolytes suggest incipient Addisonian crisis, the initial treatment is 20–25 mg hydrocortisone/m^2/day equivalent to 2.5 mg twice daily in a full-term infant; the equivalent parenteral dose can be given if the infant is vomiting. Add 25–50 μg of fludrocortisone daily with 2–4 g NaCl daily in salt losers.

THE INFANT (OFTEN MALE) WHO PRESENTS WITH ADRENAL COLLAPSE

Any male infant who suddenly collapses with vomiting, pallor or hypotension during the first 10 days of life should be suspected of having CAH, especially if his nipples, scrotum or penis appear to be too pigmented. The infant will usually have hyponatraemia and hyperkalaemia, and is often profoundly hypoglycaemic.

Treatment

1. Give IV normal saline and glucose as necessary (150 ml/kg/24 h). Plasma infusion may be necessary for resuscitation.
2. Give, 50 mg hydrocortisone IV immediately. Oral fludrocortisone 25–50. 1 microg can then be added.
3. Severe hyperkalaemia can be treated as outlined on p. 375.
4. Set in train the investigations outlined above for CAH.

OTHER NEONATAL ADRENAL PROBLEMS

Adrenal haemorrhage

This may occur in any seriously ill neonate, but is characteristically associated with perinatal asphyxia. Adrenal haemorrhage may present as a loin mass or incidentally during ultrasound evaluation of the abdomen. The adrenal may calcify. Surprisingly adrenal haemorrhage rarely causes clinical problems, but if identified it is prudent to check blood glucose levels and to measure the plasma cortisol.

Perinatal steroid therapy

Repeated maternal dexamethasone therapy or high dose steroid treatment for maternal conditions such as rheumatoid arthritis can, rarely, cause fetal and neonatal Cushing's syndrome. These babies have a reduced response to ACTH, but few clinical problems result from it.

Large doses of steroids are now used to treat CLD (p. 209) and babies can develop classic side effects including reduced growth, hypertension and hyperglycaemia. When steroids are withdrawn the baby usually has an essentially normally responsive hypothalamo-pituitary-adrenal axis, but if in doubt a short Synacthen test should be carried out, using 36 microg/kg of ACTH. We give steroids to cover surgery in infants who have been treated with prolonged courses of steroids.

THYROID PROBLEMS

CONGENITAL HYPOTHYROIDISM

The incidence is about 1 in 3500 due to thyroid dysgenesis or agenesis (usually sporadic) or goitrous cretinism (autosomal recessive or environmental). Antenatal detection is not possible and postnatal screening is routine.

Neonatal hypothyroidism screening is now routine in many parts of the world, and this means that the diagnosis is now usually established before the infant presents with prolonged jaundice, lethargy, poor feeding or constipation.

Infants detected on neonatal screening with TSH levels above 10 units/ml should have the diagnosis confirmed by T_3 (and T_4) measurements before starting on treatment. Since transient neonatal hypothyroidism may occur, especially in preterm infants, all such patients need to be reinvestigated at 12 months of age to reconfirm the diagnosis of hypothyroidism.

In a neonate with goitre, check for maternal ingestion of goitrogens (iodides, antithyroid drugs). Unless goitrogens were the cause, or the mother comes from an area with endemic cretinism, the infant will need to be investigated for one of the rare autosomal recessive inherited forms of goitrous cretinism. However, so long as any hypothyroidism is treated, this assessment can wait until he is older.

Once neonatal hypothyroidism is suspected, after taking all the appropriate samples for investigation, start the infant on 10 microg/kg of L-thyroxine daily, given as a single daily dose.

TRANSIENT HYPOTHYROIDISM

Small sick neonates have depressed thyroid function (low T_4, low free T_4 and poor TSH response), and the sicker and smaller they are the more abnormal the thyroid function. It has been suggested that this results in more severe respiratory illness and a poorer prognosis on follow up. These claims are being evaluated in current trials, but as yet there is no justification for routine thyroxine supplementation in ill VLBW neonates.

The VLBW baby can absorb iodine from topical antiseptics through the skin. This may cause hypothyroidism as well as damage to the skin. These babies may also acquire transient hypothyroidism from the iodine load of intravenous preparations used to opacify long lines. Such preparations should therefore not be used in neonatal intensive care.

NEONATAL THYROTOXICOSIS

This condition is due to transplacental passage of thyroid-stimulating IgG immunoglobulins, and develops in infants born to mothers who currently have Graves' disease, or who had it in the past but are now euthyroid as a result of treatment. Only 1–3% of babies delivered to mothers with this past history develop symptoms but the disease can be life-threatening.

The neonate is usually less than 2.5 kg at birth and may develop all the signs of thyrotoxicosis, including:

1. tachycardia progressing to heart failure;
2. exophthalmos and lid lag;
3. extreme jitteriness;
4. vomiting, diarrhoea and poor weight gain;
5. sweating;
6. goitre (with a bruit) which may obstruct the trachea.

The disease may be very severe, and can present at any time up to 6 weeks of age. Initial therapy is with propranolol 2 mg/kg/24 h, and propylthiouracil 10 mg/kg/24 h. Lugol's iodine 1 drop three times a day is also useful, and prevents release of thyroid hormones. The disease is usually easily controlled, and with the disappearance of maternal IgG in the neonatal plasma, antithyroid drugs can be discontinued after 4–6 months. On follow-up, however, many of these infants are found to have a low IQ and craniostenosis.

FURTHER READING

Cheetham, T.D. and Barnes, N.D. (1999) Endocrine disorders. In: *Textbook of Neonatology*, 3rd edn. Rennie, J.M. and Roberton, N.R.C. (eds), Churchill Livingstone, Edinburgh, pp. 957–985.

17

DISORDERS OF GLUCOSE HOMEOSTASIS

- *A brief period of asymptomatic hypoglycaemia is virtually universal in babies.*
- *Term babies mount a brisk response and can use alternative fuels, and there is no evidence that the episode is harmful.*
- *There is no evidence that asymptomatic hypoglycaemia is followed by any adverse sequelae; the same is not true for symptomatic hypoglycaemia.*
- *Symptoms that suggest hypoglycaemia which is likely to cause brain damage include apnoea, seizures and coma.*
- *Screening for hypoglycaemia is indicated in certain high risk groups including premature babies, growth retarded babies, infants of diabetic mothers, and babies who have suffered from intrapartum asphyxia.*
- *Symptomatic hypoglycaemia in a normally grown, term baby is unusual and full investigation including insulin assay is indicated.*

GLUCOSE METABOLISM IN THE NEWBORN

The fetal blood glucose concentration is in equilibrium with, and is usually about 80% of, the maternal value. Glucose is transferred to the baby by facilitated diffusion, and is stored after metabolism as fat and glycogen. Human subcutaneous and body fat is deposited from 28–30 weeks gestation onwards, and glycogen reserves are built up from 36 weeks, especially in the liver and myocardium.

The blood glucose concentration falls rapidly during the first two hours of life when it is the main energy source. Simultaneously, since the enzymes of glycogenolysis (release of glucose from stored glycogen) are present and active, hepatic glycogen stores fall rapidly. During this period of glucose utilization the respiratory quotient is 1.0.

At the same time, gluconeogenesis from glycerol, alanine, lactate and pyruvate is switched on by the hormonal changes which follow delivery, and the neonate can use ketones and lactate for brain metabolism. After the first few hours, the baby switches to fatty acids as his principal energy source, and his respiratory quotient falls to 0.7. Glucose production continues from both glycogenolysis and gluconeogenesis (glucose production in the liver), producing 4–6 mg glucose/kg/min.

After birth there is a rapid rise in glucagon and catecholamine levels, but insulin levels remain low usually less than 20 mu/ml (135 pmol/l). The result is that newborn babies, particularly if they are premature, have impaired glucose tolerance in response to both intravenous and oral glucose loads, but this may also be due to insulin resistance.

Conversely, some neonates who become hypoglycaemic appear incapable of switching off insulin production and retain "normal" but inappropriately high insulin levels.

NORMAL VALUES

This topic has been a matter of intense debate in recent years. It is clear that blood glucose levels fall immediately after birth in all babies (Fig 17.1), sometimes to levels below 1.5 mmol/l (27 mg%). This brief period of hypoglycaemia is "physiological", cannot be significant and should not be treated. Thereafter blood glucose levels rise steadily for the first few days. As with all biochemical data values fall into three groups:

1. *Normal.* The data in Fig 17.1 are now widely accepted. After the first 24 hours the values are between 2.2 and 5.5 mmol/l (40–100 mg%) for both term and preterm babies. During the first 24 hours the lower range is down to 1.5 mmol/l (27 mg%).
2. *Abnormal but harmless.* These are values outside the normal range that require treatment but which when corrected do no harm. This concept applies to hyperbilirubinaemia, hypocarbia and hyperkalaemia, for example, but for some reason people have difficulty in accepting that it also applies to hypoglycaemia. This range is between 2.6 and 10 mmol/l (pp. 31, 32).
3. *Harmful.* As with hyperbilirubinaemia there is no absolute cut-off between dangerous and safe levels and there may be an "area under the curve" phenomenon in which degree and duration of hypoglycaemia interact. Hawdon and Aynsley-Green (1999) suggest a functional definition: "the level of blood glucose at which body function, particularly that of the brain, is compromised". Damaging hypoglycaemia is always associated with neuroglycopenia (*v.i.*); in other words it is symptomatic.

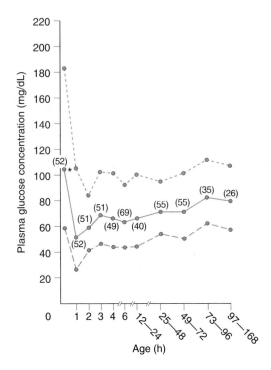

Figure 17.1 Predicted plasma glucose values during the first week of life in healthy term neonates appropriate for gestational age; 40 mg/dl = 2.2 mmol/L. Number of samples shown in parentheses. *Mean and 95% confidence interval. (Reproduced from Srinivasan *et al.*, 1986, with permission.)

In practical clinical terms this means:

1. blood glucose must be kept above 1.5 mmol/l at all times, and above 2.0 mmol/l after the first 12 hours in both term and preterm babies;
2. if babies more than 3 days old consistently have levels below 2.5 mmol/l, a cause should be sought;
3. symptomatic hypoglycaemia is an emergency and requires intravenous treatment (*v.i.*);
4. in asymptomatic hypoglycaemia an attempt can be made to manage the problem with increased oral feeds in babies who are tolerating milk; the tempo of investigation and treatment are slower.

SYMPTOMS OF HYPOGLYCAEMIA

These include the following:

1. Those due to the catecholamine response to hypoglycaemia (pallor, sweating and tachycardia). These symptoms are unusual in neonates except those with hyperinsulinaemia (*v.i.*).
2. Signs due to the effects of hypoglycaemia on the heart, including bradycardia, hypotension, and heart failure. These signs are most often seen when hypoglycaemia accompanies hypoxic ischaemic encephalopathy and they are difficult to separate from asphyxial myocardial damage (p. 360).
3. Signs of neuroglycopenia including apnoea, convulsions or coma are signs of serious hypoglycaemia requiring urgent treatment. If in doubt the response to raising the blood glucose above 2.0 mmol/l should be tested. A prompt reduction in symptoms suggests significant symptomatic hypoglycaemia (Hawdon and Aynsley-Green 1999). The significance of "softer" CNS signs is more difficult to evaluate; for example, jitteriness is common in all babies whether or not they are hypoglycaemic.

SEQUELAE OF HYPOGLYCAEMIA

A striking feature of neonatal hypoglycaemia is that babies can have blood glucose values less than 1.1 mmol/l (20 mg%) without any symptoms, signs or sequelae, presumably because they are using ketones and lactate for brain metabolism. This fact has important clinical implications, because it means that nursery routines to detect hypoglycaemia can be designed in the knowledge that asymptomatic hypoglycaemia lasting 2–3 hours will *not* cause CNS damage. However, if hypoglycaemia is prolonged, or if there are no circulating ketones or lactate, neuroglycopenia will develop with apnoea, depression of consciousness and/or convulsions. About 30% of such babies will have severe neurological abnormalities on follow-up, including severe intellectual retardation and spastic quadriplegia.

SCREENING FOR HYPOGLYCAEMIA

Babies at risk from hypoglycaemia should be monitored as outlined in Table 17.1. A suitable method must be used. Glucose oxidase reagent sticks (Dextrostix, BM-stix) are still used because they are cheap and widely available but this method is not ideal for neonatal

Table 17.1 Screening for hypoglycaemia

Baby diagnosis	Glucose sample timing
SFD (Table 17.2)	2, 6, 12, 24, 36, 48 hours — prefeed.
Preterm	2 hours and 6–12 hourly until levels reliably above 2.5 mmol/l and tolerating feeds
HIE	On admission; 2, 6, 12, 24 hours or regularly during IPPV as for serious illness
Serious illness	6–12 hourly during illness
IDM	On admission and at 2, 6, 12, 24 hours or until two consecutive samples are above 2.5 mmol/l
Haemolytic disease of the newborn	1, 2 and 4 hours after an exchange transfusion
Fitting or excessive jittering	Immediately

screening. These sticks are designed to use a certain volume of plasma, and the high neonatal PCV and small sample size means that this is not always delivered. In addition these sticks are not accurate in the lower ranges. The search for the ideal cotside method continues. We currently use a Yellow Springs Glucometer, and have abandoned Dextrostix and BM Glycaemie stix completely.

Glucose levels are higher in plasma than blood by 13–18%, and they are higher in arterial blood than in capillary samples.

CLINICAL CAUSES OF HYPOGLYCAEMIA

In the neonatal period there are two main groups of conditions which cause symptomatic hypoglycaemia; those in which the blood glucose falls because of depleted stores of glycogen, and those that are due to hyperinsulinaemia.

HYPOGLYCAEMIA DUE TO DEPLETED GLYCOGEN STORES

Small-for-dates babies

The broad definition of a SFD baby is one who is below the third centile for birth weight at a given gestation. The detailed care of SFD babies is described in the companion volume (Roberton 1996).

SFD babies, particularly IUGR babies with poor body stores of both glycogen and fat, are at risk in two situations:

1. During labour the lower liver and myocardial glycogen stores give the baby little resistance to hypoxia, and comparatively minor insults can deplete these energy sources and cause sudden intrapartum death or handicap. Much obstetric effort is put into detecting such babies antenatally, and either monitoring them very carefully during labour or delivering them by elective caesarean section.

2. Postnatally, with no glycogen stores available to be broken down to glucose, and in the absence of fat to supply ketones as an alternative brain metabolite, hypoglycaemia and neuroglycopenia may develop.

All newborn babies should be assessed using weight-for-gestation centile tables such as that shown in Table 17.2, or charts which are appropriate for the maternal nutrition, race and the height above sea level of the local population. For many years we have used the data of Usher and McLean (1969) (Table 17.2) and have only screened for neonatal hypoglycaemia those babies whose birth weight was more than two standard deviations below the mean (2.3rd centile). Increasing the number of asymptomatic babies screened for hypoglycaemia to include those whose birth weight is between the third and the tenth centile is probably a waste of time (Jones and Roberton 1984).

Table 17.2 Birth weight by gestational age for the diagnosis of SFD babies

Gestational age* (weeks)	Birth weight below which the baby is SFD (g)
36	1890
37	2120
38	2335
39	2500
40	2615
41	2550
42	2510

* If in doubt accept the mother's estimation based on her LMP. Data from Usher and McLean (1969)

Without preventative measures the peak incidence of hypogly-caemia in IUGR babies occurs within the first 48 hours, especially between 12 and 36 hours postnatally when the body stores of glyco-gen and fat have been consumed, and the baby, particularly if breast fed, is still on a hypocaloric intake. Very IUGR babies can develop neuroglycopenia within 6–12 hours of delivery.

Prematurity

A very premature baby may develop hypoglycaemia because he was delivered before the body deposits of fat and glycogen had been laid down. Hypoglycaemia may develop at any time during the first two weeks if they are ill and the caloric intake has been inadequate. However, babies with RDS tend to have higher blood sugar levels than controls, presumably due to the high circulating levels of hormones such as adrenaline, glucagon and cortisol.

Intrapartum asphyxia

If this is severe, even normally grown term babies may be totally depleted of liver and myocardial glycogen during, or immediately following, resuscitation, and consequently become hypoglycaemic. In addition to neuroglycopenia, these babies may have congestive heart failure with cardiomegaly, muffled heart sounds, bradycardia and poor peripheral perfusion.

Breast milk insufficiency

There is a group of breast fed babies in whom feeding does not become properly established. These babies present on the third or fourth day with weight loss of more than 10–12% from birth weight, a high serum sodium concentration, and are often hypoglycaemic (Moore and Perlman 1999). After the blood glucose is restored with a feed or intravenous glucose they never become hypoglycaemic again. In general the prognosis for such babies is good.

Hypothermia

Cold babies are often hypoglycaemic, and hypoglycaemic babies will often drop their body temperature. It is therefore often impossible to know which came first. However both conditions require treat-ment.

Table 17.3 Problems in babies of diabetic mothers

Large-for-dates	Delivery problems; birth trauma, shoulder dystocia; Erb's palsy
Hepatosplenomegaly	
Congenital malformations	Cardiac, cardiac septal hypertrophy; microcolon; sacral agenesis
RDS	p. 131
Jaundice	pp. 419–421
Hypoglycaemia	v.i.
Hypocalcaemia	p. 28
Polycythaemia	p. 452

Serious illness of any type

Congenital heart disease or septicaemia may also be associated with low blood glucose levels.

HYPOGLYCAEMIA DUE TO HYPERINSULINISM

Infants of diabetic mothers

These large-for-dates babies have a very characteristic chubby plethoric (cherubic) appearance, and have an increased incidence of many complications (Table 17.3). The neonatal management of the healthy term IDM (the majority!) is described in Roberton (1996).

Throughout gestation, in equilibrium with the mother, the IDM is exposed to both high and low blood glucose values. They develop hypertrophy of the islets, and the degree of hypertrophy is dependent on the severity and duration of maternal hyperglycaemia.

Postnatally, the IDM is cut off from the constant infusion of glucose, but remains hyperinsulinaemic. This may cause a rapid fall in blood glucose immediately after delivery to levels of 0.25 mmol/l (5 mg%) or below at 90–120 minutes of age. In most IDM the anti-hypoglycaemia defences work and even profound hypoglycaemia of this degree will correct spontaneously. With meticulous antenatal control of the maternal diabetes, however, severe postnatal hypoglycaemia is now rare in IDM, and persisting hypoglycaemia that requires treatment is unusual except in IDM with other problems such as asphyxia or RDS.

If an IDM is feeding well by 12 hours of age, and has had no hypoglycaemia, he is unlikely to develop any further blood glucose problems, and these should only be checked for if the baby develops symptoms.

Haemolytic disease of the newborn

Newborn babies with rhesus HDN have marked islet hypertrophy for reasons that are not clear. Babies with cord haemoglobin levels of less than 10 g% are particularly prone to hypoglycaemia as a rebound phenomenon after exchange transfusion, since bank blood which has a high glucose content, raises the baby's glucose above 10 mmol/l (180 mg%) during the exchange and provokes further insulin release.

Maternal glucose infusion

Giving the mother glucose during labour may make both her and her fetus hyperglycaemic, which rapidly switches to hypoglycaemia after delivery when the neonatal pancreas responds by releasing insulin. This hypoglycaemia is transient, self-recovering and rarely needs therapy.

Infusion of glucose into a UAC positioned directly opposite the coeliac axis

MANAGEMENT OF HYPOGLYCAEMIA

Detection

All babies who are at risk from hypoglycaemia should have regular glucose estimations carried out as outlined in Table 17.1. If a low value is found, blood samples should be sent to the laboratory for true glucose estimation and treatment instituted at once. In a healthy term baby of normal birth weight, a sample should be centrifuged and frozen for determination of insulin levels – otherwise an opportunity to make an early diagnosis of hyperinsulinism may be lost.

Prevention

SFD and VLBW babies   If possible all such babies should be started on full-strength milk feeds by 2–4 hours of age, giving 60 ml/kg/24 h on day 1 and 90 ml/kg/24 h on day 2 (see Table 4.6(a)) to SFD babies, and smaller quantities to preterm babies (Table 4.6(b)). If the baby cannot suck, give the milk by nasogastric tube. If enteral feeding is not possible, 10% glucose plus appropriate electrolyte supplements should be given by an umbilical catheter or peripheral infusion.

Hypoxic ischaemic encephalopathy   The baby should be maintained on 10% dextrose IV until oral feeds are tolerated.

IDM   Feeding, by tube if necessary, should be started by 2 hours of age. Hypoglycaemia before that time can be ignored if the baby is asymptomatic. The blood glucose level usually rises by 4 hours of age if the baby feeds well.

Treatment

When asymptomatic hypoglycaemia (i.e. hypoglycaemia without neuroglycopenia) is detected in any of the above groups of babies who are not on IV dextrose, immediately give the next milk feed due, by tube if necessary, and check the blood glucose level 1 hour later. Continue the oral feeding if the result is now within the acceptable range. Do not give oral dextrose, but instead use milk which is more calorific, more slowly and evenly absorbed and does not irritate the stomach. If the baby is already receiving IV dextrose, the rate or concentration of the infusion should be increased.

If, despite oral feeding, the glucose 1 hour later is still less than 2.0 mmol/l (35 mg%), or if oral feeds have not been started or are not tolerated, or if neuroglycopenic symptoms develop at any time, give a single IV push of 3 ml/kg of 10% dextrose followed by an infusion of 10% dextrose, giving 60 ml/kg/24 h. Always aim to administer a total of at least 6–8 mg/kg/min of glucose to the baby by a combination of the IV and oral routes. Aim for glucose levels between 2 and 10 mmol/l   (p. 284). Intravenous dextrose must always be given with great care using a continuous infusion pump, otherwise rebound hypoglycaemia is a major hazard. Concentrations above 12.5% are best given into a secure central line because extravasation burns can be serious with highly concentrated solutions.

In the occasional baby, infusions of 15–20% dextrose are required to keep the glucose above 2 mmol/l (35 mg%) despite giving a total of 12–15 mg glucose/kg/min. Glucagon 30–100 microg/kg IM or IV may be given to such babies followed by an infusion of 5–10 microg/kg/h. A total of 100–200 microg/kg of glucagon can also be given IM in an emergency if there is difficulty or delay in starting an intravenous infusion in a symptomatic hypoglycaemic neonate.

Glucocorticoids are rarely needed. However, if they are required, 2.5 mg of hydrocortisone/kg IV should be given every 12 hours; diazoxide should only be used if there is hyperinsulinaemia. Octreotide is a synthetic somatostatin analogue which suppresses insulin release in hyperinsulinism but expert advice is required before this agent is used.

UNUSUAL CASES OF NEONATAL HYPOGLYCAEMIA

If hypoglycaemia is persistent, recurrent, or difficult to treat, and in particular if one of the obvious common causes described above is not present, then the rare conditions discussed below should be considered, and appropriate investigations carried out:

1. endocrine deficiencies, which may be multiple or single (e.g. hypopituitarism, congenital adrenal hyperplasia, hypothyroidism);
2. syndromes with hyperinsulinaemia:
   (a) Beckwith-Wiedemann syndrome;
   (b) islet cell adenoma;
   (c) idiopathic hyperinsulinism of infancy (formerly known as nesidioblastosis);
3. inborn errors of metabolism:
   (a) glycogen storage disease;
   (b) fructose intolerance: fructose 1:6 diposphatase deficiency causing lacticacidaemia;
   (c) galactosaemia;
   (d) inborn errors of fatty acid oxidation (medium chain acyl-CoA dehydrogenase [MCAD] deficiency).
4. aminoacidopathies:
   (a) maple syrup urine disease;
   (b) propionicacidaemia;
   (c) methylmalonic acidaemia;
   (d) tyrosinosis.

The work-up of such a baby is discussed by Hawdon and Aynsley Green (1999). The gene defect present in many cases of idiopathic hyperinsulinaemia has now been discovered, and the problem is a defect in the potassium channels of the beta cells of the pancreas.

NEONATAL HYPERGLYCAEMIA

NEONATAL DIABETES MELLITUS

A newborn baby occasionally develops signs of juvenile diabetes with dehydration, weight loss and polyuria. The baby is usually SFD. Hyperglycaemia, acidaemia and dehydration occur, but ketosis is rare. Some insulin is present but at inappropriately low levels for the hyperglycaemia. The disease probably represents delayed maturation of the insulin-releasing mechanism of pancreatic beta cells. These babies are exquisitely sensitive to exogenous insulin; 0.5–1.0 units twice a day is often all that is required to control the disease. Within one or two months most babies recover completely, and insulin can be discontinued (Hawdon and Aynsley Green 1999). However, insulin-dependent diabetes persists in some cases.

IATROGENIC

Babies weighing under 1.5 kg are often unable to metabolize glucose rapidly enough if the infusion rate exceeds 6 mg/kg/min (86 ml of 10% dextrose/kg/24 h), yet the fluid requirement of such babies often exceeds this volume, and 12–14 mg/kg/min is often given with TPN (p. 52). Hyperglycaemia, glycosuria and dehydration may result. When high glucose infusion rates are required to maintain calorie input during TPN babies tolerate them better if the glucose concentration is increased gradually.

If the blood glucose level exceeds 10 mmol/l (180 mg%), the infusion should be changed to 5% dextrose or a dual infusion system set up with 5% dextrose for water and 50% dextrose to deliver the required glucose. If the blood glucose does not fall rapidly on this regimen, an insulin infusion should be given, starting with 0.1 unit/kg/h. The blood glucose concentration must be monitored carefully to ensure that hypoglycaemia does not develop.

Hyperglycaemia may also be seen as a side effect of drugs used in the neonatal period, such as steroids for CLD (p. 210) and theophylline. It also occurs in stressed babies after surgery.

REFERENCES

Haddon, J. and Aynsley Green, A. (1999). Disorders of blood glucose homeostasis in the neonate. In: Rennie, J.M. and Roberton, N.R.C. (eds),

Textbook of Neonatology, 3rd edn. Churchill Livingstone, Edinburgh and London, pp. 939–956.

Jones, R.A.K. and Roberton, N.R.C. (1984) Problems of the small for dates baby. *Clinics in Obstetrics and Gynaecology* **11**: 499–524.

Moore, A.M. and Perlman, M. (1999) Symptomatic hypoglycaemia in otherwise healthy breast fed term newborns. *Pediatrics* **103**: 837–839.

Roberton, N.R.C. (1996) *A Manual of Normal Neonatal Care*. Edward Arnold, London, pp. 175–195 and 209–214.

Srinivasan, G., Pildes, R.S., Cattamachi, G., Voora, S. and Lilien, L.D. (1986) Plasma glucose values in normal neonates. *Journal of Pediatrics* **109**: 114–117.

Usher, R.H. and McLean, F.H. (1969) Intrauterine growth of live born Caucasian infants at sea level: standards obtained from measurements in 7 dimensions of infants born between 25 and 44 weeks of gestation. *Journal of Pediatrics* **74**: 901–910.

FURTHER READING

Hawdon, J. and Aynsley Green, A. (1999) Disorders of blood glucose homeostasis in the neonate. In: *Textbook of Neonatology*, 3rd edn. Rennie, J.M. and Roberton, N.R.C. (eds), Churchill Livingstone, Edinburgh, pp. 939–956.

Williams, A.F. (1997) *Hypoglycaemia of the Newborn*. World Health Organisation.

18

INBORN ERRORS OF METABOLISM

- *Cumulatively IEMs are common causes of acute neurological and metabolic deterioration in term babies <72 hours old.*
- *Consider an IEM in any baby with severe hypoglycaemia, encephalopathy or acidaemia for which there is no apparent cause after a conventional work-up.*
- *Early treatment includes IPPV, stopping enteral and parenteral feeds, normalizing glucose, pH and blood pressure.*
- *Investigation is initiated by screening tests including plasma ammonia, amino acids, and lactate together with urinary organic acids and ketones. Cases should be discussed with a specialist centre.*
- *The prognosis for babies with IEMs presenting in the neonatal period is often poor, but every effort must be made to establish the diagnosis for parental counselling, and in case antenatal diagnosis is possible in further pregnancies.*

The purpose of this chapter is to give brief accounts of the presentation and early management of some of the conditions which can be life threatening in the neonatal period. Detailed descriptions of the diseases referred to here, and many other even rarer IEMs, can be found in Scriver *et al.* (1995) and Wraith (1999). As Wraith points out, it is worth investigating ten babies to diagnose one, and whilst neonatologists are happy to adopt this approach towards infectious diseases they have difficulty sustaining it regarding IEMs. This is a rapidly advancing area; for example Smith-Lemli-Opitz syndrome was thought to be an autosomal recessive dysmorphic syndrome for many years before it was realized that there was a defect in cholesterol metabolism with very high plasma levels of 7-dehydrocholesterol.

ACUTE METABOLIC ILLNESS

There is now an enormous list of inborn errors of metabolism. Each one individually is very rare, but together IEMs confront the average

NNU with several acutely ill babies each year. The long term management of such cases is beyond the scope of this book, but the early management in the NNU is crucial if treatable conditions are to be recognized (rare) and an accurate diagnosis made in the remainder of cases so that genetic counselling and future prenatal diagnosis can be offered to parents.

CLINICAL FEATURES

The range of clinical symptoms is vast, particularly for IEMs that have a major impact on a single organ such as the liver. More commonly the presentation is with an encephalopathy coupled with multi-organ involvement that develops rapidly within 48–72 hours of birth. The history often reveals previous unexplained neonatal deaths and parental consanguinity. Table 18.1 lists the clinical and biochemical features that are common at presentation, readily identified in routine neonatal intensive care, but which if they occur together and without a ready alternative should trigger investigations for an IEM.

Table 18.1 Common presenting features of IEM and common differential diagnoses

Symptom/sign	Common condition to exclude
Encephalopathy – hypotonia, fits, coma	HIE (pp. 315–320), meningitis (pp. 245–251) CNS malformations (pp. 334–336). Exclude with history, LP, cranial ultrasound
Persistent vomiting	Bowel obstruction, sepsis. Exclude with routine tests for sepsis and abdominal XR
Metabolic acidaemia	Congenital heart disease, sepsis. IEM more likely if no response to treatment with base
Hypoglycaemia (Chapter 17)	IEM more likely if no other cause e.g. SFD, IDM, HIE
Acute liver disease – conjugated hyperbilirubinaemia	Think of alpha-1-antitrypsin deficiency; assay galactose-1-phosphate uridyl transferase (galactosaemia)
Ketonaemia, ketonuria Unusual smell (baby or urine)	Both very suspicious of IEM particularly if combined with acidaemia
Neutropenia, thrombocytopenia	Sepsis, DIC. Exclude with usual tests, pp. 449–450
Dysmorphic features	Many babies with an IEM are dysmorphic

Table 18.2 Initial investigation in a baby suspected of IEM

Blood
> Glucose
> Ammonia
> Amino acids
> Carnitine
> Lactate/pyruvate
> Urea and electrolytes, septic screen, liver function tests, blood gases

Urine*
> Reducing substances
> Ketones
> Amino acids
> Organic acids
> Orotic acid

CSF
> Lactate (if lactic acidaemia)
> Glycine/amino acids (if glycine encephalopathy)

EEG

Cranial ultrasound scan

Echocardiography

* All urine should be kept and frozen until a diagnosis is made or the baby dies; it can be used for retrospective diagnosis.

INVESTIGATION

In the first place, the investigations listed in Table 18.2 should be carried out. They are available in most hospitals with a NNU or can be completed with a 24 hour turn round time in regional laboratories. From the answers to these initial tests a more focused investigation can be initiated by sending samples (and often the baby) to supraregional units that specialize in IEMs. It is, of course, important not to miss intestinal obstruction as a cause of vomiting, or severe congenital heart disease (e.g. hypoplastic left heart, aortic atresia) as a cause of severe metabolic acidaemia.

TREATMENT

Whilst the diagnosis is being established basic intensive care should be instituted as follows:

- IPPV – controlling respiratory failure;
- IV base (bicarbonate or THAM) – controlling acidaemia;
- IV dextrose – maintain glucose above 2.6 mmol/l;
- maintain blood pressure with saline, blood or dopamine;
- control seizures with anticonvulsants.

Because many IEMs are provoked by the protein load of feeding, enteral feeds should be stopped and hydration maintained with IV dextrose for 24–48 hours. In selected cases, peritoneal dialysis or haemofiltration can be used to remove toxic metabolites (e.g. ammonia, amino acids). Exchange transfusions and "blind" megavitamin therapy are no longer recommended (Wraith 1999).

DYING BABIES

If it appears that the baby is going to die before a diagnosis can be established it is important to collect:

- all urine passed (and freeze it);
- at least 20 ml blood (freeze plasma);
- blood (? skin) for chromosomes;
- consider an urgent postmortem or immediate postmortem sampling – e.g. blood, skin biopsy, liver biopsy in consultation with a specialist in IEMs and the pathologist.

CAUSES OF SEVERE EARLY METABOLIC DISEASE

ORGANIC ACIDAEMIAS (Wraith 1999)

The commoner ones are listed in Table 18.3. These conditions present with encephalopathy, apnoea, acidaemia, hypoglycaemia and thrombocytopenia. The relevant amino acid is elevated in blood and urine. Hyperammonaemia is also found (>500 microg/dl), but less than in the true hyperammonaemias (v.i.). The treatment is that outlined above.

GLYCINE ENCEPHALOPATHY

This used to be known as non-ketotic hyperglycinaemia. The incidence is around 1 in 250 000; the condition is autosomal recessive and antenatal detection is possible. It is a primary defect of neuronal glycine metabolism, and the symptoms are due to the very

Table 18.3 Organic acidaemias; all have acidaemia and ketonaemia

Condition	Incidence	Enzyme deficiency	Treatment	Likely outcome	Prenatal detection
Maple syrup urine disease	1:200 000	Branched chain keto-acid dehydrogenase	May need IV glucose; dialysis if severe	Good chance of neurologically intact survival if diet started early	Yes
Isovaleric acidaemia (sweaty feet syndrome)	60+ cases	Isovaleric acid dehydrogenase	IV glucose, low leucine diet	Good outcome possible on low protein diet; problems with recurrent illness	Yes
Propionic acidaemia	Rare	Propionyl CoA carboxylase	IV. glucose/bicarbonate ? dialysis	Unlikely to be successful in acute neonatal form; severe handicap in survivors	Yes
Multiple carboxylase deficiency	40 cases	Deficiency of various carboxylases involved in biotin metabolism	IV glucose/bicarbonate; neonate often biotin responsive (10 mg daily)	Rarely presents neonatally	Yes
Methylmalonic acidaemia	1:40 000	Methylmalonyl CoA mutase (complex heterogenous defect)	IV glucose/bicarbonate ?dialysis. May be B_{12} responsive (1 mg daily); low protein diet	Unlikely to result in neurologically intact survival unless B_{12} sensitive.	Yes

high brain levels of glycine, which acts as an inhibitory neurotransmitter.

Glycine encephalopathy presents in the neonatal period with profound hypotonia, coma, apnoea, myoclonic seizures and hiccoughing. Glycine levels are raised in blood and urine, but the increase in CSF levels is particularly striking. A markedly raised CSF:plasma glycine ratio establishes the diagnosis. The enzyme defect can be identified on lymphocytes or liver biopsy. The condition is untreatable, although some authors have claimed improvement with dextromethorphan (an NMDA receptor antagonist).

PRIMARY LACTIC ACIDOSIS

This can be due to a variety of enzyme defects, and some cases remain unexplained. The two most commonly recognized defects are fructose 1–6 diphosphatase deficiency (c. 1:200 000), and deficiencies of pyruvate dehydrogenase complex (c. 1:200 000). They are autosomal recessive disorders but only the pyruvate dehydrogenase disorders are diagnosable antenatally.

Most cases present with lactic acidaemia and pallor, with hyperventilation in some. In others there is primarily a neurological picture with hypotonia, seizures, and delayed (or absent) neurological maturation. The plasma lactate level is >2 mmol/l, often being 10 times this value. Ideally the sample should be arterial in order to avoid problems with stasis when collecting venous blood. Urinary lactate levels are also raised. Precise diagnosis requires enzyme studies of fibroblasts or a liver biopsy. A small proportion of those with pyruvate dehydrogenase complex defects do not have a lactic acidaemia, and the underlying cause of the neurological syndrome may be difficult to establish.

While establishing the diagnosis in any group treat as described above. Nutrition should be given as a high fat, high protein, low carbohydrate diet, in particular avoiding fructose. Most cases that present neonatally are unresponsive to long-term therapy.

FATTY ACID OXIDATION DEFECTS

MCAD is the most frequently recognized of these disorders in the neonatal period. The incidence is 1 in 40 000 and the disorder is autosomal recessive. The genetic mutation has been localized to chromosome 1. Babies are hypoglycaemic and hypoketonaemic, with elevated liver enzymes. Antenatal diagnosis is possible.

PEROXISOMAL DISORDERS

Peroxisomes are subcellular organelles, and over 15 different disorders of their function have been described. Several of these diseases present in the neonatal period, usually with severe neurological abnormality often combined with abnormal facies, hepatic failure, and cataracts. Diagnosis is supported by high levels of very long chain fatty acids and/or deficiency of dihydroacetone phosphate acyl transferase in the plasma.

UREA CYCLE DISORDERS (HYPERAMMONAEMIAS)

These present as shown in Table 18.4. However, acidaemia and ketonaemia are absent and there is gross hyperammonaemia (>1000 μg/dl, equivalent to 1400 μmol/l). Other biochemical abnormalities are absent but the urea concentration is usually very low.

Emergency treatment involves reducing or stopping the protein intake, lowering the blood ammonia levels by peritoneal dialysis, and preventing ammonia release by the gut bacteria with neomycin and laxatives. Sodium benzoate (loading dose 250 mg/kg followed by 250 mg/kg/24 h by infusion) should be given to all cases. In babies with the acute neonatal form of these diseases, long-term management is problematic, and rarely successful.

Transient neonatal hyperammonaemia

This has been described occasionally in seriously ill often comatose VLBW babies who have ammonia levels above 1000 microg/dl. The cause is unknown and the babies improve steadily with vigorous treatment of the hyperammonaemia (*v.s.*).

PHENYLKETONURIA

The incidence is about 1 in 10 000. It is due to a deficiency of phenylalanine hydroxylase (or rarely dihydropteridine reductase). It is an autosomal recessive. Antenatal detection is possible; neonatal screening is routine.

Babies with PKU will not be ill during the neonatal period but will present if the screening test (Guthrie or Scriver test) is positive in a baby still in the neonatal unit. The test should only be carried out on babies who are receiving milk which gives a protein load and

Table 18.4 Urea cycle disorders

Condition and enzyme deficiency	Incidence	Genetics	Outcome	Prenatal diagnosis
Ornithine transcarbamylase deficiency	1:60 000	Sex linked dominant	Death in males with acute neonatal form; females do well with protein restriction	Yes
Argininosuccinic aciduria	Rare <1:250 000	Recessive	Long term survival possible on diet; ± amino acid supplements	Yes
Citrullinaemia	Rare <1:250 000	Recessive	Long term survival possible	Yes
Carbamyl phosphate synthetase deficiency	Rare <1:250 000	Recessive	Neonatal forms fatal	Yes
Hyperargininaemia (arginase deficiency)	20 cases	Recessive	Long term survival possible on diet with amino acid supplements	Yes

elevates the plasma phenylalanine. If the screening test is positive, before starting the diet it must be established that the hyperphenylalaninaemia detected at screening is due to genuine phenylketonuria rather than some other cause of an elevated serum phenylalanine.

GALACTOSAEMIA

The incidence is 1 in 60 000–70 000. The classical disease is caused by deficiency of galactose-1-phosphate-uridyl-transferase; rarer variants are due to absent galactokinase or galactose-4-epimerase. All types are autosomal recessives. Antenatal detection and neonatal screening are both possible.

Babies present with the following:

1. vomiting, and occasionally diarrhoea;
2. lethargy and hypotonia;
3. poor weight gain;
4. persistent jaundice;
5. hepatosplenomegaly;
6. cataracts (occasionally).

Many affected neonates become seriously ill, and they may die from septicaemia before galactosaemia is diagnosed.

A baby with suggestive symptoms *must* be receiving milk for the diagnosis of galactosaemia to be considered. Galactose will be found in the urine, but this does not react with Glucose reagent strips. Start all such babies without delay on a lactose-free milk such as Galactomin 17, while confirming the diagnosis by assay of galactose-1-phosphate-uridyl-transferase in red cells.

REFERENCES

Scriver, C.R., Beaudet, A.L., Sly, W.S. and Valle, D. (eds) (1995) *The Metabolic Basis of Inherited Disease*, 7th Edn. McGraw Hill, New York.

Wraith, J.E. (1999) Inborn errors of metabolism in the neonate. In: *Textbook of Neonatology*, 3rd edn. Rennie, J.M and Roberton, N.R.C. (eds), Churchill Livingstone, Edinburgh pp. 986–1002.

19

ORTHOPAEDIC DISORDERS

- *Neonatal fractures heal quickly and without residual deformity.*
- *Clinical screening for DDH misses many cases.*
- *Babies at risk for DDH (breech, positive family history, other skeletal malformation, any abnormal clinical finding on examination of the hip) should have an ultrasound scan of the hip joint.*
- *All clinically abnormal hips should be splinted in the neonatal period.*

FRACTURES

SKULL

With modern standards of obstetric care fractures of the skull are rarely seen. No treatment is required for a non-displaced linear fracture. Occasionally a depressed "ping-pong ball" fracture may occur, especially if the baby for some reason has a thin skull vault – craniotabes. Although some surgeons recommend that all such fractures should be elevated, if the baby is neurologically normal, and there are no fragments of bone which could damage the cortex, no treatment is required and the vault bones should be allowed to grow and remodel.

CLAVICLE

This is commonly diagnosed when evaluating a baby with Erb's palsy (p. 333). It may also present with a "crack" heard during delivery, with limitation of arm movement from pain, or with swelling from angulation of the clavicle and callus formation. No treatment is usually needed. Occasionally, if the baby is in pain, a figure-of-eight bandage can be applied. Healing is always rapid, without long-term deformity.

HUMERUS

This may be broken during extraction of the arm of a breech. It usually presents either with a "crack" heard at delivery or with pseudoparalysis due to pain. The fracture is either a proximal epiphyseal fracture or is in the mid-shaft of the bone, where it may damage the radial nerve (p. 333). Simple splinting, either with a large crepe bandage on the upper arm, or firm but not tight bandaging of the arm to the baby's thorax, is all that is required. The fracture only needs to be maintained in this way for 2–3 weeks.

These days, fractures of the long bones and ribs are much more often found in VLBW babies with osteopenia of prematurity (*v.i.*) than as a result of obstetric trauma. The fracture may result from handling, or from the baby trapping his arm between the tray and the wall of his incubator. The treatment is the same, together with more aggressive management of his osteopenia.

FEMUR

Delivery of the extended legs of a breech may be accompanied by a "crack" as the femur fractures, usually in the mid-shaft. If the diagnosis is not made at this stage, the fracture usually presents with pseudoparalysis. Despite marked displacement and angulation on X-ray, reduction is not required, and simple splinting with a bulky crepe/cotton wool bandage for 2–3 weeks is the only treatment necessary. As with the humerus, a fracture of the femur should lead one to consider osteopenia, and at birth a fractured femur can be the first clue to bone disease or a myopathy – the baby's bones are thin because he has not moved very much *in utero*.

CERVICAL SPINE

A fracture dislocation of the cervical spine may occur during vaginal delivery of a breech with an extended head or during a difficult rotational forceps delivery. This usually results in severe damage to the cervical cord, and produces a baby with a flaccid quadriplegia. If the cord is injured above the phrenic nerve, apnoea will result. Early exploration of the cervical spine is of no value. The long-term prognosis for such babies is very poor.

DISLOCATIONS

Apart from dislocation of the hip (*v.i.*) which is more accurately termed developmental dysplasia of the hip, dislocations are rare. Congenital dislocation of the knee can occur, and this is an orthopaedic emergency. The knee should be reduced and strapped.

SKELETAL MALFORMATIONS

LIMB MALFORMATIONS

Major reduction deformities of the limbs are rare. All such children should be referred early to an artificial limb centre with special interest and experience in the problems of limbless children.

TALIPES CALCANEO VALGUS

This requires no treatment other than gentle manipulations by the mother putting her baby's foot into the plantigrade position.

TALIPES EQUINOVARUS

This needs treatment if the foot cannot be moved into the plantigrade position. The initial management is to strap the foot as shown in Fig. 19.1. If this is started on day 1 or 2, a large number of cases will not require specialized orthopaedic management.

The incidence is 1 in 1000.

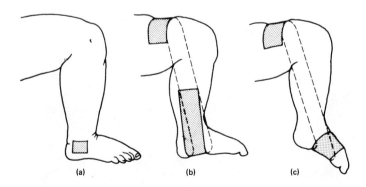

(a)   (b)   (c)

Figure 19.1 Strapping for talipes equino varus. (a) Lateral aspect showing the correct position of the leg and ankle, with both knee and ankle at a right angle. A small square of adhesive felt protects the malleolus. (b) Medial aspect showing the first length of strapping in place. (c) Medial aspect showing the second length of strapping in place. This second length is applied on top of the piece illustrated in (b), which is not shown in (c) in order to claify the details of the second length of strapping. (Reproduced from Davies *et al.*, 1972, with permission.)

DEVELOPMENTAL DYSPLASIA OF THE HIP

This malformation may either be isolated or present in a child with other abnormalities, especially spina bifida. The incidence is 1 in 600 for females and 1 in 2500 for males.

All neonatal residents must become skilled in the examination techniques used to exclude DDH in the neonatal period (Fig. 19.2). The accuracy of diagnosis has been improved by hip ultrasound. Complex classifications (Graf 1984) have been produced. Hip ultrasound examination should be performed in all babies with

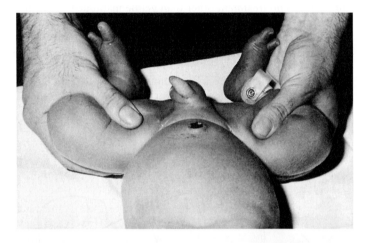

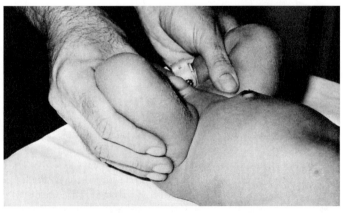

Figure 19.2 Ortolani and Barlow manoevre.

Table 19.1 Features of some skeletal dysplasias presenting at birth

Syndrome	Bony features	Outcome
Asphyxiating thoracic dystrophy (AR)	Short ribs +++	Usually lethal but can survive
Achondroplasia (AD)	Narrow chest	Good
Diastrophic dwarfism (AR)	Short tubular bones, head large	Good
Camptomelic dwarfism (AR)	Thick, short tubular bones especially first metacarpal	Good
Rhizomelic chondrodysplasia punctata (AR)	Short femora and humeri. Epiphyseal punctate calcification. Large head	Usually lethal. Low IQ
Osteogenesis imperfecta (AR)	Multiple fractures, poorly mineralized bones	Usually lethal; survivors have multiple fractures
Osteogenesis imperfecta (AD)	Thin, fractures in early life	Multiple fractures in early life — usually wheelchair bound
Hypophosphatasia (AR)	Marked bony underossification	Severe form lethal
Thanatophoric dwarfism (sporadic)	Large head. Very small chest	Lethal

abnormal hip examinations, and in those who were breech presentations, have other limb abnormalities (e.g. talipes) or have a family history of DDH. Once an abnormal hip has been identified it should be put in one of the special splints designed for this disorder.

SHORT LIMBED DWARFISM

A large number of syndromes with short limbed dwarfism are now recognized. In many of these the rib growth is also compromised, resulting in pulmonary hypoplasia, severe early respiratory distress and often death. The features of some of these conditions are given in Table 19.1.

OSTEOPENIA OF PREMATURITY (NEONATAL RICKETS) (Bishop 1999)

This condition occurs in VLBW survivors of neonatal intensive care. It is primarily a marker of the fact that it is difficult to incorporate enough calcium and phosphorus into the diet of rapidly growing babies who weigh less than 1.5 kg at birth. It is not due to vitamin D deficiency, so that the original name of rickets of prematurity is, strictly speaking, inappropriate.

Clinical features are rare. The disease usually presents radiologically with rachitic cupping visible in the ribs or at the wrists and knees, and is not usually found until 5–6 weeks of age. In severe cases there may be pathological fractures of the ribs, particularly in babies with severe persisting CLD. The calcium level is usually normal, but it may occasionally be raised (p. 30); the phosphorus concentration is low at 1 mmol/l or less, and the alkaline phosphatase markedly raised, often to values >1000 u/l.

The disease is preventable if preterm formula is used, or neonates taking EBM are given 1 mmol/kg/24 h of phosphate, and 400 units of vitamin D per day (pp. 39–40). If osteopenia does develop the baby should receive 2 mmol/kg/24 h of phosphate, and a total of 1000 units of vitamin D/day. Full recovery always occurs. If hypocalcaemia develops at any stage it should be treated with oral supplements of calcium gluconate (p. 29).

REFERENCES

Bishop, N. (1999) Metabolic bone disease. In: *Textbook of Neonatology*, 3rd edn. Rennie, J.M. and Roberton, N.R.C. (eds), Churchill Livingstone, Edinburgh pp. 1002–1008.

Davies, P.A., Robinson, R.J., Scopes, J.W., Tizard, J.P.M. and Wigglesworth, J.S. (1972) *Medical Care of Newborn Babies*. Nos 44/45. Spastics International Medical Publications, Wm. Heinemann, London.

Graf, R. (1984) Classification of hip joint dysplasias by means of ultrasonography. *Archives of Orthopaedic and Trauma Surgery* **102**: 248–255.

FURTHER READING

Faix, R.G. and Donn, S.M. (1983) Immediate management of the traumatised infant. *Clinics in Perinatology* **10**: 487–506.

Hensinger, R.N. and Jones, E. (1999) Orthopaedic problems in the newborn. In: *Textbook of Neonatology*, 3rd edn. Rennie, J.M. and Roberton, N.R.C. (eds), Churchill Livingstone, Edinburgh pp. 1063–1088.

Jones, D.A. (1998) *Hip Screening in the Newborn: a practical guide*. Butterworth-Heinemann, Oxford.

20

NEUROLOGICAL PROBLEMS

___

ASSESSMENT OF THE NERVOUS SYSTEM

Healthy newborns spend about 50 minutes of each hour asleep. This may be either quiet sleep (regular breathing, no eye movements, non REM sleep) or active sleep (irregular breathing, rapid eye movements, REM sleep). For some of the time the normal term baby is awake and alert, fixing his gaze on the examiner's face. Even when crying he is consolable and cuddly. The normal baby's movements have a fluid, elegant quality; his hands open occasionally and he can move his fingers individually. The movements are complex and variable.

Neurological assessment must *always* include measurement of the head circumference. Persistent high-pitched crying, unconsolability (irritability), paucity/poor repertoire of movement and marked jitteriness are abnormal and can indicate problems such as hypoxic ischaemic encephalopathy (pp. 315–320), meningitis (p. 245), hypoglycaemia (p. 286), drug withdrawal (p. 339), pain (p. 94) or intracranial haemorrhage (p. 324). Investigation is indicated. Alarm signals include the following:

- persisting irritability, marked jitteriness;
- difficulty in feeding;
- opisthotonus, or persistent asymmetry in posture, movements or tone;
- abnormal cry;
- states of only crying or sleeping; no quiet alert periods;
- tense fontanelle, rapidly increasing head circumference;
- seizures;
- apathy and immobility, floppiness.

CONVULSIONS IN THE NEWBORN

- *Fits in the neonatal period are often subtle.*
- *All fitting babies require full biochemical, EEG and ultrasound investigation as well as a work-up for meningitis.*

- *The current first line anticonvulsants are phenobarbitone and phenytoin, with clonazepam as the second line.*
- *Most babies who fit in the neonatal period stop fitting and can safely have their anticonvulsant treatment stopped before they go home.*
- *Fits worsen the prognosis, which largely depends on the underlying cause. Neurological sequelae are seen in 25–35% of survivors.*

INCIDENCE

The incidence of convulsions in the neonatal period is 3–6 per 1000 live births at term, and 50–100 per 1000 in preterm births.

TYPES OF CONVULSIONS

The commonest type of seizure in the neonate, both term and preterm, involves a very subtle change in activity. The baby becomes still, and there may be tiny movements of the eyes or jaw (forced blinking, eye deviation, chewing or lip-smacking), and/or changes in the breathing pattern. The period of abnormal behaviour often lasts for only 10–20 seconds. Clonic convulsions in the neonate may be focal or generalized, and boxing or cycling movements of the limbs are common manifestations of this seizure type. Babies can have short tonic seizures in which they adopt an opisthotonic decerebrate posture with extended and internally rotated limbs, and their eyes diverge outwards and downwards. They may become apnoeic with cyanosis and bradycardia. The neonate often exhibits electroclinical dissociation; that is, there is poor agreement between the stereotyped clinical manifestations of seizure and any discharge on the EEG. Only rarely are the two precisely temporally related.

AETIOLOGY AND DIFFERENTIAL DIAGNOSIS OF NEONATAL CONVULSIONS

The major causes of neonatal convulsions are listed in Table 20.1. In some babies it is comparatively easy to establish the cause of the fit (for example in babies with malformations, or the SGA baby fitting from hypoglycaemia at 12 hours of age). However, in many babies several of the factors listed in Table 20.1 may co-exist. For this reason any convulsing neonate should routinely have the following tests carried out:

Table 20.1 Causes of neonatal convulsions

Diagnosis	Age at start and type of fit	Diagnostic clues
Hypoxic ischaemic encephalopathy	2–48 hours; can be subtle, tonic or clonic	Fetal distress, need for resuscitation, obtunded, tense fontanelle, haematuria
GMH-IVH	Preterm baby, 0–72 hours; usually subtle	VLBWI; decreased PCV; increased fontanelle tension; diagnosed with ultrasound
Arterial thrombosis or "stroke" (usually middle cerebral artery)	24–72 hours, can be later. Baby remains alert between seizures, which are often focal	Well baby; can have high PCV. Diagnose with ultrasound or MRI
Meningitis	Any time and type of fit	Ill baby with signs of sepsis; LP
Hypoglycaemia	<72 hours, clonic	SFD or preterm baby. If term suggests rare cause of hypoglycaemia (see p. 293)
Hypocalcaemia	Early or late (5–8 days)	Rare now; usually seriously ill baby <48 hours old
Hypomagnesaemia	5–8 days, clonic, multifocal	Associated with low calcium and high phosphate
High or low serum sodium	Any age, usually clonic	Ill babies
Kernicterus	Any time, any type	Jaundice
Congenital CNS malformation	Any time, any type	Increasingly recognized with imaging. Can be small head, etc.
Fifth day fits	Around the fifth day, usually clonic	Normal investigation results
Benign familial neonatal seizures	Usually 3–7 days. Brief clonic seizures	Family history (autosomal dominant). Normal investigations, but microdeletion on chromosome 20
Benign neonatal sleep myoclonus	5 days on; only in sleep; only myoclonic jerks	Normal investigations, exclude inborn errors
Maternal drug withdrawal	Usually less than a week, clonic	Maternal history, hair or urine analysis
Rare inborn errors (e.g. pyridoxine deficiency)	Usually <72 hours; any type of fit	Can be a family history of previous sudden neonatal death.

- blood glucose, electrolytes and urea;
- blood gases;
- calcium and magnesium;
- white blood count and differential;
- blood culture;
- lumbar puncture;
- EEG whenever possible;
- ultrasound brain scan.

On the basis of these tests and the history of, for example, asphyxia, hypoxic episodes or maternal drug ingestion, an accurate diagnosis can be made in most babies. Any baby with seizures in whom the suggested first line investigations do not yield a diagnosis should have MR imaging performed. Stroke, in particular, is often ultrasound-negative.

Very occasionally babies convulse because they suffer from rare inborn errors of metabolism. In general, these babies are acidotic and show other neurological abnormalities (p. 297). In acutely ill babies, the routine outlined on p. 298 should be followed. In less ill neonates, urinary amino acid chromatography should always be carried out.

A small number of babies have a blameless clinical history, are well between fits, and all the above investigations are negative. Some of these fall into the category of "fifth day fits" or "benign familial epilepsy" for which the prognosis is excellent.

TREATMENT OF NEONATAL CONVULSIONS

Turn the baby on his side and secure the airway (intubate and give IPPV if apnoea, cyanosis or bradycardia develop). Gently aspirate the pharynx if inhalation of milk or vomit has occurred. Give oxygen by mask if the baby is cyanosed but breathing. This should be done very carefully in babies at risk from ROP.

Take blood for a laboratory and ward estimation of glucose while anticonvulsants are being obtained, and give 3 ml/kg of 10% dextrose IV if the result is below 2.6 mmol/l.

Use phenobarbitone as the first-line anticonvulsant. Give 20–30 mg/kg IV depending on whether or not the baby is ventilated; larger doses cause apnoea. If phenobarbitone does not work then the following should be tried, in order: phenytoin 10–20 mg/kg IV (only if there is no myocardial ischaemia), clonazepam 100 micrograms per kg, lignocaine 4 mg/kg then 3 mg/kg/h (not if phenytoin has been given already).

In most babies with neonatal convulsions, maintenance anticonvulsant therapy (usually with phenobarbitone 5 mg/kg/24 h) should be started and continued for several days. In general babies who recover to a normal neurological state before going home do not need maintenance anticonvulsants, but anticonvulsants should be continued in babies in the following situations:

- babies who are not neurologically normal at discharge after hypoxic ischaemic encephalopathy or meningitis;
- babies with other persisting clinical or EEG abnormality;
- babies with underlying CNS malformation.

HYPOXIC ISCHAEMIC ENCEPHALOPATHY

- *HIE causes permanent damage to the central nervous system in 1 in 2000 to 1 in 5000 births.*
- *Prevention of HIE depends in part on obstetric care.*
- *Neonatal care in HIE involves maintenance of homeostasis, and control of seizures; there is as yet no specific neuroprotective regimen which has been shown to be of benefit.*
- *Predicting outcome is difficult in the first 24 hours; it is usually best to maintain full intensive care during this period.*
- *Predicting outcome accurately is aided by the results of EEG, neuroimaging, and careful clinical assessment of the worst grade of encephalopathy, which is usually reached by 48 hours.*

The characteristic neurological syndrome seen in term babies after a period of perinatal asphyxia is called hypoxic ischaemic encephalopathy. The underlying insult is usually a combination of hypoxia and acidosis during late fetal life. The insult can be an acute, profound hypoxia lasting 10–25 minutes (e.g. cord prolapse, uterine rupture) or a chronic partial hypoxia lasting for an hour or more (e.g. cord entanglement, uterine hyperstimulation) (pp. 64–68). The diagnosis must be based on more than just a low Apgar score, for which there are many other causes (p. 63). However, in the delivery room the Apgar score may be the only piece of information available. After successful resuscitation, it is helpful to consider the following factors (Table 20.2) when deciding whether to admit a baby to the NNU for observation (Portman *et al.* 1990). The clinical picture evolves over the first 12 hours, and babies who go to the postnatal ward must be observed carefully because they can, and often do, develop symptoms between 12–72 hours after birth.

Table 20.2 The Portman score for postasphyxia morbidity (Portman *et al.* 1990)

	0 points	1 point	2 points	3 points
5 min Apgar score	>6	5–6	3–4	0–2
Base deficit from arterial blood gas in first hour (mmol/l)	<10	10–14	15–19	>19
CTG	Normal	Variable decelerations	Severe variable or late decelerations	Prolonged bradycardia

≥ 6 points: severe morbidity; positive predictive value 78%

DIAGNOSIS OF HIE

The severity of HIE has been divided into three grades which corre-
late well with prognosis (Tables 20.3 and 20.4). About 6 per 1000
babies in the UK suffer some form of HIE with grades II and III
each affecting one in a 1000, and the severity of the illness mirrors
the severity of the previous hypoxic ischaemic insult. Worldwide, the
incidence of HIE is known to be high in developing countries, and
the disorder makes a large contribution to the burden of childhood
disability.

If the insult was mild, all that usually happens is that the baby will
be wide-eyed and irritable, making a rapid recovery within a few
days. With more severe injury, for example following full cardiopulmonary resuscitation with a prolonged Apgar score of 0 the fits can
often be multiple and difficult to control. Alternatively the baby
may never breathe, and may be ventilator-dependent and have an
isoelectric (flat) EEG. Grades II and III HIE are the commonest
cause of seizures in term babies (Table 20.1), but if the positive
features of fetal distress, birth depression, multiple organ system

Table 20.3 Clinical grade of hypoxic ischaemic encephalopathy (From Levene *et al.* 1986)

Grade I (mild)	Grade II (moderate)	Grade III (severe)
Irritability "hyperalert"	Lethargy	Comatose
Mild hypotonia	Marked abnormalities in tone	Severe hypotonia
Poor sucking	Requires tube feeds	Failure to maintain spontaneous respiration
No seizures	Seizures	Prolonged seizures

Table 20.4 Risk of death or severe handicap in survivors of hypoxic ischaemic encephalopathy according to the worst clinical grade reached (from Peliowski and Finer 1992)

HIE grade	Risk of death or severe handicap in survivors		
	Percentage	**Likelihood ratio**	**95% confidence interval**
I Mild	1.6	0.05	0.02–0.15
II Moderate	24	0.94	0.71–1.23
III Severe	78	10.71	6.71–17.1

involvement are lacking then a search must be made for one of the other diagnoses. The seizures of HIE are often very subtle and typically occur at a postnatal age of 12 hours with a range of 3–48 hours.

Other organ systems are involved, and there may be hypoglycaemia and marked hypotension from myocardial depression. The chest X-ray may show a large heart and there may be ECG changes of ischaemia. Renal failure with oliguria and haematuria is also common.

INVESTIGATION OF HIE

Imaging

Ultrasound and CT scanning show a featureless brain with loss of the normal sulci and gyri with compressed ventricles when there is cerebral oedema. Evidence of cerebral oedema is not predictive of outcome (v.i.) but does support a clinical diagnosis of HIE. Damaged thalami and lentiform nuclei produce abnormal signals on MR images, and there can be abnormal MR signal in the motor strip, the perirolandic cortex (Rutherford et al. 1996). MR is more sensitive than ultrasound in detecting these abnormalities, although when basal ganglia changes are severe enough to be imaged with ultrasound the prognosis is usually poor.

EEG

The EEG in HIE has an abnormal background, often with multifocal seizures of varying morphology. The background EEG is of diagnostic and prognostic value. An attenuated (flat) EEG recorded in the first 12 hours can recover, but a persistently attenuated or discontinuous EEG in a term baby is a poor prognostic indicator. A normal or mildly abnormal EEG in the first 12 hours means either that the diagnosis is wrong, or the baby will recover completely from his very mild insult.

Doppler ultrasound estimation of cerebral blood flow velocity

Doppler ultrasound studies of the cerebral circulation reflect the problem of maximally dilated cerebral arteries, with a high cerebral blood flow velocity and a particularly high diastolic velocity. The Pourcelot Index (PI) is calculated from the formula PI=(peak systolic – end diastolic velocity)/peak systolic velocity. A value less than 0.55 reliably predicts a poor outcome, although the abnormality does not develop until the second 24 hours of life.

TREATMENT OF HIE

Although both clinically and on MR spectroscopy studies, brain function would appear to deteriorate during the first 24 hours in many babies, as yet there is no therapy available that modifies this progression. Reducing cerebral oedema with steroids or mannitol has no influence on the neurological outcome. Brain cells have been killed by the asphyxial insult, and controlling the cytotoxic cerebral oedema which results does not bring them back to life. Further apoptotic cell death occurs in the 24–48 hours after delivery (secondary energy failure, excitotoxic amino acid release). Whether oxygen free radical scavengers, magnesium sulphate, brain cooling or calcium channel blockers will help remains speculative. Babies with HIE usually have damage to other body systems. The common effects and management of each are summarized in Table 20.5.

All one can do is to manage the complications as suggested, and then sit back and wait. Most babies begin to improve by 48–72 hours of age. Their fits are controlled, their tone improves, and any evidence of raised intracranial pressure resolves. Fluid balance can be very tricky, and many babies become oedematous from a combination of renal failure, SIADH, heart failure, lack of movement and the leaky capillaries of the critically ill neonate (p. 22). These babies do not respond well to a fluid challenge and they should be managed with fluid restriction, diuretics and inotropic support.

Anticonvulsants should be stopped once the fits cease, as ongoing unnecessary treatment contributes to the hypotonia and feeding difficulty and makes the baby hard to assess. The following clinical features are worrying, and add prognostic information to that obtained from investigation.

Table 20.5 Organ systems affected in HIE

Organ system	Manifestation of dysfunction	Management
CNS	Seizures; apnoeas; raised intracranial pressure; intracranial bleeding; nerve palsies	v.s. p. 333
Respiratory	Respiratory distress due to surfactant deficiency; ARDS; apnoea; PPHN; pulmonary haemorrhage; meconium aspiration	Ventilate; measure blood gases; correct acidosis; see Chapter 11
Cardiovascular	Shock; hypotension; cardiomegaly; heart failure; ECG evidence of ischaemia	Ventilate; give inotropes; fluid restriction; diuretics
Renal	Oliguria; haematuria; proteinuria; myoglobinuria; renal failure	Fluid restriction; careful monitoring; consider dialysis if CNS prognosis considered good
Haematological	DIC; raised white cell count; raised nucleated red cell count	Vitamin K; fresh frozen plasma; cryoprecipitate; cover for infection
Metabolic	Hypoglycaemia; hypocalcaemia; hyponatraemia	Replace lost ions; careful fluid balance
Gastrointestinal	Ileus; necrotising enterocolitis	Start enteral feeds cautiously; treat NEC as on p. 387–388
Hepatic	Elevated transaminases/ammonia; prolonged coagulation times; jaundice	Vitamin K; support coagulation; phototherapy/exchange transfusion as indicated p. 427–430

- Persisting fits or apnoeas.
- Prolonged hypotonia and apathy.
- Prolonged hypertonia.
- Persisting failure to suck feeds.

PROGNOSIS IN HIE

In babies who seize and reach grade II–III hypoxic ischaemic encephalopathy, a more accurate individual prognosis can be given if an EEG is obtained between 12 and 72 hours, together with ultrasound imaging/Doppler studies and MRI scans. Accurate early prognostication can be helpful if withdrawal of intensive care is being considered, but care is needed in the interpretation of these tests. Intensive care should never be withdrawn on the basis of Apgar scores alone, or because of the sole finding of cerebral oedema on an ultrasound scan. Poor prognostic features include the following:

- EEG background with an isoelectric pattern after 12 hours of age;
- EEG background with "burst suppression" pattern after 12 hours of age;
- neuroimaging evidence of bilateral basal ganglia involvement;
- MR imaging showing absent signal from myelin in the posterior limb of the internal capsule;
- Doppler CBF velocity studies showing a high diastolic velocity, making the Pourcelot index less than 0.55;
- prolonged grade II and any grade III HIE with a marked delay in establishing sucking or in acquiring normal tone.

The following features are **not** helpful in the prognosis of HIE:

- Neuroimaging evidence of cerebral oedema.
- The number or type of clinical or electrical seizures.
- The degree of renal impairment.
- The cord pH.
- The Apgar score at less than 10 minutes of age.
- Early clinical assessment; later assessment is useful (*v.s.*).

Many clinicians offer to withdraw ventilatory support if the EEG shows marked abnormalities, the baby is ventilated with clinical grade III encephalopathy, the Doppler CBF velocity studies are abnormal and the diagnosis is certain to be HIE. Even if care is withdrawn appropriately parents should be warned that the baby might not die. Prognosis is not accurate enough for intensive care not to be instituted, or for it to be withdrawn before 48 hours of life.

FOCAL VASCULAR LESIONS

NEONATAL STROKE

Neonatal cerebral artery infarction may occur if a vessel is blocked by an embolus or thrombus. The baby presents with fits, but is usually alert between the episodes and even during them. Cranial ultrasound may be normal but can show midline shift and an abnormal area of echodensity, most commonly in the left middle cerebral artery territory. MRI may be necessary to make the diagnosis. Investigation should include a search for the inherited thrombotic disorders, such as protein C or protein S deficiency or the factor V Leiden mutation. Treatment is conservative, and the outcome is usually surprisingly good.

CEREBRAL VENOUS THROMBOSIS

Thrombosis of the cerebral veins can occur as a result of dehydration, infection, skull trauma or the inherited thrombotic disorders. The diagnosis may be more common than is suspected and can be confirmed by CT or MRI scan. Treatment with thrombolytic therapy has been tried but the results are not encouraging.

EXTRACRANIAL HAEMORRHAGE

SUBGALEAL (SUBAPONEUROTIC) HAEMORRHAGE

The subgaleal space is a large potential space beneath the aponeurotic membrane, and a large amount of blood can collect here before the diagnosis is made (Fig. 20.1). Ventouse delivery increases the risk of this form of bleeding. Babies present with a boggy swelling which crosses the suture lines, and the head circumference can increase by several centimetres in less than 24 hours. In severe cases the baby can collapse with shock before the source of the bleeding is realized, and the mortality is 17–25%. Treatment with blood and volume replacement is effective, and the outlook for babies who are successfully treated is excellent.

INTRACRANIAL HAEMORRHAGE

- *Serious intracranial haemorrhage is rare at term. Babies with subdural or intracerebral haemorrhage should be evaluated in consultation with neurosurgeons. SAH is common, causes minimal symptoms, and has a good prognosis.*
- *GMH-IVH occurs in up to 20% of VLBWI. The incidence can be minimized by antenatal steroids and attention to maintaining homeostasis in critically ill neonates. We do not use any specific drug prophylaxis.*

- *Uncomplicated GMH-IVH is frequently asymptomatic and has few sequelae.*
- *Complicated GMH-IVH includes post haemorrhagic ventriculomegaly, progressive hydrocephalus and periventricular venous infarction. Serious long term neurological sequelae are frequent in such babies.*
- *Other than treating hydrocephalus, no treatment is available for these serious complications.*

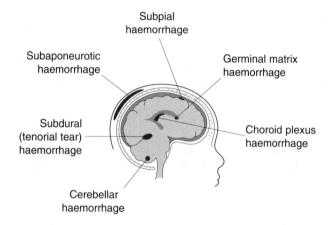

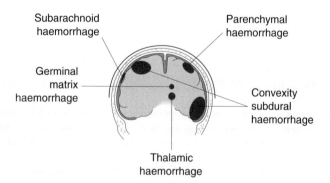

Figure 20.1 Sites of intracranial haemorrhage. Modified from Levene 1999 with permission.

Bleeding can occur at many sites (Fig. 20.1). Presentation is usually with seizures, but fever can occur, although the first sign of the problem may be the associated coagulopathy (bruising, bleeding) or shock. Intracranial haemorrhage is detected in 3–5% of apparently healthy term babies with neuroimaging, but the significance of subclinical bleeding is not yet clear.

SUBDURAL HAEMORRHAGE

This often arises from the anterior end of the insertion of the falx cerebri into the tentorium cerebelli, where the great cerebral vein and the inferior saggital sinus combine to give the straight sinus (Fig. 20.1). This area is easily damaged, and the vessel walls can be torn during a difficult delivery of the fetal head. Subdural bleeds can also result from tearing of the bridging veins over the vault, where the bleeding coagulates to cause a convexity subdural haemorrhage.

Signs

These are usually those of associated severe asphyxia (*v.s.*), of raised intracranial pressure, or blood loss. Although the anterior fontanelle is often bulging, this is primarily due to cerebral oedema. The diagnosis can be confirmed ultrasonically, although the subdural space is not always well visualized with this technique and a CT or MR scan is often required.

Treatment

Any coexisting asphyxia should be treated (*v.s.*). A large subdural haemorrhage can be drained by subdural tap (p. 489) or with formal neurosurgical intervention, but consideration needs to be given to the prognosis of any accompanying HIE. Small subdural collections, consisting of little more than a film of blood over the cortex, cannot be aspirated without further traumatizing the cortex which is pressed up against the inside of the skull. They should therefore be left alone.

SUBARACHNOID HAEMORRHAGE

This form of haemorrhage is probably much more common than is generally realized, with small amounts of capillary or venous subarachnoid bleeding occurring during many mildly traumatic or asphyxial deliveries. The condition is often asymptomatic, but may present with fits, jitteriness or irritability during the first few days. The CSF obtained is uniformly bloodstained. A cerebral ultrasound scan should be performed to exclude other types of ICH, but subarachnoid bleeding cannot usually be detected with ultrasound.

Symptomatic treatment of the fits or co-existing birth asphyxia is all that is required. There is no need to do repeat lumbar punctures to drain CSF, and the prognosis is good.

GERMINAL MATRIX-INTRAVENTRICULAR HAEMORRHAGE
AND ACCOMPANYING INTRAPARENCHYMAL LESIONS

This type of intracranial bleeding is found in 20% of babies who weigh less than 1.5 kg at birth. Around 90% of these bleeds appear for the first time within 72 hours of birth, and up to 20% will extend during the next few days.

GMH-IVH may occur spontaneously in a comparatively asymptomatic baby weighing less than 1 kg at birth, but is most commonly seen in babies who weigh less than 1.5 kg at birth and who have been hypoxic, hypotensive (Appendix C), hypercarbic (p. 140) and acidaemic in association with apnoea, severe birth asphyxia, pneumothorax or RDS. The underlying problem is thought to be an alteration in cerebral blood flow causing bleeding into the fragile capillary bed of the germinal matrix. Fluctuations in blood pressure, or of blood flow in this area associated with the baby fighting the ventilator are thought to be important. Vasodilatation associated with hypercarbia is a contributory factor.

Classification (De Vries and Rennie 1999)

In the past, the term "periventricular haemorrhage", abbreviated to PVH, was widely used to embrace germinal matrix haemorrhage, intraventricular haemorrhage and haemorrhage into the brain parenchyma. In our view, the term PVH should be abandoned as it is now known that not all parenchymal lesions are haemorrhagic, nor are they all periventricular. The Papile classification, which was based on CT scan appearances, is outmoded. According to the Papile system grade I described a haemorrhage confined to the subependymal region, grade II referred to bleeding into the ventricular cavity but not distending it, grade III described an intraventricular bleed

Table 20.6 Description of neonatal intracranial lesions seen early in life with ultrasound

Description	Generic term
Germinal matrix haemorrhage	GMH-IVH
Intraventricular haemorrhage without ventricular dilatation	GMH-IVH
Intraventricular haemorrhage with acute ventricular dilatation (measure the ventricle)	GMH-IVH and ventriculomegaly
Intraparenchymal lesion – describe size, location, degree of echogenicity and permanently record the image	IPL

with ventricular enlargement and grade IV denoted any parenchymal lesion. There are several disadvantages to this system, including the fact that grade IV "lumps" together all parenchymal lesions, whereas modern neuroimaging can distinguish many different types, and that the evolution of a parenchymal lesion often provides the best clue to which type of lesion it is. We prefer to refer to these as intraparenchymal lesions (IPLs). Using ultrasound it is not possible to make a definitive pathological diagnosis so the terms "grade IV intraventricular haemorrhage" and "parenchymal extension of intraventricular haemorrhage" should be abandoned. As yet there is no universal agreement on how to classify GMH-IVH or intraparenchymal lesions. Table 20.6 provides a suggested classification.

Pathology

The bleeding arises in the germinal matrix, a structure which is abundant over the head of the caudate nucleus and can also be found in the periventricular zone. The germinal matrix involutes early in the third trimester, making GMH-IVH rare in babies over 32 weeks gestation and 1.5 kg birth weight. The venous drainage of the deep white matter occurs via a fan shaped leash of vessels which drain into a vessel lateral to and below the germinal matrix (the vena terminalis). Obstruction of this vein is thought to be responsible for the common accompaniment of a fan-shaped white matter lesion on the same side as a GMH-IVH. These lesions are intraparenchymal venous infarctions which often become haemorrhagic and develop into a porencephalic cyst.

An IVH can occur at term. When it does, the baby has often been delivered by forceps or Ventouse (Towner *et al.* 1999). Other causes include vitamin K deficiency bleeding (pp. 447–449) or a coagulopathy associated with HIE.

Signs

In about half of the cases, mostly those with an uncomplicated GMH, the haemorrhage develops without causing any clinical signs. With bigger haemorrhages, babies often become limp and unresponsive, and may then develop short tonic fits with decerebrate posturing and a divergent squint.

If babies are breathing spontaneously they may become apnoeic, and are difficult to resuscitate because they have become hypotensive and acidaemic. Some of these changes are due to blood loss, but they are also due to reflex changes in the pulmonary vasculature following an abrupt rise in intracranial pressure (Malik 1977). Very characteristically the babies' PCV will drop by 5-10% after a few hours, and they often look pale and peripherally vasoconstricted. However, only if the GMH-IVH is very large does the neonate develop a tense anterior fontanelle or an acute increase in his head circumference.

Diagnosis

GMH-IVH is readily diagnosed with cerebral ultrasonography, and many neonatal units routinely screen all VLBW admissions this way (Fig 20.2(a)). A GMH can be recognized as an echogenic area between the caudate nucleus and the ventricle, and an IVH as an echogenic clot within the normally echolucent ventricle (Fig. 20.2(b)). Unilateral IPL accompanying GMH-IVH (Fig. 20.2(c)) is usually globular and on the same side, evolving over a period of weeks into a porencephalic cyst.

Prevention

Recognition of the importance of good general care, with attention to control of blood pressure and blood gases, gentle handling, gentle ventilation, combined with the benefits of antenatal steroids and postnatal surfactant, has produced a welcome decline in the incidence of GMH-IVH over the last decade. The interrelationship between clinical disturbance and GMH-IVH is one of the major justifications for the minimal handling concept (Chapter 8) and yet another reason for only sucking out endotracheal tubes if this is

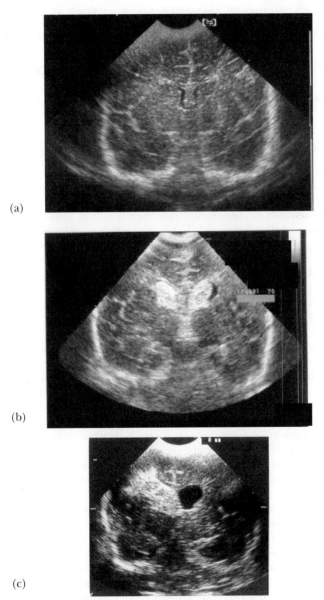

Figure 20.2 (a) Normal ultrasound scan, (b) IVH and (c) IPL accompanying GMH-IVH.

absolutely necessary (p. 154), and designing ventilator techniques which reduce the incidence of pneumothorax (p. 182).

The current low incidence of GMH-IVH and IPL that is seen in many units means that the use of specific prophylaxis has fallen. The most promising drug in this respect is indomethacin, but the long term outcome studies did not show benefit. Our current practice does not include routine drug prophylaxis against GMH-IVH.

Treatment and management of complications

Babies with GMH-IVH are often asymptomatic and neither receive nor need treatment. In those who do deteriorate, anaemia, acidaemia and hypotension usually respond promptly to blood transfusion and dopamine, and this often results in spontaneous resolution of the acidaemia. If it does not, infusions of base should be given. Fits should be controlled with phenobarbitone and coagulation abnormalities corrected. There is no specific treatment for GMH-IVH.

About 30% of babies with GMH-IVH develop post haemorrhagic ventricular dilatation (PHVD) on ultrasound scan; the larger the initial GMH-IVH the greater the risk of developing PHVD. When the initial bleed forms a cast of the whole ventricle, PHVD is a certainty. Enlargement of the ventricles can be imaged with ultrasound long before clinical symptoms or excessive head growth occur. In about 50% of babies with PHVD the condition is transient; the remaining 50% go on to develop hydrocephalus requiring treatment. Distinguishing between these groups is the key to management. In many babies the PHVD is mild and asymptomatic, and will resolve. Progressive hydrocephalus is very likely if the CSF pressure is more than 15 cm of water; the upper limit of normal pressure in the newborn is about 7 cm of water. Once the diagnosis has been made, a lumbar puncture should be done to measure the pressure, to exclude low grade infection as a cause of the ventricular enlargement, and to measure the CSF protein concentration in case a shunt is required.

Once PHVD has been recognized serial measurements of ventricular size and head circumference are mandatory. There are many measurement systems available, but we recommend the Levene ventricular index (Fig. 20.3). This linear measure, of the width of the lateral ventricle on a coronal ultrasound scan in the plane of the third ventricle, has proved robust and repeatable. There is no

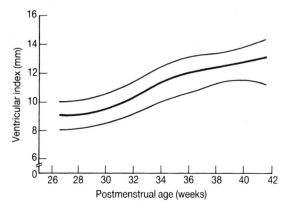

Figure 20.3 Normal range for the ventricular index (from Levene 1981).

evidence that early drainage of CSF or diuretic treatment alters the natural history of PHVD. Repeated ventricular taps are not recommended as they can result in multiple needle tracks through the brain.

Absolute indications for CSF drainage, either with a ventriculo-peritoneal shunt or via a reservoir if the baby is too frail or the CSF protein concentration is too high for a definitive procedure, include the following:

- symptoms such as apnoea, seizures, irritability or vomiting associated with a CSF pressure of more than 10 cm water;
- a head circumference enlarging at twice the normal rate for more than two weeks, or crossing two centile lines.

Prognosis

The prognosis for babies with uncomplicated GMH-IVH is good. Babies with PHVD which is non-progressive are at increased risk (by about 50%) of neurodevelopmental sequelae, whereas those who require shunting do less well. Babies with an IPL which evolves into a porencephalic cyst are at high risk of a hemiplegic cerebral palsy, with or without developmental delay. However, there is no certainty about this prognosis and many babies with large porencephalic cysts do surprisingly well.

PERIVENTRICULAR LEUKOMALACIA

- *Bilateral occipital PVL diagnosed with ultrasound in the neonatal period predicts cerebral palsy with virtually 99% certainty.*
- *PVL is not reliably diagnosed with neonatal ultrasound; later MRI detects far more cases.*
- *The aetiology of PVL is unclear; underperfusion of the periventricular white matter and the effects of cytokines (released during infective processes) on the oligodendroglia are thought to be important.*
- *There is no treatment of proven value to prevent PVL or which can modify its prognosis once changes are seen on ultrasound or with MR imaging; antenatal steroids may help.*

The term PVL was first coined to describe the "white spots" seen at autopsy in the periventricular white matter. In recent years it has been realized that in some cases the diagnosis can be made in life, either with ultrasound or MRI. Ultrasound remains a relatively insensitive technique for the detection of PVL, but there is a well recognized sequence of changes through a persisting periventricular "flare", via cystic cavities to periventricular loss of myelin which carries a poor prognosis. This is because damage to the deep white matter in the centrum semiovale is the main reason for spastic diplegia in ex-preterm babies. Damage to the myelin precursor cells (oligodendroglia) leads to a permanent reduction in myelin which can be imaged years later with MRI. Ultrasound scanning can detect evidence of white matter damage by detecting cystic change, but is relatively insensitive and cannot detect more subtle diffuse damage. The incidence of cystic PVL diagnosed with ultrasound is about 3% in VLBWI. A persistent "flare" or oedema in the periventricular white matter which is not followed by cystic change is thought to represent more subtle damage, and is diagnosed with ultrasound in up to 26% of preterm cohorts. Cohort studies using MR imaging are just emerging, and they suggest that white matter injury may be even more common than this. PVL and IPL (*v.s.*) can co-exist and bleeding may occur into an area of previous ischaemia.

PATHOGENESIS

This is less well understood than that of GMH-IVH, and PVL is less tightly linked to gestational age. Hypoxia-ischaemia or toxic injury to the oligodendroglia are thought to be important. There are associations between bacterial infection, both antenatal and postnatal, and white matter injury. Hypotension may be a factor but convincing evidence is lacking. Hypocarbia is important and levels below 3 kPa should be avoided (p. 140). Twins are at high risk, particularly those with twin-twin transfusion syndrome (pp.433–435) or where one twin has died.

DIAGNOSIS

There are few clinical signs, although some babies exhibit abnormal neurological behaviour and/or abnormal movement patterns. Ultrasound can detect cystic change in the white matter, and "flares" but autopsy studies confirm that many areas of diffuse gliosis are missed by ultrasound imaging.

PREVENTION AND TREATMENT

In contrast to GMH-IVH, for which many intervention studies have been performed both before and after delivery, hardly any data are available with regard to the prevention of PVL. However, antenatal steroids reduce postnatal PVL. Prevention of systemic hypotension is considered to be important. Adjusting ventilatory settings in order to avoid severe hypocarbia can be recommended. There is no treatment.

PROGNOSIS

Bilateral occipital cystic PVL is a depressingly reliable predictor of spastic diplegic cerebral palsy. Small anterior cysts, and cysts confined to the parietal region appear to have a better outlook. Studies are in progress regarding the prognosis of prolonged flare which does not progress to cyst formation. There may be an association with later childhood clumsiness.

NEONATAL HYPOTONIA

The common causes of a baby being very floppy during the neonatal period include the following:

- aftermath of birth asphyxia;
- prematurity;
- sepsis, including NEC;

- drug depression;
- hypoglycaemia;
- any severe illness with hypoxia and acidaemia.

These diagnoses are usually obvious and the hypotonia disappears as the baby recovers.

If these common causes of hypotonia can be excluded, there are a large number of rare differential diagnoses (Table 20.7). These babies usually require sophisticated biochemical, electrophysiological or morbid anatomical investigation, and should be referred to an appropriate centre. Most NNU's should be capable of managing neonatal myasthenia which can be diagnosed with a Tensilon test. Give 1 mg edrophonium chloride intravenously, the first 0.1 mg very slowly. If the baby's condition is due to transplacental passage of maternal acetylcholine receptor antibodies, then an exchange transfusion can be carried out. If this is not the case, treatment with pyridostigmine (5–10 mg every 4 hours) should be started. This topic has been fully reviewed by Dubowitz (1980).

Table 20.7 Causes of hypotonia

Condition	Differential diagnosis
Spinal cord injury	Usually breech delivery. Diagnose with MRI
Werdnig-Hoffman disease and variants	Absent tendon jerks; tongue fibrillation; EMG and muscle biopsy
Neonatal polio	Rare less than 2 weeks of age; culture stools; throat swab
Myasthenia gravis	Maternal history (not always); Tensilon test
Congenital myopathies e.g. central core disease, nemaline myopathy	EMG; muscle biopsy (see Dubowitz 1980)
Myotonic dystrophy	Examine mother. Baby often oedematous with respiratory difficulty; EMG and muscle biopsy
Malformation syndrome e.g. Down, Prader-Willi	Characteristic facies; other abnormalities; see Chapter 30
Inborn errors of metabolism e.g. glycogenoses, organic acidaemia	See Chapter 18
Benign congenital hypotonia	Diagnosis reached by exclusion

NERVE PALSIES

FACIAL PALSY

In the majority of cases of neonatal facial palsy the facial nerve has been injured by being compressed against the ramus of the mandible during a forceps delivery, and the facial weakness rapidly resolves during the first week. Difficulty with feeding may occasionally occur, and the baby should then be tube-fed until facial power returns. If a facial palsy occurs in a baby who was not delivered by forceps, then the lesion is either a nuclear agenesis – in which case evidence of other cranial nerve palsies is usually present (Möebius' syndrome); or the facial nerve had been squashed *in utero* between the mandible and some part of the maternal pelvis. The prognosis for recovery of function in the latter cases is poor.

ERB'S PALSY

The incidence of Erb's palsy is 1–2 per 1000 deliveries, and there is an association with macrosomia and shoulder dystocia. The upper cords of the brachial plexus C(4)56(7) may be torn by excessive traction when there is difficulty in delivering the anterior shoulder, or in extracting the head in a breech delivery. The clavicle is often fractured as well.

Virtually all movement at the shoulder joint is lost, and the baby cannot flex his elbow. His arm lies limply at his side in the 'waiter's tip' position. The biceps jerk is absent. The phrenic nerve may also be involved, and diaphragmatic paralysis should be sought in all babies with these arm abnormalities.

Most cases recover spontaneously, and no form of treatment has been shown to be of any benefit in the early neonatal period. If weakness persists beyond the first week, physiotherapy should be started to prevent joint contractures. Advances in microsurgical technique mean that surgical repair of the plexus should be considered if there is no return of biceps function by three months (Hunt 1988; Gilbert *et al.* 1991). This is because in these cases the prognosis for attaining full function is significantly impaired.

OTHER PERIPHERAL NERVE INJURIES

The radial nerve may be injured if the humerus is fractured during delivery, causing wrist drop. No specific treatment is required.

Damage to the lower cord of the brachial plexus (C78, T1 – Klumpke palsy) may occur when the arms of a breech are delivered. The baby has weakness in the muscles of the forearm and hand. This lesion is rare.

CENTRAL NERVOUS SYSTEM MALFORMATIONS

Diagnosis of malformations such as lissencephaly and schizencephaly has increased with the availability of MR scanning, and in some of these conditions the gene deletion or homeobox gene mutation is now known. Conversely, neural tube defects have become very rare in modern neonatal practice. Prenatal prophylaxis of neural tube defects with folic acid is feasible (MRC 1991) and antenatal detection is possible with ultrasound.

ANENCEPHALY

This is a uniformly fatal condition, although some babies live for a few weeks or even months. No attempt should be made to resuscitate a baby with anencephaly. The disorder is now rarely seen, since antenatal diagnosis is easy and most parents opt for termination.

ENCEPHALOCELE (CRANIUM BIFIDUM)

These are usually occipital and are comparatively rare. They may be part of complex multisystem malformations which are usually fatal shortly after birth.

Encephaloceles are usually skin covered, but when they are large, death may result from trauma to the lesion during an unexpectedly difficult delivery.

The prognosis for most babies is poor. With small lesions, which may just be meningoceles which contain no neural tissue, the prognosis is better, and complete neuroradiological and neurosurgical appraisal should be carried out after delivery.

HOLOPROSENCEPHALY

In this condition there is a single monoventricle. Sometimes there is the associated sign of a single nostril, or cyclops. The prognosis is poor.

SPINA BIFIDA WITH MENINGOCELE OR MENINGOMYELOCELE

Meningocele

Babies with these skin covered lesions which contain no neural tissue pose few immediate problems. They usually have small defects, and these can be repaired during the neonatal period or later. Orthopaedic problems are rare, and only about 10% of these babies develop hydrocephalus.

Meningomyelocele

These defects, in which the neural plate is exposed or is only covered with a thin film of easily ruptured leptomeninges, may occur in the cervical, thoracic or lumbar regions. Undiagnosed lesions are now rare. Immediately after delivery, an exposed lesion should be covered with a sterile, non-adhesive dressing to protect it from physical injury and to minimize the chance of infection. The baby should be admitted to the NNU for assessment by an experienced paediatrician and neurosurgeon, and the following features should be noted (Lorber 1972):

1. birth weight and gestation;
2. general condition (e.g. vigorous, neurologically depressed, shocked);
3. associated malformations (e.g. heart murmur, imperforate anus);
4. size, level and condition of the lesion;
5. severity of the neurological deficit, aiming to identify the lowest cord segment with detectable motor and sensory function;
6. sphincter function;
7. associated orthopaedic malformation (e.g. CDH, talipes);
8. degree of kyphoscoliosis – all babies should have a lateral spinal X-ray;
9. head circumference, shape, fontanelles, degree of hydrocephalus – all babies should have skull X-rays and a cerebral ultrasound;
10. eye movements and position.

Treatment

Treatment is surgical. The back is closed and a VP shunt inserted. There may still be a case for selective non-treatment if the prognosis is deemed to be very poor, but now that most severe lesions are detected antenatally liveborn cases are very rare. If the parents have elected to continue the pregnancy in such a case they will usually have already decided in favour of active surgical management.

LISSENCEPHALY/SCHIZENCEPHALY

The diagnosis is usually made by imaging during investigation of seizures or abnormal head size. These disorders involve either smooth brain (lissencephaly) or involve a cleft in the brain around the Sylvian fissure (schizencephaly).

AGENESIS OF THE CORPUS CALLOSUM

This diagnosis is made antenatally or postnatally by ultrasound, and confirmed on MR imaging. There is an association with trisomy 8, but often the abnormality is an isolated problem. The prognosis is then uncertain, but perhaps 50% of children are normal.

ISOLATED HYDROCEPHALUS

Hydrocephalus that is present at birth, or which develops during the neonatal period, may be due to congenital infection, congenital malformations or an acquired condition such as intracranial haemorrhage or meningitis.

A baby whose head circumference is increasing abnormally quickly should be referred for neuroradiological and neurosurgical assessment. In many cases, such as those with stenosis of the aqueduct or interventricular foramina and no other cerebral abnormality, the prognosis for long-term handicap-free survival is excellent after the insertion of a shunt.

REFERENCES

De Vries, L.S. and Rennie, J.M. (1999) Preterm brain injury. In: *Textbook of Neonatology*, 3rd edn. Rennie, J.M. and Roberton, N.R.C. (eds), Churchill Livingstone, Edinburgh pp. 1252–1271.

Dubowitz, V. (1980). The floppy infant. *Clinics in Developmental Medicine* No. 76. Spastics International Medical Publications. William Heinemann, London.

Gilbert, A., Brockman, R. and Carlioz, H. (1991) Surgical treatment of brachial plexus palsy. *Clinical Orthopaedics* **264**: 39–47.

Hunt, D. (1988) Surgical management of brachial plexus birth injuries. *Developmental Medicine and Child Neurology* **30**: 824–828.

Levene, M.I. (1981) Measurement of the growth of the lateral ventricles in pre-term infants with real-time ultrasound. *Archives of Disease in Childhood* **56**: 900–904.

Levene, M.I. (1999) Intracranial haemorrhage at term. In: *Textbook of Neonatology*, 3rd edn. Rennie, J.M. and Roberton, N.R.C. (eds), Churchill Livingstone, Edinburgh pp. 1223–1231.

Levene, M.I., Sands, C., Grindulis, H. and Moore, J.R. (1986) Comparison of two methods of predicting outcome in perinatal asphyxia. *Lancet* **i**: 67–68.

Lorber, J. (1972) Spina bifida cystica: results of treatment of 270 consecutive cases with criteria for selection for the future. *Archives of Disease in Childhood* **47**: 854–873.

Malik, A.B. (1977) Pulmonary vascular response to increase in intracranial pressure. *Journal of Applied Physiology* **42**: 335–343.

Medical Research Council (1991) Prevention of neural tube defects. Results of the Medical Research Council Vitamin Study. *Lancet* **338**: 131–137.

Peliowski, A. and Finer, N.N. (1992) Birth asphyxia in the term infant. In: *Effective Care of the Newborn Infant.* Sinclair, J.C. and Bracken, M.B. (eds), Oxford University Press, Oxford pp. 249–279.

Portman, R.J., Carter, B.S., Gaylord, M.S., Murphy, M.G., Thieme, R.E. and Merenstein, G.B. (1990) Predicting neonatal morbidity after perinatal asphyxia: a scoring system. *American Journal of Obstetrics and Gynecology* **162**: 174–182.

Rutherford, M., Pennock, J.M., Schwieso, J., Cowan, F. and Dubowitz, L.M.S. (1996) Hypoxic ischaemic encephalopathy: early and late magnetic resonance imaging findings in relation to outcome. *Archives of Disease in Childhood* **75**: F145–F151.

Towner, D., Castro, M.A., Eby-Wilkens, E. and Gilbert, W.M. (1999) Effect of mode of delivery in nulliparous women on neonatal intracranial haemorrhage. *New England Journal of Medicine* **341**: 1709–1714.

FURTHER READING

Levene, M.I., Lilford, M.I., Bennett, M.J. and Punt, J. (eds) (1995) *Fetal and Neonatal Neurology and Neurosurgery*, 2nd edn. Churchill Livingstone, Edinburgh and London.

Volpe, J.J. (2001) *Neurology of the Newborn*, 5th edn. Saunders, Philadelphia.

Section on neonatal neurology. In: *Textbook of Neonatology*, 3rd edn. Rennie, J.M. and Roberton, N.R.C. (eds), Churchill Livingstone, Edinburgh, 1203–1311.

21

DRUG WITHDRAWAL

Illicit drug use continues to increase, with the worrying associations between intravenous drug addiction, alcohol misuse, HIV and hepatitis B or C infection, unemployment/poverty, squalid accommodation, parental imprisonment and social isolation continuing to present a threat to babies who are being cared for by these chaotic families. A wide spectrum of drugs taken by the mothers in addition to narcotics, can induce abstinence syndrome in their babies (Table 21.1).

During pregnancy the aim is to reduce fetal exposure to fluctuating drug levels, and in general this means replacing heroin with methadone. Babies who are born to drug abusing mothers are often preterm and small-for-dates, but are protected against RDS, because many of these drugs mature the surfactant synthesizing enzymes.

Table 21.1 Drugs described as being associated with a neonatal withdrawal syndrome (From Rivers 1999)

Drug	Time of onset of withdrawal
Heroin	0–96 hours (peak 12–24 hours)
Methadone	12–72 hours (peak 24–48 hours); can be up to 2 weeks
Short acting barbiturates	0–24 hours
Longer acting barbiturates	>7 days
Diazepam	2–6 hours
Chlordiazepoxide	3 weeks
Tricyclic antidepressants	0–12 hours
Propoxyphene	<24 hours
Pentazocine	<24 hours
Codeine	<24 hours
Dihydrocodeine (DF118)	<48 hours
Alcohol	<24 hours

Table 21.2 Signs of opiate withdrawal

Jitteriness, irritability, shrill cry
Hyperactivity, poor sleeping, wakefulness
Excessive sucking, hyperphagia
Seizures
Diarrhoea, vomiting, reflux
Snuffles, sneezing, salivation
Tachypnoea
Yawning, hiccoughs
Sweating, fever

OPIATE WITHDRAWAL SYNDROME

Between 60 and 90% of babies born to opiate using mothers develop withdrawal, usually in the first 24 hours. The clinical features of those who do develop symptoms are summarized in Table 21.2. The typical baby is intensely irritable and miserable with jitteriness, poor sleeping, crying, snuffles and feeding problems. These babies frantically suck at their hands, and are excessively alert and agitated. Despite all the sucking they are not good at co-ordinating swallowing, and vomiting and diarrhoea are frequent. If the drug use is concealed, analysis of urine can be done to make the diagnosis.

An important part of the management of these babies is good nursing care, swaddling, a quiet environment and small frequent feeds. Several scoring systems have been devised, and one such chart is reproduced as Fig. 21.1. At any time the baby may score 0 or 1 for each item, with a maximum total score of 10.

Babies who score more than 6 on two occasions more than 2–4 hours apart should be treated. We use oral morphine or the intravenous form of methadone given orally. This prevents seizures, and has superseded the older treatments involving chlorpromazine, phenobarbitone, paregoric and diazepam. The dose of oral morphine is 0.5 mg/kg/dose given four times a day, and the dose can be increased to 0.75 mg/kg/dose. Wean by 0.05 mg/dose every 2–3 days. Methadone can be used in a dose of 0.1 mg/kg/dose four times a day; increase by 0.05 mg/kg/dose if symptoms are not controlled. Reduce the dose slowly, by 10–20% a day once control is achieved (i.e. score <5).

WITHDRAWAL CHART

Irritability								
Scratching								
Wakefulness								
Shrill cry								
Tremors								
Hypertonicity								
Convulsions								
Pyrexia >38°C								
Tachypnoea >60								
Vomiting								
Diarrhoea								
Yawning								
Hiccoughs								
Salivation								
Stuffy nose								
Sneezing								
Sweating								
Dehydration								
SCORE								
TIME								
DATE								

Figure 21.1 Drug withdrawal chart. Score 1 if item is present and if it is absent. (Reproduced from Rivers, 1999, with permission.)

COCAINE

Maternal abuse of cocaine causes major problems for the fetus, mainly due to the vasoconstrictor and hypertensive effects of this drug. These damage tissues by ischaemia and vascular disruption, and their effects include fetal cerebral infarction or haemorrhage, bowel atresia, limb reduction defects and renal tract dilatation. In addition, as with opiates, these babies may be born prematurely and SFD, and have a reduced incidence of RDS. More specifically, abruptio placenta occurs in a high proportion of pregnancies (Jones 1991).

CANNABIS/MARIJUANA

Day and Richardson (1991) reviewed the extensive literature on this subject. If maternal cannabis use has any deleterious effects on the fetus or on the neonate they are small.

ALCOHOL

Although binge drinkers are likely to produce babies with fetal alcohol syndrome or abstinence syndrome a study from Scotland among women without associated problems like malnutrition and drug abuse showed no ill effects from social alcohol consumption during pregnancy (Forrest *et al.* 1991).

REFERENCES

Day, N.L. and Richardson, G.A. (1991) Perinatal marijuana use: epidemiology, methodologic issues and infant outcome. *Clinics in Perinatology* **18**: 77–91.

Forrest, F., Florey, C. du V., Taylor, D., McPherson, F. and Young, J.A. (1991) Reported social alcohol consumption during pregnancy and infants' development at 18 months. *British Medical Journal* **303**: 22–26.

Jones, K.L. (1991) Developmental pathogenesis of defects associated with prenatal cocaine exposure: fetal vascular disruption. *Clinics in Perinatology* **18**: 139–146.

Rivers, R. (1999) Infants of drug addicted mothers. In: *Textbook of Neonatology*, 3rd edn. Rennie, J.M. and Roberton, N.R.C. (eds), Churchill Livingstone, Edinburgh pp. 443–451.

FURTHER READING

Prenatal drug exposure and child outcome. *Clinics in Perinatology*, March 1999, Volume 26, no. 1.

Rivers, R. (1999) Infants of drug addicted mothers. In: *Textbook of Neonatology*, 3rd edn. Rennie, J.M. and Roberton, N.R.C. (eds), T Churchill Livingstone, Edinburgh pp. 443–451.

22

CONGENITAL HEART DISEASE IN THE NEONATAL PERIOD

━━━

- *Innocent murmurs are very common in babies.*
- *The features of an innocent murmur are that the baby is well, the murmur is systolic with normal heart sounds and does not radiate, and the pulses are normal.*
- *Many babies with significant cardiac disease have no murmur.*
- *The investigation of choice is an echocardiogram.*
- *Babies who present in shock with acidosis and mottled peripheries can have left heart outflow problems such as coarctation of the aorta or aortic atresia.*

The incidence of congenital heart disease is slightly less than one in a hundred live births. One-third of these babies have severe defects which present in the neonatal period with either cyanosis, cardiac failure, low output shock or an arrhythmia. The risk of CHD is increased in the following situations:

- a parent or sibling has CHD;
- the baby has a syndrome or malformation known to be linked with CHD (e.g. Down syndrome, Turner syndrome, Di George syndrome, exomphalos, TAR);
- the mother has diabetes, or collagen vascular disease, or has exposed the fetus to teratogens (e.g. alcohol, phenytoin, lithium);
- the fetus is found to be hydropic or to have an arrhythmia.

Increasingly the diagnosis of CHD is made antenatally by specialized detailed ultrasonography, but the detection rate of the routine 18 to 20 week fetal anomaly scan remains poor. The four chamber view obtained detects less than 50% of CHD and a "normal" result cannot provide total reassurance. Coarctation and VSD are easily missed. Early diagnosis of CHD is vital because the outlook for these children has improved dramatically since the first ductal ligation was performed almost 60 years ago.

THE FETAL CIRCULATION

There are two key differences between the fetal and the neonatal circulation:

- The fetus supplies blood to the low resistance, high flow placental bed.
- During fetal life only 10% of the cardiac output goes to the lungs, and the pulmonary vascular bed is a relatively high resistance, low-flow circuit.

There are three vascular structures which close soon after birth. These are:

- *the ductus venosus,* which channels some of the returning oxygenated blood travelling in the umbilical vein from the placenta through the liver, into the IVC and hence into the right atrium (Fig. 22.1);
- *the foramen ovale,* which is a flap valve opening between the atria which allows 33% of the blood returning to the right heart to be diverted to the left atrium and hence to the aorta;

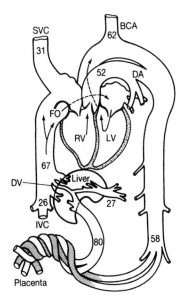

Figure 22.1 The fetal circulation. The numbers represent the SaO$_2$ in fetal lambs.

- *the ductus arteriosus*, which in fetal life has right to left flow and diverts blood from the pulmonary artery into the descending aorta before it reaches the lungs.

Oxygenated blood returns from the placenta via the umbilical vein to the fetus. Once it reaches the fetal body, some blood passes through the liver to the hepatic vein and IVC, and the remainder bypasses the liver by travelling through the ductus venosus to enter the IVC. Within the right atrium blood flowing from the IVC is separated into two parts. Approximately 33% passes through the foramen ovale, into the left atrium, left ventricle, and ascending aorta (Fig. 22.1). This ensures that the coronary arteries and the brain receive blood with the highest PaO_2. The remainder of the IVC flow passes into the right ventricle and pulmonary artery.

Deoxygenated blood returning from the upper part of the fetal body returns through the SVC into the right atrium and almost all of it passes into the right ventricle. Most of the output of the RV passes from the PA through the ductus arteriosus into the descending aorta, where it is joined by blood ejected from the left ventricle. The ductus is kept patent in utero by circulating and locally produced prostaglandins.

CHANGES IN THE CIRCULATION AT BIRTH

At birth, the site of oxygen uptake changes from the placenta to the lungs. This occurs as follows:

1. The baby takes his first breath, pulmonary vascular resistance falls and pulmonary blood flow increases. Delay in this normal fall results in PPHN (p. 189–194).
2. The umbilical cord is clamped, the ductus venosus begins to close (closure is complete in 76% of normal newborns by the 7th day, (Fugelseth *et al.* 1997). The IVC flow falls and the systemic vascular resistance rises.
3. The increased pulmonary blood flow increases the pulmonary venous return and raises the left atrial pressure. The differential pressure between the left and right atria tends to close the foramen ovale, though bidirectional shunting across the foramen ovale is common in the normal neonate. Right to left shunting can become evident clinically if the right atrial pressure is higher than normal.
4. The ductus arteriosus closes owing to the rise in PaO_2 and a fall

in circulating prostaglandin levels. By about twelve hours of age the ductus arteriosus is functionally closed in 90% of normal neonates. Closure may be delayed in conditions associated with hypoxaemia (e.g. RDS p. 136, cyanotic CHD *v.i.*, PPHN p. 191). Complete obliteration of the ductus takes up to one year.

PRESENTATION OF HEART DISEASE

Symptomatic heart disease in the neonate presents as cyanosis, shock or heart failure, or less commonly as a combination of two of these. Asymptomatic heart disease may come to light because of the incidental finding of a murmur or weak pulses, or because of the association with another diagnosis, for instance Down syndrome.

Precise diagnosis of anatomical lesions depends upon specialist investigations. The initial clinical assessment will often not point to a definite diagnosis. Rather it should be directed at answering the following specific questions:

1. Does the baby have heart disease?
2. How seriously ill is he?
3. Does he need immediate treatment?
4. Does he need referral for further investigation?

HISTORY

The history is of limited value in the diagnosis of CHD in the neonate, but it should be determined whether there is a family history of CHD, or a maternal history of diabetes mellitus or other maternal conditions that might affect the neonate's heart (e.g. systemic lupus erythematosus). Any maternal illness and/or drug ingestion during pregnancy should also be noted. There may be poor feeding, excess weight gain, or sweating in the baby.

EXAMINATION

The most important part of the examination of neonates with suspected heart disease is observation. If possible, the examination should be when the baby is quiet and settled.

Look for:

1. Cyanosis. This is surprisingly easy to miss, especially in neonates with dark skin pigmentation. Look carefully at the tongue and

mucous membranes. Use a pulse oximeter (p. 103) if in any doubt. Remember that cyanosis depends on the presence of more than 5 g% deoxygenated haemoglobin, so it is more obvious in plethoric babies and may not be detectable in anaemic babies. Normal babies can become cyanosed whilst crying but the colour does not persist.

2. Dyspnoea. Count the respiratory rate, but what is more important is to observe the pattern of breathing. Look for recession and grunting. Tachypnoea with no or moderate recession is the common pattern of breathlessness due to heart failure.

3. Look for the apex beat; is there a hyperdynamic praecordium?

4. Note dysmorphic features that would indicate a syndrome of which heart disease could be part (e.g. Down, Turner, Noonan syndromes).

Feel for:

1. The heart rate, from either a peripheral pulse or the cardiac impulse. Heart failure may be due to a paroxysmal tachycardia, or less commonly a bradycardia. Fast heart rates can be difficult to count accurately, so if necessary run off an ECG rhythm strip to confirm the rate.

2. The strength of the pulses in all four limbs and the carotids. If the baby is quiet, the brachial, femoral and axillary pulses can all be felt. If all of the pulses are weak or absent, then there may be severe left heart disease with a poor cardiac output. Weak femoral pulses with good volume upper limb pulses suggest an abnormality of the aortic arch such as a coarctation or interruption. If there is any doubt about the pulses it is important to measure the systolic blood pressure in all four limbs. Care needs to be taken to obtain accurate blood pressure measurements. It is important that the baby is quiet. Use cuffs which cover two-thirds of the upper arm, ideally with a Doppler probe to detect the pulse. Oscillometric measurements are useful, but are not always reliable. Make sure that the measurements are reproducible before you accept them.

3. Peripheral perfusion. Test capillary refill, which should be <3 seconds. Note clammy mottled skin, which is often a sign of significant heart disease in a neonate.

4. The size of the liver. Oedema is rare in neonates, but hepatic enlargement is commonly seen. Measure, in cm, how far the liver edge extends below the costal margin at the mid-clavicular line.

5. Thrills. Praecordial thrills are nothing more than loud murmurs.

They always indicate heart disease, although the degree of loudness is not a measure of the severity of the defect.

Listen for:

1. Murmurs. Transient (innocent) systolic murmurs in the neonatal period are common (*v.i.*). The commonest cause is a mild degree of branch pulmonary artery narrowing which resolves with growth and disappears by the age of 6 months (Arlettaz *et al.* 1998). Innocent murmurs are not associated with any other signs of heart disease. The murmurs of ventricular septal defects are often heard only after the neonatal period, when the drop in pulmonary vascular resistance has caused sufficient shunt across the defect to cause turbulence.

     Serious heart disease may exist without any murmurs being detected in the first weeks of life.

2. The heart sounds. Splitting of the second heart sound is said to be detectable in 50% of neonates by 4 hours and in 80% by 48 hours. In practice clinical determination of the splitting of the second sound in neonates is often unreliable.

3. Any other added sounds or ejection clicks. A gallop rhythm is frequently heard in babies with heart failure.

INVESTIGATIONS

Echocardiography has revolutionized the ability to diagnose and manage CHD. Consequently, the chest X-ray and ECG have become less important. Echocardiography is readily available and non-invasive. If there is any doubt about whether or not a neonate has significant CHD, an echocardiogram should be carried out without delay.

CHEST X-RAY

The chest X-ray is seldom diagnostic in CHD. Nevertheless, it is still an essential base line investigation. The position of the heart, abdominal situs, the heart size and pulmonary vascularity should be assessed. On some films it is possible to determine the side of the aortic arch and the bronchial situs. A cardiothoracic ratio of more than 60% is outside the normal range in the neonatal period.

ECG

For information on how to interpret the neonatal ECG, including the criteria for ventricular hypertrophy and the axis, see Appendix D.

ECHOCARDIOGRAPHY

Echocardiography is usually the definitive investigation in structural heart disease in the neonate. Babies have excellent echocardiographic "windows", so that detailed anatomical views can be obtained of the whole of the heart and most of the major vessels. The main exceptions are the aortic arch, which cannot be imaged very well in a minority of cases and the peripheral pulmonary arteries, which are hidden by the surrounding lung tissue. Cross-sectional echocardiography is supplemented by Doppler measurements of blood flows within the heart and great vessels and by direct colour Doppler imaging of blood flows. Diagnosis is now so precise that it is rarely necessary to perform any additional imaging studies in neonates before undertaking treatment by surgery or transcatheter procedures.

DIFFERENTIAL DIAGNOSIS

An approach to the differential diagnosis of babies with probable heart disease is given in Figs 22.2–22.4 (modified from Franklin *et al.* 1991).

HEART MURMURS IN ASYMPTOMATIC BABIES

Heart murmurs are commonly heard during the neonatal examination (*v.s.*). The exact prevalence varies widely, and depends on the postnatal age and skill of the examiner. The incidence of murmurs detected ranges from 6 to 759 per 1000 neonatal examinations (Ainsworth *et al.* 1999 (6:1000), Arlettaz *et al.* 1998 (21:1000), Braudo and Rowe 1961 (750:1000), Hallidie-Smith 1960 (759:1000)).

The most helpful "further investigation" of a baby with a murmur is an examination by an experienced observer. A chest X-ray and ECG were traditionally performed, but add little to this clinical assessment in distinguishing those babies with significant CHD.

Innocent murmurs have several positive features (Arlettaz *et al.* 1998):

- the murmur is grade 1-2/6 and heard at the left sternal edge without radiation;
- there are no audible clicks;

- the pulses are normal;
- the baby is otherwise well.

Suspicious features on examination such as:

- murmur grade 3/6 or more, radiating to the back or upper left sternal edge;
- pansystolic murmur;
- murmur extending into diastole;
- harsh quality;
- abnormal second heart sound;
- early or mid-systolic click.

Suspicious features mean that the baby should remain in hospital, a chest X-ray and ECG should be obtained, and an early cardiological opinion with echocardiography sought. See Figs 22.2–4. Otherwise the baby can go home to be reviewed in outpatients in a few weeks. We no longer perform a CXR or ECG in this situation. Give general advice to the parents with instructions to return early if the baby feeds poorly, fails to gain weight, or is breathless.

CHD PRESENTING AS SHOCK WITH ACIDOSIS

Babies with poor left heart function (hypoplastic left heart syndrome, p. 357; interrupted aortic arch, severe coarctation of the aorta, p. 356) frequently present with shock during the first few days of life. The baby feeds poorly, grunts, has cold peripheries, and progresses to become mottled with a generally low volume pulse. Investigation reveals a profound metabolic acidosis and there can be confusion with a diagnosis of inborn error of metabolism (p. 297). It is important to exclude treatable CHD as early as possible in this situation because some of these babies have an excellent chance of intact survival with surgery.

CHD PRESENTING AS HEART FAILURE

SIGNS OF HEART FAILURE

Neonates with heart failure usually present with breathlessness on feeding and increasing lethargy. The babies are either lethargic or irritable, and may be cold, pale and sweaty, with grunting, indrawing

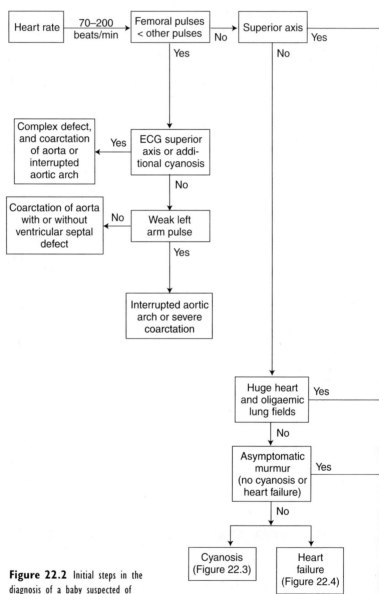

Figure 22.2 Initial steps in the diagnosis of a baby suspected of congenital heart disease (modified from Franklin *et al.* 1991).

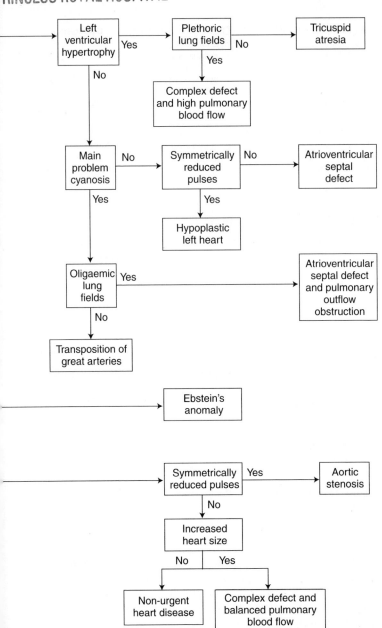

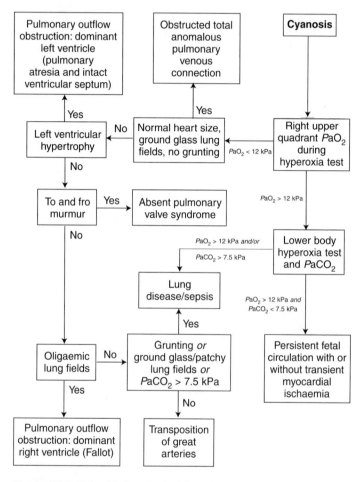

Figure 22.3 Differential diagnosis of a baby with cyanosis (modified from Franklin *et al.* 1991).

and possibly cyanosis. The respiratory rate will be increased to >60 breaths/min; tachypnoea may be the only sign of mild heart failure. There may be pulmonary crepitations, and a tachycardia of at least 150 beats/min. The severity of heart failure can be assessed by the degree of hepatomegaly. Weight gain in excess of 30 g/kg/24 h suggests fluid retention (Table 22.1).

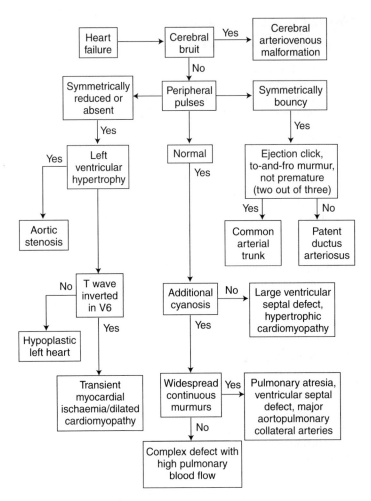

Figure 22.4 Differential diagnosis of CHD where heart failure is present (modified from Franklin *et al.* 1991).

Feel the peripheral pulses, and listen to the heart to see if there is a gallop rhythm, as well as the signs that are characteristic of the individual defect. The CXR will show an increased cardiothoracic ratio, and may show increased pulmonary vascular markings, possibly pulmonary oedema.

Table 22.1 Symptoms of congestive cardiac failure in neonates

- Tachypnoea over 60/min with or without a grunt
- Pallor and sweating during feeds
- Taking more than 30 minutes to feed
- Tachycardia over 150 beats/min
- Hepatomegaly over 2 cm or progressive enlargement
- Cardiomegaly, cardiothoracic ratio greater than 60% on CXR
- Gallop rhythm
- Weight gain in excess of 30 g/24 h
- Failure to thrive

CAUSES OF HEART FAILURE

In premature babies, heart failure can be caused by the following:

1. persistent ductus arteriosus;
2. ventricular septal defect);
3. metabolic causes – hypoxia, hypoglycaemia, hypocalcaemia, hypomagnesaemia.

In full-term babies from birth to one week, one of the following is likely to be the cause of the heart failure. These are predominantly diseases of the left side of the heart:

1. aortic atresia;
2. severe aortic valve stenosis;
3. coarctation of the aorta;
4. interrupted aortic arch;
5. transient myocardial ischaemia of the newborn;
6. cardiomyopathies (e.g. Coxsackie B myocarditis);
7. arrhythmias (tachycardias or bradycardias);
8. arteriovenous fistulae (e.g. cerebral or hepatic);
9. atrioventricular valve incompetence;
10. arterial valve incompetence;
11. obstructed anomalous pulmonary venous drainage;
12. combined complex lesions.

After the first week, as the pulmonary vascular resistance falls, left to right shunts become an important cause of heart failure, these include the following:

1. VSD;
2. PDA;
3. truncus arteriosus;

4. non-obstructed anomalous pulmonary venous drainage;
5. atrioventricular septal defect.

TREATMENT OF HEART FAILURE IN THE NEWBORN

1. Correct all associated metabolic problems and apply the routines of neonatal cardiorespiratory care described in Chapter 11.
2. Make sure that the baby has an adequate calorie intake; use NG feeding if he cannot take an adequate volume for himself. Additives to milk are often needed.
3. Nurse the baby in the neutral temperature range (p.10).
4. Administer diuretics: give frusemide first. If more than once daily frusemide is required, add spironolactone in the same dose as frusemide. A check should be kept on the electrolytes, particularly in premature babies.
5. Consider ACE inhibitors (e.g. captopril). These reduce the work of the heart and may reduce the size of a left to right shunt. Neither ACE inhibitors nor digoxin should be used if there is any outflow obstruction on the left side of the heart. Consequently neither of these drugs should be used without cardiological assessment and advice.
6. Digoxin. The demarcation between the therapeutic and toxic dose is narrow, and the response to the drug varies markedly, but neonates require lower doses than older children. Rapid digitalization should not be required. Digoxin should only be used on the advice of a cardiologist, and is rarely beneficial.
7. If heart failure cannot be controlled medically, surgical correction of the lesion offers the baby the only hope of survival. It is essential that the anatomical diagnosis be obtained in all babies presenting in heart failure. If the heart failure is severe arrange early transfer to a specialist centre.

INDIVIDUAL CONDITIONS WHICH CAN CAUSE HEART FAILURE OR SHOCK (Fig. 22.4)

PERSISTENT DUCTUS ARTERIOSUS

In premature babies usually recovering from RDS, a symptomatic PDA presents with a progressive increase in $PaCO_2$, an increasing inspired oxygen requirement and the need for more vigorous IPPV

(p. 172). In babies who are not on IPPV, PDA presents with increasing dyspnoea, increasing oxygen requirements or apnoeic episodes.

On examination, the pulses are bounding with a hyperactive praecordium, tachycardia and often a gallop rhythm. A systolic, or continuous, murmur is maximal at the first left intercostal space; and a mid-diastolic murmur at the apex may be audible. The CXR may show an increased heart size and pulmonary plethora, but the ECG is not helpful.

Echocardiography has shown that the ductus is patent in many preterm babies whether or not they are symptomatic. In symptomatic babies, echocardiography shows normal anatomy, but an enlarged left atrium and left ventricle indicative of a left to right shunt. It is usually possible to see the ductus in suprasternal notch views and to demonstrate flow across it with colour Doppler. The significance of a PDA detected with echocardiography must be assessed in the light of the clinical picture.

Treatment consists of controlling pulmonary oedema by respiratory support with CPAP or IPPV plus PEEP, and fluid restriction initially to 60–90 ml/kg. Fluids can be increased by 10 ml/kg per day, provided that there is no oedema and the urine osmolarity is in excess of 200 mosmol/kg, until a slow but steady weight gain is attained. Frusemide can be given, but there are theoretical reasons and some clinical evidence to suggest that frusemide promotes ductal patency. Indomethacin in a dose of 0.1 mg/kg per day for 6 days or 0.2 mg/kg, 8–12 hourly for three doses can achieve closure, but to be effective it needs to be given early – preferably less than 8 days after birth. In these circumstances indomethacin has a response rate of nearly 80%. A third of babies relapse. Often when they relapse no further treatment is required because they have been successfully weaned from ventilation, but in babies who are still ventilator dependent a further course can be tried. Indomethacin is less effective in babies who, irrespective of gestation, are more than 3 weeks old. Surgical closure should be considered in babies who remain ventilator dependent and who prove to be unresponsive to indomethacin. Indomethacin should always be used first, unless it is contraindicated. Contraindications include thrombocytopenia, renal failure, or NEC.

COARCTATION OF THE AORTA

Severe forms of coarctation, often with marked tubular hypoplasia of the aortic isthmus, present with heart failure. The symptoms arise when the ductus begins to close, and this can occur on the first day or during the first week of life. Less severe forms may be detected because of weak or absent peripheral pulses in an asymptomatic baby.

The abnormality of the peripheral pulses may be masked by persistence of the ductus arteriosus. However, Doppler measurements of systolic blood pressure usually show more than a 20 mmHg difference between the upper and lower limbs. The upper limb hypertension may not be present if there is a large VSD giving a low resistance run off into the pulmonary circulation. There may be a gallop rhythm and either no murmur or the systolic murmur of a VSD, atrioventricular valve incompetence or aortic stenosis. Differential pulses between the two arms suggest an aberrant origin of one subclavian artery.

Chest X-ray shows a large heart with pulmonary venous congestion. The ECG shows either biventricular or right ventricular hypertrophy. Cross-sectional echocardiography will demonstrate the associated lesions and shows narrowing of the aortic arch in the isthmal area, often with a shelf projecting from the posterior wall of the aorta. The coarctation shelf is usually preceded by a hypoplastic segment, and the transverse aorta may be hypoplastic too. Aortic valve abnormalities are present in 25% of cases.

Urgent transfer to a cardiac centre is required. Pending transfer treatment for heart failure should be started, and the baby should be ventilated for transfer. Start an infusion of prostaglandin E_2 to maintain ductal patency. Consider starting an infusion of dopamine (5 microg/kg/min) to improve renal perfusion.

Early surgical repair of the coarctation is performed. This may be combined with repair of any associated lesions, such as a VSD. Coarctation repair can be combined with pulmonary artery banding for complex defects with an unrestricted pulmonary blood flow.

Repair of the coarctation leads to a rapid improvement of the heart failure. Recurrence of the coarctation is not uncommon, so careful surveillance of these babies is essential. Repair often leads to a reduced pulse in the left arm. This can cause difficulties with subsequent blood pressure measurements.

AORTIC ATRESIA (HYPOPLASTIC LEFT HEART)

Babies with this condition are of normal birth weight and gestational age, but cardiac failure with shock and varying degrees of cyanosis appear soon after birth. Poor or absent peripheral pulses in all areas and mottled peripheries are characteristic. There is a marked metabolic acidosis. Auscultation reveals a loud single second heart sound. A soft ductal murmur may be present. Chest radiography shows marked cardiomegaly, with pulmonary congestion – a "globular heart". The ECG shows right axis deviation, right atrial hypertrophy, right ventricular hypertrophy, with a qR pattern over the right praecordial leads. If this condition is suspected it is essential that an early echocardiogram is obtained so that the parents can be advised of the diagnosis. If necessary the condition of the baby can be improved by a prostaglandin infusion pending definitive diagnosis.

Cross-sectional echocardiography will confirm the diagnosis. The mitral valve is small or imperforate, and the left ventricular cavity small, often with a thick wall with endocardial fibroelastosis. The aortic valve is an imperforate membrane, with a small valve ring and a small ascending aorta that may be little larger than a coronary artery, and nearly always is less than 6 mm in diameter. The descending aorta is of normal size, and the aortic arch tapers towards the heart as the head and neck vessels come off. A large patent ductus connecting the main pulmonary artery with the descending aorta is the only source of systemic blood flow.

Most cardiac centres offer, rather than recommend, treatment for this condition. Treatments are being undertaken in a very few centres (neonatal heart transplantation, the Norwood operation). These remain very controversial. Without treatment the condition is fatal, usually within a few days.

AORTIC VALVE STENOSIS

When this is severe, it presents with cardiac failure and a low output state. There may be hypotension and acidosis, which are more severe the tighter the stenosis. The pulses are all of small volume. There is an ejection systolic murmur at the second right intercostal space, conducted to the carotid vessels. The lack of an ejection click reflects the severe obstruction in this age group. The second heart sound is closely split or often single. If the carotid artery is palpated routinely during clinical examination for a thrill, then few cases of aortic stenosis should be missed.

Chest X-ray shows a large heart with pulmonary venous congestion. The ECG shows left ventricular hypertrophy – differentiating it from aortic atresia – occasionally with ST segment depression, and T wave inversion. Cross-sectional echocardiography shows a thickened, usually dysplastic, aortic valve that may be bicuspid. The ascending aorta may be smaller than usual but is more than 6 mm in diameter. The left ventricle is thick walled, often with endocardial fibroelastosis, and may show reduced contractility. Doppler can be used to measure the gradient across the aortic valve, but at this age, gradient is not an indication of severity as low velocity may reflect poor ventricular function and reduced cardiac output.

The prognosis for this condition is critically dependent on the function of the left ventricle, which can be seen to deteriorate during fetal life. Overall, when aortic stenosis presents in the neonatal period there is a mortality of about 50%. Early referral to a specialist centre is essential. Treatment is usually by balloon dilation of the aortic valve. Pending transfer, treat the heart failure and acidosis appropriately. If the failure and low output state are severe, an attempt to reopen the ductus with a prostaglandin infusion is indicated. Ventilate the baby for transfer, and consider starting a dopamine infusion.

VENTRICULAR SEPTAL DEFECT

This is the commonest form of CHD and a large defect can cause heart failure in the first weeks of life. Most VSDs do not present at this time, and the murmur appears later as the right heart pressure falls. There is a harsh systolic murmur and the chest X-ray shows a large heart with pulmonary plethora. The ECG may show biventricular hypertrophy. Medical treatment for heart failure should be tried, but babies who do not respond need early surgery.

ATRIOVENTRICULAR CANAL DEFECT

This condition is associated with Down syndrome. There is a complex intra-atrial and ventricular septal defect.

PULMONARY ATRESIA WITH VSD AND MAJOR AORTO-PULMONARY COLLATERAL ARTERIES

In this condition the pulmonary circulation is usually supplied by a PDA with or without MAPCAs. The pulmonary arteries are often underdeveloped. Pulmonary atresia with a VSD presents in a similar fashion to tetralogy of Fallot (*v.i.*). There will be no murmur from the right ventricular outflow tract, but continuous murmurs from major pulmonary collateral arteries may be present. PA with a VSD and MAPCAs is usually treated like severe tetralogy. The prognosis depends upon the presence and size of the pulmonary arteries. If central pulmonary arteries are present, the first step is usually an aortopulmonary shunt. The condition is associated with Di George syndrome and 22q11 deletions.

TRUNCUS ARTERIOSUS (CAN PRESENT WITH CYANOSIS AND HEART FAILURE)

This defect consists of a single arterial trunk that leaves the heart through a single semilunar valve and supplies the aorta, the pulmonary trunk and the coronary arteries. A subarterial VSD is always present. The baby is usually not obviously cyanosed, but a hyperoxia test is abnormal. The pulses are bounding because of the run off to the lungs through the pulmonary arteries. The first heart sound is normal. There is an ejection click in 50% of cases, an ejection systolic murmur is heard at the upper left sternal border, but may be very quiet, and there is a loud single second sound, which represents truncal closure. An early diastolic murmur of truncal valve insufficiency, which is diagnostic if present, is a bad prognostic sign. There is tachypnoea, and heart failure develops usually in the third or fourth week.

Initial management consists of vigorous treatment of heart failure.

HEART MUSCLE DISEASE

Several forms of cardiomyopathy can produce heart failure in the neonatal period. These include the following:

- hypoxic ischaemic myocardial injury
- anomalous origin of the left coronary artery
- viral myocarditis (p. 254)
- hypertrophic cardiomyopathy
- hypoglycaemia.

The most common conditions that cause neonatal hypertrophic cardiomyopathy are maternal diabetes and steroid treatment for CLD. These two conditions do not usually give rise to symptoms and need no treatment. Hypertrophic cardiomyopathy of the autosomal dominant variety, or in association with Noonan syndrome may be progressive and give rise to symptoms because of outflow tract obstruction and poor ventricular compliance or serious arrhythmias. More rarely, the cause is a glycogen storage disease or a mitochondrial abnormality. The management is difficult and controversial. Inotropes and vasodilators may be detrimental as they can accentuate the left ventricular outflow obstruction. There may be a role for beta blockade in some cases, under supervision of a paediatric cardiologist.

CYANOTIC HEART DISEASE
(see Fig. 22.2 and Fig. 22.3 for differential diagnosis)

DIAGNOSIS

Cyanosis with minimal dyspnoea in a baby should suggest the possibility of cardiac disease, particularly if the CXR does not show the evidence of respiratory disease (Table 11.5). In some forms of congenital heart disease there may be no murmur. Furthermore, because of the high oxygen affinity of fetal haemoglobin, babies with cyanotic heart disease involving common mixing of systemic and pulmonary venous return within the heart are often not cyanosed in early life. If there is a suspicion of cyanosis then the presence of hypoxaemia must be confirmed by an arterial blood gas analysis. Pulse oximetry is second best (*v.i.*).

Hyperoxia test (see p. 118)

This test was described before echocardiography was widely available, but it still has a place in the assessment of a baby with suspected CHD, especially if echocardiographic skills are a long ambulance journey away.

A PaO_2 of less than 20 kPa (150 mmHg) when the baby is breathing 100% oxygen is very suggestive of cyanotic CHD unless there is severe lung pathology. A PaO_2 greater than 33 kPa (250 mmHg) excludes virtually all types of cyanotic CHD. Pulse oximetry will not provide the same assurance because a baby can achieve 100% saturation at PaO_2 levels well below 20 kPa. A very low PaO_2 with a normal $PaCO_2$ suggests a cardiac cause of right to left shunting. An elevated $PaCO_2$ strongly suggests lung disease (Chapter 11). Always consider the possibility of septicaemia (p. 239), particularly in a hypotensive baby or if there are apnoeic episodes.

RIGHT TO LEFT SHUNTS IN NEONATES WITH NORMAL HEARTS

There are two related conditions that can cause right to left shunts and therefore cyanosis in neonates with structurally normal hearts.

Persistent pulmonary hypertension of the newborn (see pp. 189–194)

Transient myocardial ischaemia

Myocardial ischaemia accompanying HIE is quite common, and hypoglycaemia can cause transient myocardial dysfunction. Clinical signs include the murmur of tricuspid repurgitation and there may be hypotension and/or heart failure. The ECG can show ST segment changes. Treatment is with inotropic support and fluid restriction.

RIGHT TO LEFT SHUNT CAUSED BY STRUCTURAL HEART DEFECTS (Fig. 22.3)

Transposition of the great arteries

The incidence is 1 in 3000 live births. The aorta arises from the right ventricle and the pulmonary trunk from the left, which produces persistent hypoxia, the severity of which is dependent on whether there are associated shunts through the foramen ovale, the ductus arteriosus or septal defects.

The predominant physical sign is cyanosis. In uncomplicated cases there are often no murmurs. A ventricular septal defect is the most common associated abnormality, followed by pulmonary stenosis. The ECG is normal during the first few days but later shows moderate right ventricular hypertrophy with upright T waves in V_1. At birth the CXR is usually normal. The classic CXR of an "egg-shaped" heart with a narrow vascular pedicle is seen rarely and is a relatively late finding. Pulmonary plethora is observed when a large ductus or a VSD is present.

Cross-sectional echocardiography shows the posterior great artery arising from the left ventricle to be the pulmonary trunk. The aorta arises in parallel with it anteriorly from the right ventricle. During the first few days of life, the ductus arteriosus closes and the baby becomes lethargic, mottled and tachypnoeic with severe hypoxia and acidosis, rapid deterioration and death. The severity of hypoxia depends upon the potential for mixing across the foramen ovale and the presence and size of any VSD. When the diagnosis is suspected a prostaglandin infusion should be commenced, and the baby must be referred to a specialist centre. Nowadays, most centres undertake an arterial switch operation within a few days of diagnosis. Balloon septostomy enlarges the foramen ovale and helps to stabilize the situation by mixing the circulations and is still likely to be needed if there is a poor response to prostaglandins or if early surgery cannot be done.

Tetralogy of Fallot

In this defect there is a large VSD and infundibular pulmonary stenosis, often associated with pulmonary valve and pulmonary arterial stenosis. Cyanosis is present from birth in about 25% of cases and deepens with crying, but the clinical course depends on the severity of the pulmonary stenosis. The harsh ejection systolic murmur of infundibular stenosis tends to diminish with very severe narrowing and may disappear completely during "cyanotic spells". Splitting of the second heart sound may be heard if the obstruction is mild, but it becomes single with progressive narrowing.

The chest film is often diagnostic in that there is a normal cardiothoracic ratio with a decrease in pulmonary vascularity and a small or absent pulmonary trunk contour giving a "pulmonary artery bay" or "boot shaped heart". A right sided aortic arch is seen in 30% of cases.

The ECG shows right axis deviation and right ventricular hypertrophy with an upright T wave in V_1. The R wave is tall in V_1 with an rS pattern in V_6. Cross-sectional echocardiography shows a large aortic root overriding a subaortic VSD and the interventricular septum. The infundibular part of the septum deviates anteriorly into the RV outflow tract creating infundibular pulmonary stenosis. The severity of the pulmonary stenosis can be estimated with Doppler. The pulmonary valve ring and pulmonary arteries are reduced in size to a variable degree. With severe infundibular and valve narrowing, echocardiographic differentiation from pulmonary atresia with a VSD is difficult, but in tetralogy, colour Doppler will usually show the anterograde flow across the right ventricular outflow tract.

If arterial hypoxia is severe a prostaglandin infusion may be required, pending transfer to a specialist centre. Treatment there is governed by the size of the pulmonary arteries. If they are large, complete correction with VSD closure and resection of infundibular stenosis is possible. Some centres prefer initial management with a Blalock shunt to encourage growth of the pulmonary arteries before total correction at a later stage. Hypercyanotic spells are uncommon in neonates. If they occur, they should be treated by IV morphine or propranolol, oxygen, ventilation and sedation, and an immediate referral for surgery should be made.

Pulmonary atresia with intact ventricular septum

This condition is sometimes referred to as "hypoplastic right heart", since a characteristic feature is a small, dysplastic, right ventricle.

These babies all present with cyanosis in the newborn period. The pulmonary blood flow is always dependent upon flow through the ductus. There is usually persistent cyanosis from birth, which deepens as the ductus flow diminishes. The outflow of venous blood from the right atrium is obstructed which can lead to marked hepatic enlargement. Auscultation reveals a single second sound and either no murmur, or a ductus, or a tricuspid regurgitation murmur.

The ECG usually shows a QRS axis between + 120° and –30°, right atrial hypertrophy and paucity of right ventricular forces with a dominant S in V_1. The CXR shows a normal sized or large heart depending on the degree of right atrial dilation secondary to tricuspid incompetence. There is decreased vascularity and an absent main pulmonary artery shadow creating a pulmonary artery bay. The aortic arch is usually on the left side.

Cross-sectional echocardiography shows an enlarged right atrium. In 85% of babies the right ventricle is very small but thick walled, often with endocardial fibroelastosis. The tricuspid valve is often small and dysplastic. The pulmonary valve is usually an imperforate membrane with a good-sized main pulmonary artery; but at the other extreme there may be absence of the outlet portion of the right ventricle and of most of the pulmonary trunk. Colour Doppler often shows marked tricuspid incompetence. The absence of flow across the pulmonary valve differentiates the condition from severe pulmonary valve stenosis. Immediate transfer to a specialist centre, with prostaglandin infusion to maintain duct patency is essential.

Surgical treatment involves an aortopulmonary shunt, with valvotomy if possible, and atrial septostomy may be necessary. The prognosis is proportional to right ventricular size, and the size of the central pulmonary arteries, but is often poor.

Pulmonary valve stenosis

When this is severe, it often presents with a loud systolic murmur along the upper left sternal edge and radiating to the back. The second sound is single and a pulmonary ejection click is usually absent. Cyanosis and hepatic enlargement appear with right ventricular failure, often associated with tricuspid regurgitation. This usually occurs during the first week of life. Sinus tachycardia and a low output state may be present.

The ECG shows right atrial and right ventricular hypertrophy, with ST segment depression over the right ventricle suggesting suprasystemic pressure in the right ventricle. The CXR shows a normal sized or large heart depending on the degree of right atrial enlargement, and reduced or normal pulmonary vascularity. Poststenotic dilatation of the main pulmonary artery is not seen in the neonatal period.

Cross-sectional echocardiography reveals right atrial enlargement and a thick-walled right ventricle that may be normal sized or small, often with bright subendocardial echoes suggesting endocardial fibroelastosis. The pulmonary valve is often a thick, dysplastic membrane but may be thin and doming. Pulmonary arteries are normal sized or small. Colour Doppler reveals a high velocity jet across the pulmonary valve and possibly tricuspid regurgitation. The gradient across the pulmonary valve can be estimated from the Doppler trace, but this is not a reliable measurement of severity, especially if the ductus is open.

Anti-failure treatment should be instituted. In a neonate the circulation may be duct dependent and a prostaglandin infusion should be considered. Urgent referral for surgery or transcatheter balloon dilation of the pulmonary valve is essential.

Tricuspid atresia

Tricuspid atresia generally presents with cyanosis from birth, unless the pulmonary blood flow is increased. The high right atrial pressure causes an enlarged liver. Approximately 50% of cases have a systolic murmur at the lower left sternal edge, but 25% have no murmurs. The second sound is single.

Chest X-ray shows a square heart with cardiac enlargement in proportion to the pulmonary blood flow. There is a prominent superior vena cava and right atrium, and the pulmonary artery segment may be absent. Lung fields are usually oligaemic. The ECG usually shows left axis deviation (usually $-30°$ to $-60°$), and extreme paucity of right ventricular forces (more pronounced than pulmonary atresia). Right atrial hypertrophy is usually present.

Cross-sectional echocardiography most commonly shows a total absence of the valve, with the right atrium separated from the ventricles by a wedge of atrioventricular sulcus tissue, and rarely a thin imperforate membrane is seen. The blood reaches the left side of the heart through an ASD, with the atrial septum bulging from right to left. If the ASD is small (restrictive) there is marked dilatation of the inferior vena cava and hepatic veins. The right ventricular cavity is diminutive or absent in 70% of cases. There may be associated pulmonary atresia, in which case pulmonary blood flow is dependent on the ductus arteriosus. In 70% of babies the pulmonary artery arises from the small RV and the aorta from the LV. In these cases the pulmonary blood flow is usually reduced, because of obstruction at the level of the VSD, or within the cavity of the small RV. In contrast, in a minority of cases, there is ventriculo-arterial discordance (transposition of the great arteries) in association with tricuspid atresia. The pulmonary artery arises from the LV, causing excessive pulmonary blood flow. The aorta arises from the RV, and this may be associated with subaortic stenosis and coarctation.

If the baby is severely hypoxic start a prostaglandin infusion. Treatment with diuretics is unwise until the degree of obstruction at the level of the atrial septum has been determined. If there is a restrictive ASD an atrial septostomy must be performed. The surgical approach depends upon the anatomy. Reduced pulmonary blood flow is managed with an aortopulmonary shunt. If the pulmonary blood flow is high, pulmonary artery banding may be required. In the older child definitive treatment by a Fontan procedure (right atrial to pulmonary artery conduit) may be possible. In reality, only about 50% of cases survive to have a Fontan procedure, and the long term prognosis for survivors of surgery is uncertain.

Ebstein's malformation

This is a rare cause of cyanosis in the newborn, but milder, often asymptomatic, cases are not rare. The tricuspid valve is dysplastic and may be both stenotic and incompetent. The right atrium is often very markedly dilated. This can lead to pulmonary hypoplasia and it is upon this that the prognosis of neonates presenting with this condition chiefly depends. The chest X-ray shows a very large heart and reduced pulmonary perfusion. The ECG shows paucity of RV forces with a dominant S wave in V_1; the malformation predisposes to supraventricular tachycardias and the delta waves of Wolff-Parkinson-White syndrome may be seen. Echocardiography confirms the diagnosis, showing an abnormal apical displacement of the tricuspid valve, particularly the septal leaflet. Treatment is supportive, including a prostaglandin infusion and administration of oxygen. With the postnatal fall in pulmonary vascular resistance the pulmonary blood flow gradually improves and in many cases the hypoxia resolves. There are few surgical options for the neonate with Ebstein's malformation and intractable hypoxia.

Total anomalous pulmonary venous drainage

The non-obstructed type presents as heart failure in pink babies over one week of age, but the obstructed types cause early cyanosis and feeding difficulties. The clinical severity is determined by the degree of obstruction to the pulmonary venous return. TAPVD mimics respiratory disease and can cause confusion with rising CO_2 and some response to an increase in F_IO_2.

The site of return of the anomalous veins may be supracardiac, cardiac or infracardiac; obstruction is particularly common and severe in the infracardiac group. Most commonly the pulmonary veins all enter a confluence behind, but separate from, the left atrium. Obstruction can occur at a number of sites including the pulmonary vein orifices, the confluence, or on passage through the liver. In the latter situation the cyanosis gets dramatically worse when the ductus venosus shuts.

There is a loud first heart sound and narrow fixed splitting of the second heart sound. A pulmonary ejection systolic murmur and a tricuspid flow murmur may be present, but with severe obstruction a loud pulmonary component of the second sound may be the only clue. Another clue may be the paradoxical finding of well oxygenated blood from an umbilical venous catheter with deoxygenated blood from an umbilical artery catheter. The respiratory rate is increased, with dyspnoea proportional to the severity of obstruction. Hepatomegaly is present in most types of infracardiac drainage. A chest X-ray shows a small heart with increased vascularity and venous congestion. With infracardiac drainage a total white-out of the lung fields may be seen, and an erroneous diagnosis of lung disease is often made. Some babies present later on with chestiness and failure to thrive. In the first days of life the ECG is usually normal.

Cross-sectional echocardiography shows a small left atrium with no pulmonary veins entering it, and large right-sided chambers. The pulmonary venous confluence is seen behind the left atrium and often an ascending or descending vein can be demonstrated. Colour Doppler is of great value in tracing the flow of pulmonary venous blood. When there is infracardiac obstructed drainage, hugely dilated portal veins are seen within the liver.

Obstructed anomalous venous drainage is one of very few serious heart conditions presenting in the first few days of life that does not respond to a prostaglandin infusion. Urgent surgery to redirect the pulmonary veins to the left atrium is essential.

ARRHYTHMIAS IN THE NEONATAL PERIOD

ATRIAL ECTOPICS

These are very common, and they resolve within 3 months in 90% of cases. Atrial ectopics can be a marker for SVT, and may occasionally cause a ventricular bradycardia because they occur in a refractory period and conduction is blocked.

PAROXYSMAL SUPRAVENTRICULAR TACHYCARDIA

This occurs once in every 25 000 children. The heart rate during attacks ranges from 180 to over 300 beats/min, and the QRS complex is normal. Episodes usually begin and end abruptly. The child presents in heart failure with pallor, irritability and poor feeding. The diagnosis is made from the ECG. Look for an abnormal P wave axis or P wave morphology, or for a shortened PR interval and for the presence of delta waves (suggesting WPW syndrome) on the ECG during sinus rhythm. Death may occur if untreated for 48–72 hours. There is a 20% recurrence rate.

Treatment

The blood sugar level, electrolytes and acid–base status should be checked and corrected. Vagal stimulation, such as an ice bag to the face or immersion of the baby's face in cold water for a maximum of 10 seconds, is often successful. Attacks will usually respond to intravenous administration of adenosine, repeated after 20 minutes, if necessary (Fig. 22.5). In refractory cases an infusion of amiodarone over 20 minutes may be successful. If the baby is shocked, consider using synchronized DC cardioversion, starting with 1 joule/kg. Flecainide can be considered but verapamil is contraindicated in the newborn.

Maintenance treatment may not be indicated if the attacks are rare, short and easily stopped; but if they are not the baby should be treated with digoxin for 6–12 months. If the child has remained free from attacks at this age, an attempt should be made to tail off drug treatment unless there is documented WPW syndrome. Oral main-

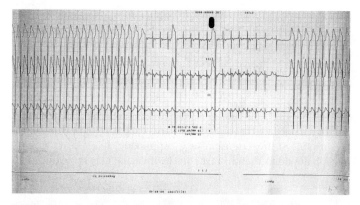

Figure 22.5 SVT responding to an injection of adenosine and relapsing.

tenance treatment with other drugs in patients refractory to digoxin should be supervised by specialists.

VENTRICULAR ECTOPICS

Like atrial ectopics (*v.s.*), these are common and usually harmless. Review the baby in 6 weeks and check the QTc interval (p. 509). If this is prolonged, then 24 hour monitoring is indicated to look for ventricular tachycardia.

CONGENITAL HEART BLOCK

Congenital heart block occurs once in 20 000 liveborn babies. Around 30% of cases of congenital atrioventricular block are associated with congenital heart disease, commonly atrioventricular septal defects and atrioventricular discordance (congenitally corrected transposition). Evidence of systemic lupus is commonly found in mothers of other cases. The babies present with bradycardia, often noted while still *in utero*, with Stokes-Adams attacks, or even with cardiac failure. There is usually an ejection murmur in the aortic area, and a mid-diastolic murmur at the apex, even without a structural heart abnormality.

Many babies are asymptomatic and do not require treatment. Mild congestive heart failure may respond to diuretics. Symptomatic cases require treatment with an isoprenaline infusion to raise the heart rate, followed by pacing. The indications for pacing in asymptomatic babies are controversial, but a mean heart rate below 50 beats/min or the presence of runs of ventricular tachycardia on a 24 hour ECG recording have been cited.

HYPERTENSION

Sustained significant hypertension, with a systolic BP above 100 mm Hg (Appendix C), requires treatment. Propranolol and captopril are useful. If hypertension is symptomatic (e.g. heart failure, encephalopathy) then intravenous hydralazine may be required.

REFERENCES

Ainsworth, S., Wyllie, J.P. and Wren, C. (1999) Prevalence and clinical significance of cardiac murmurs in neonates. *Archives of Disease in Childhood* **80**: F43–F45.

Arlettaz, R., Archer, N. and Wilkinson, A.R. (1998) Natural history if innocent murmurs in newborn babies: controlled echocardiographic study. *Archives of Disease in Childhood* **78**: F166–F170.

Braudo, M. and Rowe, R.D. (1961) Auscultation of the heart – early neonatal period. *American Journal of Disease in Children* **101**: 67–78.

Franklin, R.C.G., Maccartney, F.J., Bull, K. and Speigelhalter, D.J. (1991) Evaluation of a diagnostic algorithm for heart disease in neonates. *B.M.J.* **302**: 935–939.

Fugelseth, D., Lindemann, R., Liestol, K., Kiserud, T. and Langslet, A. (1997) Ultrasonographic study of ductus venosus in healthy neonates. *Archives of Disease in Childhood* **77**: F131–F134.

Hallidie-Smith, K.A. (1960) Some auscultatory and phonocardiographic findings observed in early infancy. *BMJ* **i**: 756–759.

FURTHER READING

Archer, N. (1999) Cardiovascular disease. In: *Textbook of Neonatology*, 3rd edn. Rennie, J.M. and Roberton, N.R.C. (eds), Churchill Livingstone, Edinburgh, pp. 673–713.

Archer, N. and Burch, M. (1998) *Pediatric Cardiology: An introduction.* Chapman & Hall Medical, London.

Freedom, R.M., Benson, L.N. and Smallhorn, J.F. (eds) (1992) *Neonatal Heart Disease.* Springer-Verlag, London.

Wernovsky, G. and Rubenstein, S.D. (2001) Cardiovascular disease in the neonate. *Clinics in Perinatology* Vol 28 No 1 March, whole issue.

23

GENITOURINARY AND GYNAECOLOGICAL PROBLEMS

- *Renal failure in the neonate is diagnosed when the urinary output is <0.5 ml/kg/h in the first day and <1.0 ml/kg/h thereafter with a rising serum creatinine.*
- *Differentiating prerenal from intrinsic renal failure can usually be done on the basis of the clinical findings and plasma and urine biochemistry. A saline load is rarely helpful, and may be hazardous in the oedematous oliguric baby.*
- *Conservative treatment with control of fluid balance and hyper-kalaemia is sufficient in most cases as the oliguria is usually short-lived. Dialysis should be considered if ARF is persistent.*
- *Babies with renal malformations detected prenatally or neonatally require assessment and follow up in all cases.*
- *Male infants with bilateral ureteric dilatation and a thick walled bladder on ultrasound have urethral valves until proved otherwise and must be investigated urgently.*

URINE

Most babies pass urine at or immediately after birth; 97% will have done so within 24 hours and all normal babies pass urine within 48 hours. Breast fed infants, who have a relatively low intake for the first 24–48 hours, pass little urine during this period. Following this 40–60 ml/kg/24 h are produced. Passing less than 12 ml/kg/24 h (0.5 ml/kg/h) on day 1 and less than 24 ml/kg/24 h (1 ml/kg/h) thereafter is certainly abnormal and requires investigation. The commonest cause of oliguria is pre-renal failure (Table 23.1). Polyuria is defined as a urine flow of more than 7 ml/kg/h. Polyuria can be caused by a reduced ADH concentration (diabetes insipidus) or resistance to ADH in the renal tubules (nephrogenic diabetes insipidus) but is more commonly seen in the polyuric phase of renal

Table 23.1 Causes of renal failure in the neonate (adapted from Modi 1999)

Pre-renal	Intrinsic renal	Post-renal (obstructive)
Systemic hypovolaemia Any severe illness with shock Fetal or neonatal haemorrhage Drugs (e.g tolazoline) Operative fluid loss	*Malformation* (e.g. PCKD) *Maternal drugs* (captopril, indomethacin) *ATN, ACN* in severe illness	*Malformation* (valves, PUJ obstruction, recessive polycystic disease) *Extrinsic compression* (tumour)
Renal hypoperfusion Severe illness e.g. RDS, asphyxia Drugs (e.g. indomethacin)	*Renal vein/artery thrombosis* *Pyelonephritis* *DIC*	*Neurogenic bladder* (from HIE, or spina bifida)

failure or in the diuretic phase of RDS (p. 142). Babies can concentrate their urine to about 500 mosmol/kg H_2O (preterm) and 700 mosmol/kg H_2O (term), but this is much less than the adult value of 1400 mosmol/kg H_2O. Providing there is no glycosuria, proteinuria or haematuria this corresponds to a specific gravity of 1002 to 1030. The pH of neonatal urine is usually between 5 and 8. For more information on neonatal renal function see p. 17–20.

HAEMATURIA

This is comparatively common in very sick infants as a result of one of the conditions listed below. Haematuria is often misdiagnosed when a female infant has had a small vaginal haemorrhage, and occasionally haematuria is diagnosed incorrectly when there are pink urate crystals on the nappy. Causes of haematuria include the following:

1. Bleeding tendency, particularly DIC (p. 449–450). This is probably the commonest cause of haematuria in very sick infants with RDS, septicaemia or NEC who are receiving intensive care.
2. Emboli from umbilical artery catheters, or with CONS sepsis (endocarditis) in association with long lines.
3. Trauma – particularly after suprapubic bladder aspiration.
4. Hypoxic ischaemic encephalopathy with associated tubular or cortical necrosis.
5. Renal artery or vein thrombosis (*v.i.*).
6. Urinary infection (p. 251).

7. Malformation, particularly from the wall of a trabeculated bladder in the presence of urethral valves (p. 405–406), or with hydronephrosis.
8. Other very rare causes of neonatal haematuria include:
   (a) drugs;
   (b) tumours;
   (c) polycystic disease of the kidneys – the kidneys are often palpable and uraemia may be present.

Haemoglobinuria is very rare in the newborn except in the presence of DIC with intravascular haemolysis.

In most of the conditions listed above the differential diagnosis is comparatively straightforward on clinical grounds, but if any doubts remain renal ultrasound is the investigation of choice.

PROTEINURIA

The normal newborn infant may excrete up to 1 g albumin/l during the first 24–48 hours of life, but the level falls rapidly after that time.

Proteinuria in the neonatal period is rare as a primary finding. It is common in association with any of the severe illnesses such as septicaemia, hypoxic ischaemic encephalopathy, hypotension and DIC which compromise renal perfusion and in some cases also cause haematuria. Massive proteinuria occurs in congenital nephrotic syndrome.

RENAL FAILURE

Acute renal failure can be defined either biochemically or in terms of urine flow. Blood urea levels are unhelpful, but a serum creatinine concentration above the normal range for gestation and postnatal age (100–130 µmol/l) (Appendix F) and/or a rising creatinine during the first few days suggests renal failure. Creatinine usually falls steadily after birth. Any infant passing less than 0.5 ml/kg/h of urine with a rising serum creatinine is in renal failure.

Most cases of ARF occur in neonates who have hypoxic ischaemic encephalopathy, or who are being ventilated because of sepsis or RDS. In some of these babies renal failure is prerenal due to over-enthusiastic fluid restriction (p. 23), but in others, acute tubular necrosis or renal cortical necrosis may have occurred. Causes of ARF in the neonate are listed in Table 23.1.

DIAGNOSIS

Most of these conditions can be established by taking the history, examining the baby (including catheterization of the bladder if necessary), and performing a renal and bladder ultrasound scan. The important differential diagnosis is then between prerenal uraemia and renal failure. This differentiation can usually be made clinically, and confirmed by simultaneous measurements of serum and urinary sodium and osmolarity (Table 23.2). However, the biochemical discrimination is less clear-cut in VLBW babies who have poor kidney function to start with and in whom sodium excretion rates may have been increased by frusemide.

If uncertainty persists the "fluid challenge" test beloved of nephrologists involves volume expansion with 15 ml/kg of normal saline with a simultaneous bolus of 2 mg/kg of frusemide. This test can be useful but is clearly ill advised in a hypotensive, oedematous ventilated 1 kg baby who is already requiring inotropic support. Such infants cope badly with a fluid load.

TREATMENT

If ARF is prerenal the correct treatment is volume expansion with blood or electrolyte solutions, maintaining a urine output above 1 ml/kg/h and giving frusemide 2–4 mg/kg (which can be repeated daily if it is effective).

If there is intrinsic renal failure, the following regimen should be instituted:

1. Weigh the baby at least twice daily.
2. Restrict fluid administration to insensible loss (20–30 ml/kg in a term baby) plus urine output. If the neonate is oedematous

Table 23.2 Biochemical indices which differentiate prerenal from intrinsic renal failure

	Prerenal	Renal
Urinary Na (mmol/l)	<10	>40
Urine/plasma osmolarity	>2	<1.1

replace insensible loss only. Flush arterial lines with the smallest possible volume of solution and remember to add this to the daily intake. Do not give potassium-containing solutions; add calcium to the IV fluid only if necessary; give enough sodium to keep the plasma level in the range 135–145 mmol/l.

3. Measure plasma electrolytes and acid–base status at least twice a day.
4. Measure blood glucose every 12 hours and correct hypoglycaemia.
5. Correct metabolic acidaemia with bicarbonate if the Na^+ is less than 130 mmol/l. Use THAM if the Na^+ is greater than 130 mmol/l.
6. If the potassium exceeds 7 mEq/l, give resonium enemas, usually as the Ca^{++} salt. Give 0.5 g/kg 6 hourly as a high rectal enema. For treatment of even higher levels of potassium see next section.
7. Treat *hypo*tension with dopamine up to 15 microg/kg/min. Treat *hyper*tension with hydrallazine 0.2–0.3 mg/kg 4–6 hourly.
8. Consider dialysis in appropriate cases (*v.i.*).

Of these problems the most important one is hyperkalaemia, which at levels above 8–9 mmol/l can cause severe cardiac disturbance and death. This can be treated in an emergency by:

1. giving IV salbutamol 0.4 mg/kg over 20 minutes;
2. giving 10% calcium gluconate (2 ml/kg/IV over 5–10 minutes) with ECG monitoring;
3. giving sodium bicarbonate (2 mEq/kg) over 5–10 minutes;
4. setting up a glucose/insulin infusion while preparing to perform peritoneal dialysis. Give 0.5 g dextrose/kg IV over 30 minutes using a concentrated solution if possible. Give IV insulin in the infusion in the ratio of 1 unit of insulin per 3 g of dextrose.

Most infants remain stable on this regimen, and start to pass urine within 48–72 hours. However, dialysis should be instituted if there is:

1. a severe metabolic acidaemia (H^+ >80 nmol/l) (pH <7.10) not controlled by administration of alkali;
2. hyperkalaemia not responding to medical therapy and causing episodes of ventricular tachycardia or ventricular fibrillation;
3. severe oedema and fluid overload;
4. intractable hypoglycaemia.

Peritoneal dialysis

This can be done using the Guy's Hospital paediatric peritoneal dialysis cannula (Wallace) with the Avon infant peritoneal dialysis set. The peritoneal cannula should be inserted as described on p. 491–492.

Most babies who require peritoneal dialysis are fluid overloaded, and one of the purposes of the procedure is to remove excess fluid. Although in the past there has been anxiety about the suitability of commercial dialysis solutions this has proved to be unfounded and peritoneal dialysis can be started using the conventional isotonic dialysis solutions with 1.36% dextrose. If this does not remove enough fluid the dextrose concentration can be increased. Add potassium 4.0 mmol/l once the baby's level is below this.

The dialysate should be heparinized (1 unit/ml) and warmed. Each dialysis cycle should be with 30–40 ml/kg of fluid run in over 5–10 minutes. Ideally this should be allowed to dwell in the peritoneal cavity for 20–30 minutes. In practice many infants on PD are ventilated and do not tolerate the diaphragmatic splinting which occurs when the peritoneum is full of dialysate, so the dialysate has to be run in and out sequentially with no "resting" phase.

Dialysis should be continued until the fluid balance is satisfactory and/or the potassium concentration is below 6 mmol/l. Once this has been achieved, and if the conservative treatment of renal failure outlined above is maintained, the baby will probably only need peritoneal dialysis for about 8 hours a day until renal function returns, although this may take up to 3 weeks.

Haemofiltration

Neonatal haemofiltration is also possible. Free-flowing arterial and venous access is essential and even the low volume 10 ml Gambro unit requires the baby to be able to sustain a mean BP of 40 mmHg for filtration to be successful. It is, therefore, more often useful in term than preterm babies. Pumps can be used to assist flow around the circuit in hypotensive babies but experience with these is limited.

URINARY TRACT INFECTION (p. 251)

CONGENITAL NEPHROTIC SYNDROME

This is extremely rare but may present with hydrops or the clinical stigmata of nephrotic syndrome. The causes are:

1. "Finnish" congenital nephrotic syndrome;
2. congenital syphilis, or CMV (that due to syphilis is treatable);
3. renal vein thrombosis.

The treatment is to maintain serum albumin and try diuretics. The prognosis for babies with an untreatable underlying cause is poor.

RENAL MALFORMATIONS

PRENATALLY DIAGNOSED RENAL MALFORMATIONS

Renal malformations are identified by antenatal ultrasound in about 1 in 800 pregnancies; about a fifth of childhood renal malformations are now detected this way. The commonest problem identified antenatally is dilatation of the renal tract, but renal agenesis, malpositioned or multicystic kidneys are also found. All babies with an antenatally diagnosed problem should have a renal ultrasound scan within a week, and if the antenatal dilatation of the renal pelvis (pyelectasis) was 15 mm or more this scan should be done urgently, before the baby goes home from the maternity unit. This serves to identify those babies with problems that require early intervention, for example those with urethral valves. The yield of investigating babies with prenatal dilatation of the renal tract is as follows:

5–10 mm	approximately 3% with abnormality
10–15 mm	approximately 50% with abnormality
>15 mm	approximately 94% with abnormality

All babies who have antenatal dilatation of the renal tract diagnosed must be discharged on trimethoprim prophylaxis (2 mg/kg at night) even if the early postnatal scan is normal. This is because there is relative oliguria in the first days of life and a single normal scan is not sufficient to rule out a problem. A repeat scan at 4–6 weeks should be obtained and further investigations organized in those babies who, on the second scan, are confirmed to have pyelectasis because reflux will be found in about 20%. The commonest causes are PUJ obstruction, VUJ obstruction, or reflux. Further investigation includes a MCU and a MAG 3 isotope study to examine function and the degree of obstruction of the renal tract. Opinions differ about whether or not all babies who *ever* had antenatal dilatation should have an MCU and isotope studies performed, whatever the postnatal findings. Our current practice is to discharge those who have normal ultrasound scans at 6 weeks and a year and have remained well, stopping the trimethoprim after the 6 week normal scan. Some paediatric urologists recommend full investigation for all cases. It is now clear that vesico-ureteric reflux is a familial disease, so if there is a family history of VUR a MCU should be offered even if both postnatal scans are normal.

Pelvi-ureteric junction (PUJ) obstruction

This is diagnosed with MAG 3 renography, which confirms "hold-up" at the PUJ level and provides information about renal function. The latter is the key to management. Minimal dilatation is usually defined as 5–12 mm, moderate as 12–20 mm, and severe as >20 mm. Most cases of PUJ obstruction with mild to moderate dilatation of the renal tract and normal renal function will not deteriorate and can be watched safely. Those with severe dilatation are at risk of deteriorating renal function, and these children should be watched carefully with repeat isotope renograms and referred for consideration of pyeloplasty. Antibiotic prophylaxis should be continued.

Vesico-ureteric junction obstruction (VUJ obstruction)

This condition is also a common cause of antenatal pyelectasis. These babies have a megaureter. Management is similar to that of PUJ obstruction and the two conditions can co-exist. Again, conservative management is indicated when the renal function is stable and the child is asymptomatic because the problem can resolve spontaneously. Antibiotic prophylaxis is recommended. Uretero-coeles are commoner in girls, and a prolapsed ureterocoele can cause obstruction of a (commonly associated) duplex system upper pole and cause VUJ obstruction. Most ureterocoeles respond to simple puncture carried out in the neonatal period.

Urethral valves (see p. 405–406)

These are a very important cause of pyelectasis in males.

Vesico-ureteric reflux

This is diagnosed with MCU done either because of follow-up of an abnormal antenatal renal scan or because of a diagnosis of UTI. Unfortunately no other test is available to make this diagnosis in infancy although progress can be followed with isotope studies once the child is continent. These babies must remain on trimethoprim prophylaxis against infection. A DMSA scan should be done to look for renal scars. Most cases do not require re-implantation of the ureters, but those with break-through infections or deteriorating renal function should be considered for surgery. The natural history of reflux diagnosed in the neonatal period is that it will resolve, but prophylaxis needs to be continued until it does.

POTTER'S SYNDROME (RENAL AGENESIS PLUS PULMONARY HYPOPLASIA)

In Potter's syndrome there is oligohydramnios during pregnancy and the fetal membranes show amnion nodosum. The baby has a squashed face, hypertelorism, epicanthic folds, micrognathia, low-set ears and large, floppy hands and feet.

This condition presents at birth with severe dyspnoea due to pulmonary hypoplasia and the infants usually die within two to three hours. In those in whom the pulmonary abnormality is less severe, survival for 24 to 48 hours may occur.

At postmortem the baby is anephric or has grossly abnormal, vestigial or multicystic kidneys, and the lung volume is usually less than 25% of normal.

RENAL VASCULAR THROMBOSIS

Renal arterial thrombosis is rare except as a complication of UACs.

Renal vein thrombosis usually presents with haematuria and a loin mass in ill term babies often in association with maternal diabetes, fetal asphyxia or congenital heart disease. Cases with inherited disorders resulting in a thrombotic tendency are being increasingly recognized, for example factor V Leiden deficiency. There is no evidence that anything other than conventional intensive care has any influence on outcome. Anticoagulation with heparin is usually offered, and may prevent spread of the thrombus to the other renal vein or embolization. The affected kidney usually becomes atrophic. The outcome in unilateral disease is good, but up to a half of bilateral cases die, with hypertension and renal failure occurring in some survivors.

RENAL MASSES

Loin masses in the neonate due to kidney enlargement are usually caused by the following:

1. hydronephrosis with or without outflow obstruction of any type;
2. cystic dysplasia/multicystic disease;
3. polycystic disease – infant or adult variety;
4. renal vein thrombosis (*v.s.*);
5. tumours;
6. adrenal haemorrhage or tumour.

Investigations should include:

1. electrolytes, urea and creatinine, urinary electrolytes;
2. blood pressure;
3. urine for chemistry, cytology, culture;
4. renal ultrasound;
5. DTPA, MAG 3, isotope scans;
6. IVU;
7. micturating cystogram;
8. renal arteriography and aortography.

Depending on the diagnosis, appropriate therapy can be instituted. Hydronephrosis will usually require surgical correction. With cystic dysplasia, the prognosis depends on the amount of normal renal tissue that is present. Unilateral disease or local cysts may be resectable.

POLYCYSTIC DISEASE

The classification of polycystic disease is complex (Hildebrandt 1999). Both autosomal dominant and autosomal recessive forms may present in the neonatal period with marked kidney enlargement. The prognosis for the AR form is poor. The AD form, which is often associated with hepatic cysts and congenital hepatic fibrosis, has a reasonably good prognosis. Ultrasound cannot distinguish between the two.

MULTICYSTIC DYSPLASTIC KIDNEYS

These are quite commonly detected antenatally. Postnatal management should include MCU because 20% of cases have reflux into the other kidney, which becomes a single kidney once the multicystic one shrivels up. This is the eventual fate of all these kidneys, and there is controversy as to whether or not they should be surgically removed because of a risk of malignancy in the residuum. Most paediatric urologists in the UK do not remove these kidneys.

NEPHROCALCINOSIS

Nephrocalcinosis is commonly diagnosed in VLBW babies on diuretics, particularly those who have received TPN. The crystals are calcium oxalate or calcium urate, and they eventually resolve. In term babies, nephrocalcinosis can occur secondary to renal tubular acidosis or primary oxalosis.

RENAL TUBULAR ACIDOSIS

This is defined as a metabolic acidosis resulting from the inability of the kidney to excrete hydrogen ions or to reabsorb bicarbonate. There is an inappropriately high urinary pH given the systemic acidosis. RTA can occur as a genetic defect, secondary to nephrocalcinosis, or be due to drugs. Treatment is with sodium bicarbonate 2–3 mEq/kg/day orally in divided doses.

FANCONI SYNDROME

In renal Fanconi syndrome a generalized proximal tubular dysfunction results in proximal renal tubular acidosis as well as urinary loss of phosphate, glucose, amino acids and low molecular weight proteins. Cystinosis is the most frequent cause of inherited Fanconi syndrome in babies.

GYNAECOLOGICAL PROBLEMS

Acute gynaecological problems, other than the child with ambiguous genitalia (p. 275–276), are very rare in the neonatal period. Ovarian cysts may be detected antenatally by ultrasound. If these cysts are large they can be aspirated percutaneously otherwise a watching brief is recommended. Occasionally the cysts can tort and produce a "chocolate cyst".

An imperforate hymen, if noted in the neonatal period, should be evaluated clinically and with ultrasound. Surgical correction can be carried out electively.

Vaginal haemorrhage, which is an oestrogen withdrawal bleed, is very common and does not require investigation or treatment so long as there are no other clinical abnormalities and the bleeding stops within a few days.

REFERENCES

Hildebrandt, F. (1999) Renal cystic disease. *Current Opinion in Pediatrics* **11**: 141–151.

Modi, N. (1999) Renal function, fluid and electrolyte balance and neonatal renal disease. In: *Textbook of Neonatology*, 3rd edn. Rennie, J.M. and Roberton, N.R.C. (eds), Churchill Livingstone, Edinburgh, pp. 1009–1037.

FURTHER READING

Dhillon, H.K. (1999) Antenatally diagnosed hydronephrosis. In: *Pediatric Surgery and Urology: Long term outcomes.* Stringer, M.D., Oldham, K., Mouriquand, P.D. and Howard, E.R. (eds), Saunders, London, pp, 479–486.

Modi, N. (1999) Renal function, fluid and electrolyte balance and neonatal renal disease In: *Textbook of Neonatology*, 3rd edn. Rennie, J.M. and Roberton, N.R.C. (eds), Churchill Livingstone, Edinburgh, pp. 1009–1037.

24

GASTROENTEROLOGICAL PROBLEMS

- *The aetiology of NEC is complex. Most cases occur in preterm babies who have suffered from gut hypoperfusion and have been fed milk, especially formula milk.*
- *Treatment of NEC involves resting the gut for 7–10 days, using TPN, antibiotics and full intensive care.*
- *Perforation or failure to improve within 7–10 days is usually an indication for a laparotomy in NEC.*
- *Bilious or faeculent vomiting and bleeding per rectum in babies must always be investigated, but not all causes are serious.*

The many malformations of the gastrointestinal tract which cause intestinal obstruction in the neonatal period are described in Chapter 25.

NECROTIZING ENTEROCOLITIS

NEC is a serious disease that primarily affects preterm or SGA babies, and which occurs almost exclusively in NNUs. The disease usually involves the terminal ileum and the colon, but lesions can occur anywhere from the stomach to the rectum, and multiple areas may be involved. The incidence varies, but is around 3% in VLBWI. Clusters of cases are relatively common, and the disease can affect term babies.

SYMPTOMS AND SIGNS

NEC should always be suspected in babies with abdominal distension, bilious aspirate or vomiting, blood in the stool and signs of infection (p. 230–231). NEC is most common in the second week of life, but late cases can occur. The staging of NEC is shown in Table 24.1. Histological proof may be obtained at laparotomy or autopsy.

Table 24.1 Staging of disease in NEC (Bell *et al.* 1978)

Stage 1: suspect
- History of perinatal stress.
- Systemic signs of ill-health: temperature instability, lethargy, apnoea.
- Gastrointestinal manifestations: poor feeding, increased volume of gastric aspirate, vomiting, mild abdominal distension, faecal occult blood (no fissure).

Stage 2: confirmed
Any of features of stage 1 plus:

- Persistent occult or gross intestinal bleeding, marked abdominal distention.
- Abdominal radiograph: intestinal distension, bowel wall oedema, unchanging bowel loops, pneumatosis intestinalis, portal vein gas.

Stage 3: advanced
Any of the features of stage 1 or 2 plus:

- Deterioration in vital signs, evidence of shock or severe sepsis, or marked gastrointestinal haemorrhage.
- Abdominal radiograph shows any of features of stage 2 plus pneumoperitoneum.

Some babies have a slow insidious onset of NEC and do not progress beyond the "suspect" stage with abdominal distension and mild systemic illness. In others, the disease progresses and the infant becomes paler and more mottled, the abdominal distension increases, the stools are bloodier and the baby may vomit. Eventually an ileus develops, no stools are passed, and the vomit becomes bilious or faeculent. Bowel sounds are absent, and the distended abdomen may be tender. At this stage ascites may develop, and bowel perforation occurs in some cases. There may be redness and induration of the abdominal wall overlying areas of involved gut, and flank lividity appears in advanced cases. This progression may take several days or there may be a fulminant course leading to death within a few hours. In babies with severe disease apnoea, hypotension and jaundice occur early in the course of the illness.

INVESTIGATION

In addition to the usual tests which are indicated for suspected infection (p. 232–234), request a plain X-ray of the abdomen with a lateral horizontal film taken with the infant lying on his left side, to detect fluid levels and free intraperitoneal gas. Remember gas collects round the liver in babies who are lying down, and can also appear in the lesser sac. In mild cases the X-rays will be normal, though occasional fluid levels may be seen; there may be some dilated bowel loops, and the gut wall may be rather thicker than usual. A fixed dilated loop of gut may remain in the same position in different X-ray views, and for several days and this is an abnormal finding. Oedema of the gut wall can give rise to an abnormal shadow from the junction between it and the peritoneal fat. As the disease progresses, gas bubbles (the pathognomonic feature of NEC) appear first in the bowel wall and eventually in the liver, where they are sometimes seen within the biliary tree. Ascites may be present, and when an intestinal perforation occurs free gas will be seen within the abdomen. Barium studies or diagnostic paracentesis are rarely necessary for the diagnosis.

DIFFERENTIAL DIAGNOSIS

The history, clinical examination and the X-ray findings are very characteristic. Babies with other causes of intestinal obstruction – including congenital malformation – never show intramural gas, and rarely pass bloody stools. A pneumoperitoneum from air tracking down from the mediastinum is usually associated with high-pressure IPPV for lung disease (p. 185), and there are none of the other signs of intra-abdominal sepsis. Bleeding PR from some local cause such as fissure-in-ano must be excluded (p. 391).

AETIOLOGY

(See Fig. 24.1.)

NEC begins in the mucosa with oedema, haemorrhage and microvascular sludging. The disease is multifactorial (Fig. 24.1) with the most important risk factors being prematurity and its complications, intrauterine growth restriction (particularly with reversed flow in the fetal umbilical artery), and oral feeding. All the factors on the left of the diagram tend to diminish mucosal blood flow. The ischaemic mucosa is very susceptible to gut infection with gas-forming organisms, and the presence of milk in the gut provides a substrate for these organisms. In all babies there is a tendency for undigested carbohydrate to pass into the colon, where bacterial fermentation lowers the intraluminal pH. Carbohydrate fermentation explains the high breath hydrogen levels that are found in these babies.

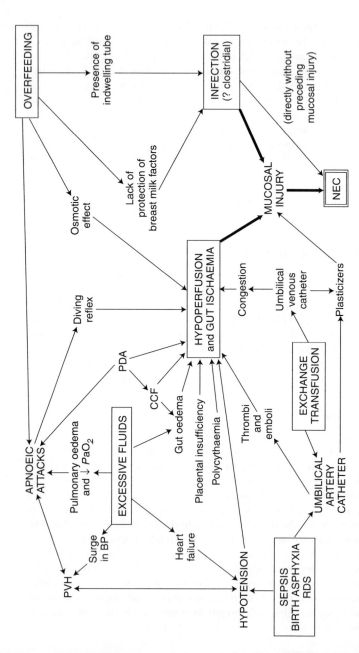

Figure 24.1 Aetiological factors in NEC. Major factors are enclosed in boxes. (From Lucas and Roberton, 1982.)

PREVENTION

Many of the important aetiological factors are preventable, particularly the avoidance of asphyxia or apnoea, but NEC is not a totally preventable disease. The disease is virtually unknown in babies who have not been fed. Some neonatologists interpret this as an indication to inflict TPN on all sick babies, and avoid enteral feeds entirely until IPPV is discontinued, UAC are removed, and blood gases are normal. This approach is not justified, but convalescent babies should not be fed until bowel sounds are present and meconium has been passed, and feeds should be discontinued at the earliest signs of milk being retained in the stomach or abdominal distension (p. 46). We wait at least a week before starting feeds if reversed end-diastolic flow was demonstrated in the umbilical artery with Doppler ultrasound before birth (p. 44). Breast milk should be used to start feeding if available because there is some evidence that it is protective against NEC. If pre-term formula has to be used, it should be started as 1/4 or 1/2 strength feeds for a day or two, and full strength formula only given once the dilute preparation is tolerated. An alternative is to build up feeds to full volume using term formula and to switch to preterm formula when feeding is established. Milk feeds should be increased at the rate of about 20 ml/kg/day; this often means increasing the feed volume by as little as 1 ml each day. Prophylactic oral administration of immunoglobulins, colonizing the gut with the "right" sort of bacteria, and non-absorbable antibiotics have all been suggested, but none of them are of proven benefit.

TREATMENT

A "drip and suck" regimen must be started to rest the baby's gut. Remove all umbilical cannulae and give total parenteral nutrition through a central venous catheter (Chapter 5). Treat hypotension, anaemia and respiratory failure as outlined on p. 137 *et seq*. These babies lose a lot of protein-rich fluid as ascites, and frequent blood and/or plasma transfusions are an important part of therapy. Ampicillin, gentamicin and metronidazole should be given intravenously.

This regimen should be continued for at least 7–10 days. Lateral abdominal X-rays should be taken daily, or more frequently following any clinical deterioration, in order to detect bowel perforation as soon as possible, in which case laparotomy should be carried out. Laparotomy should be considered in babies who show no response to conservative treatment, and in whom ileus and ascites persist for more than 4–5 days.

At laparotomy, involved segments of gut will be resected. If the baby is in good condition primary anastomosis can be performed, but if the baby's condition is parlous during the laparotomy, affected bowel is excised and a defunctioning proximal "ostomy" is made

In very unstable babies, an alternative to laparotomy is to insert soft peritoneal drains and wait. Surgery is almost always needed eventually if these babies survive. With the current high standard of neonatal anaesthesia and surgery even the smallest and sickest babies can withstand surgery, making drainage a less attractive option.

If widespread disease is present, totally necrotic bowel is excised and the peritoneum washed out, with the intention of doing a repeat laparotomy when much "suspect" bowel is often seen to be viable. To preserve as much bowel as possible it may be necessary to fashion several "ostomies" which can be joined up when the baby is over the severe toxaemic stage of his illness, after checking the patency of the distal gut with contrast radiography.

Enteral feeding, ideally with EBM can be restarted after 7–10 days, but only if the abdominal X-ray is normal, bowel sounds are present and there is minimal aspirate up the N/G tube. Feeds should then be increased very slowly – often at rates about half those given in Table 4.6b. Long-term TPN may need to continue until enteral feeding is established.

SEQUELAE

The mortality is about 20% among those babies who perforate, but should be less than 10% in those who do not. About 10% of babies develop a further typical attack of NEC. In a further 5–10%, particularly if they did not come to laparotomy, the area of gut involved becomes stenosed. These cases develop signs of intestinal obstruction without enterocolitis 2–6 weeks after the original illness. Barium studies at this stage demonstrate the stricture which may need to be resected with primary reanastomosis of the bowel. VLBW babies who survive NEC have a higher incidence of neurological sequelae at follow up than control babies of similar gestation.

ISOLATED BOWEL PERFORATION

Various parts of the bowel may perforate spontaneously during neonatal intensive care. Gastric perforation may occur spontaneously, as a result of a nasogastric tube, or in association with face mask ventilation. Isolated ileal or colonic perforations without NEC may be the result of ischaemia due to drugs such as indomethacin or emboli from umbilical artery catheters. It is not unknown for the bowel to be perforated by paracentesis tubes inserted to drain a pneumoperitoneum or ascites.

In all these situations the baby will develop a peritonitis as bowel contents leak out, and he will have abdominal distension. Plain X-ray of the abdomen will confirm free intraperitoneal air.

The treatment is laparotomy and closure of the perforation or resection of the localized area of bowel.

SHORT BOWEL SYNDROME

This is likely to occur after surgery for NEC, volvulus or other gut malformations if less than 40 cm of small bowel is left, particularly if the ileocaecal valve has been resected, and short bowel syndrome may occur (but with a much better long term prognosis) with 50–100 cm of residual small bowel.

Survival has been achieved with as little as 10–15 cm of jejunum and an intact ileo-caecal valve, or 25–40 cm without it. The prognosis has improved over the last 20 years, and the cornerstone of management is careful TPN. TPN is maintained whilst providing some enteral nutrition ("feeding the gut" or "trophic feeding") and waiting for the bowel to grow and adapt. It cannot be stressed enough that the bowel will never adapt if enteral feeds are not given; far better to continue at a slow rate than to keep stopping and starting. Enteral feeds need to be started and increased at an extremely slow rate. Milks which are easily digested and absorbed such as pregestimil or nutramigen are usually used. Stool output can increase dramatically as feeds are increased and needs to be watched carefully. Agents such as H_2 antagonists (ranitidine), antimotility agents (loperamide), and bile acid binders (cholestyramine) can be helpful. A paediatric gastroenterologist must supervise difficult cases. Small bowel transplantation is possible, but is a last resort.

GASTRO-OESOPHAGEAL REFLUX

This may be a problem in babies with persistent apnoeic attacks, and may complicate CLD. Reflux is also frequent in children who are brain damaged after hypoxic ischaemic encephalopathy. The diagnosis can be made clinically, on the basis of oesophageal pH studies, or a barium swallow. Therapy involves nursing the baby head up and thickening the feed with a commercial agent such as carobel or Thick-and-Easy. The Committee on the Safety of Medicine in the UK currently blacklists cisapride. There have been few trials to confirm the efficacy of cisapride, and it has been shown to increase the QT interval in some babies, particularly those who are being treated simultaneously with macrolide antibiotics, anti-fungals or who are hypokalaemic.

NEONATAL APPENDICITIS

This may mimic NEC with disease localized to the right iliac fossa. Haematuria and/or pyuria suggest that the damaged organ is lying on the bladder. The condition is only usually recognized at laparotomy carried out for NEC or a perforation.

THE BABY WITH PERSISTENT VOMITING

All babies can be expected to vomit once or twice a day. Only if the vomiting is bile stained, faeculent, bloody or becomes persistent is investigation required. Haematemesis is considered below.

The serious causes of persistent vomiting in the neonate include the following:

1. neonatal intestinal obstruction from any cause (p. 396 *et seq*);
2. ileus in association with severe illness, e.g. birth asphyxia or RDS;
3. septicaemia, including meningitis;
4. necrotizing enterocolitis (*v.s.*);
5. rare metabolic causes, e.g. galactosaemia (Chapter 18) and CAH (Chapter 16);
6. raised intracranial pressure, e.g. hydrocephalus, intracranial haemorrhage.

The first four are usually associated with bilious vomiting, and the diagnosis is usually easy to establish by simple clinical, laboratory and X-ray methods.

It is also important not to forget the common causes of vomiting in older babies. These include:

1. gastroenteritis;
2. upper respiratory tract infections and otitis media;

3. urinary infection;
4. pyloric stenosis.

These can present during the neonatal period, particularly in very low birth weight babies who remain in the NNU for several weeks. It is important to exclude urinary tract infection in this situation.

A large number of entirely normal newborn babies, however, just vomit! – and it may be bilious (Lilien *et al.* 1986). Immediately after birth this is often ascribed to having swallowed blood or meconium stained amniotic fluid, or to the baby being "mucousy". In our view there is no longer any place for stomach washouts in babies. If the baby has a problem this will only serve to delay diagnosis and treatment, and if he is normal he should not be subjected to this unpleasant procedure.

If a baby continues to vomit in the absence of clinical abnormalities, it is safest to set up an intravenous infusion, give nothing orally and aspirate the stomach regularly for 24–48 hours before trying oral feeds again. If these are still vomited a barium meal is indicated.

PERSISTING DIARRHOEA

In the baby with frequent loose stools and failure to thrive without gastroenteritis consider the following:

1. Cow's milk protein intolerance.
2. Cystic fibrosis.
3. Immune deficiency syndromes (e.g. Schwachman's syndrome).
4. Congenital monosaccharide or disaccharide deficiency.
5. Congenital chloride or sodium diarrhoea.
6. Congenital microvillous atrophy.
7. Autoimmune enteropathies.

Conditions 2–6 can be autosomal recessive conditions so a family history may help. The first two conditions can be evaluated in any neonatal service, but the last five require specialist referral for diagnosis and management.

HAEMATEMESIS, MELAENA AND BLOODY STOOLS IN THE NEWBORN

Minor degrees of these disorders are very common, and the following conditions should be excluded before embarking on complex studies of the clotting system or diagnosing serious intra-abdominal disease:

1. swallowed maternal/placental blood at delivery;
2. swallowed maternal blood from a cracked nipple;
3. local trauma (e.g. from a nasogastric tube, laryngoscopy, over-vigorous laryngeal suction);
4. fissure-in-ano.

It is important to test whether the blood is maternal (swallowed) or fetal, and this can be done using Apt's test for fetal haemoglobin. When 1% sodium hydroxide is added to a dilute solution of the bloody effluent in water, fetal haemoglobin remains pink, whereas adult haemoglobin denatures and goes brown.

The serious differential diagnoses for haematemesis or blood in the stools are as follows:

1. necrotizing enterocolitis (v.s.);
2. haemorrhagic diatheses of various types, including haemor-rhagic disease of the newborn, and DIC (pp. 449–450);
3. steroids;
4. rare causes:
    (a) trauma (e.g. broken rectal thermometer);
    (b) Meckel's diverticulum;
    (c) malrotation;
    (d) peptic ulceration;
    (e) rectal polyps/haemangiomas;
    (f) colitis;
    (g) intussusception;
    (h) gut reduplication.

These should only be sought if the other much commoner conditions have already been excluded, and bleeding persists.

REFERENCES

Bell, M.J., Ternberg, J.L., Feigin, R.D. *et al.* (1978) Neonatal necrotising enterocolitis: therapeutic decisions based upon clinical staging. *Annals of Surgery* **187**: 1–7.

Lilien, L.D., Srinivasan, G., Pyati, S.P., Yeh, T.F. and Pildes, R.S. (1986) Green vomiting in the 1st 72 hrs in normal infants. *American Journal of Diseases of Children* **140**: 662–664.

Lucas, A. and Roberton, N.R.C. (1982) The care of the low birthweight infant. In: *Recent Advances in Obstetrics and Gynaecology*. Bonnar, J. (ed.), Churchill Livingstone, Edinburgh and London, pp. 115–160.

FURTHER READING

Neu, J. (ed.) (1996) Neonatal Gastroenterology. In: *Clinics in Perinatology*. W B Saunders, Philadelphia, Vol 23 Number 2.

Newell, S. (1999) Gastrointestinal Problems. In: *Textbook of Neonatology*, 3rd edn. Rennie, J.M. and Roberton, N.R.C. (eds), Churchill Livingstone, Edinburgh and London, pp. 744–764.

Wilkinson, A.R. and Tam, P.K.H. (eds) (1997) Necrotising enterocolitis. In: *Seminars in Neonatology*. W B Saunders, London, Volume 2 Issue 4.

25

SURGICAL PROBLEMS

The majority of neonates requiring surgery should be referred to a Regional Neonatal Surgical Unit. The presenting features of the more commonly encountered problems are described, with advice on immediate management. Detailed descriptions of operative management are not appropriate but the post-operative care for all the bowel disorders is outlined at the end of the chapter.

PRENATAL DIAGNOSIS

The increasing expertise in the prenatal diagnosis of many congenital anomalies forewarns obstetricians and neonatologists and allows appropriate counselling of parents and planning for the delivery of the baby and subsequent management. Some anatomical abnormalities can only be inferred from a prenatal scan – an example is oesophageal atresia which may be suspected if a stomach bubble is not visible. Babies with multiple anomalies may have some but not all diagnosed prenatally – necessitating careful assessment post-natally.

CLEFT LIP AND CLEFT PALATE

The incidence is one in 600. These abnormalities range from the bifid uvula to the complete bilateral cleft lip with cleft palate.

Having excluded other congenital abnormalities (e.g. Trisomy 13, oesophageal atresia), it is important that mother and baby remain together providing the baby's general condition permits. She should be involved in overcoming any initial feeding difficulties, using special teats, or spoon feeding if breast feeding is impossible or unsuccessful. Individual surgeons will have their own preference for timing the repair of the lip and palate. Advances in the post-operative care of the neonate permits lip repair within the first few days of life to be carried out safely. Either prenatal or early postnatal consultation with a plastic surgeon allows consideration of this option and a clear plan of management removes uncertainties for the parents. The use of specially moulded palatal prostheses is an option. The prosthesis is designed to enable the baby to feed normally and to promote normal maxillary growth.

Showing the parents serial photographs of previously treated babies will confirm the excellent results that are now achieved and further reassure them.

TUMOURS OF MOUTH AND PHARYNX

Rare, usually benign, tumours – including congenital epulis, dermoids, teratomas and epignathus – may be visible at birth. They may cause respiratory obstruction, which may be intermittent and positional. Swallowing difficulties and excessive nasal mucus should also suggest pharyngeal obstruction.

Intubation or tracheostomy may be necessary to maintain the airway. Prompt surgery is necessary after appropriate imaging, and is usually curative but can be technically very demanding and requires very experienced post-operative care.

OESOPHAGEAL ATRESIA AND TRACHEO-OESOPHAGEAL FISTULA

The incidence is one in 3500. 85% have a blind-ending upper oesophagus-oesophageal atresia, the lower oesophagus joining the trachea in the region of the carina (TOF). Oesophageal atresia without a fistula occurs in 7% of cases, and other varieties of the malformation occur rarely, including isolated fistula without oesophageal atresia.

DIAGNOSIS

Inability to swallow may result in polyhydramnios prenatally. Postnatally the baby will have frothy saliva coming from the mouth, associated with coughing, choking and cyanotic episodes. The isolated tracheo-oesophageal fistula is more likely to become apparent on feeding, when coughing and choking will occur often associated with abdominal distension resulting from an excess of air in the intestine.

A wide-bore radio-opaque (FG 10 or 12) tube should be passed. Small tubes curl in the capacious upper oesophagus and give a false impression of normal passage to the stomach. In oesophageal atresia the tube will meet resistance 9–11 cm from the nose or lips. An X-ray will confirm the tip of the tube lying in the upper oesophagus (T2–T4 level). The X-ray should include the abdomen. If gas is present in the bowel a TOF must exist. If the abdomen is gasless the diagnosis is likely to be a pure oesophageal atresia. Contrast studies to confirm the diagnosis of oesophageal atresia are not necessary.

At least 50% of these babies will have other abnormalities (imperforate anus, cardiac, vertebral, skeletal and genitourinary).

MANAGEMENT

The airway must be maintained, and frequent suction of the pharynx should achieve this. Continuous suction using a Replogle double lumen tube placed in the upper oesophagus is ideal, but the alternative of a wide-bore tube left *in situ* and aspirated every 10 minutes is acceptable. The baby should be nursed prone or on his side. Provided the saliva is being removed adequately, a head-up position to prevent reflux of gastric contents via the TOF is ideal.

In the majority of cases of oesophageal atresia with TOF, division of the fistula and primary anastomosis of the oesophagus will be possible. In some cases, particularly the pure oesophageal atresia, primary anastomosis is not feasible because too large a gap exists between the ends of the oesophagus. Formation of a feeding gastrostomy, with delayed anastomosis, or formation of a cervical oesophagostomy with eventual oesophageal replacement, is then employed.

The results of treatment are excellent in good-sized babies without associated major anomalies. Small babies or those with major anomalies continue to show an appreciable mortality (10–20%).

INTESTINAL OBSTRUCTION

An infant with RDS, septicaemia, early NEC, cerebral irritation following birth asphyxia, electrolyte disturbance or severe HDN may develop abdominal distension, bile-stained vomiting and constipation.

A careful history and examination will usually distinguish these cases of functional obstruction from true mechanical obstruction; the plain abdominal X-ray shows uniform distension of the bowel with air, but few if any fluids levels.

Management is directed towards correcting the underlying problem. A good-size (FG 6 or 8) *in situ* nasogastric tube should be aspirated frequently and left on free drainage. If meconium has never been passed, and several days have elapsed, it may be necessary to stimulate the colon by gently irrigating the rectum with a few millilitres of saline because the meconium may become inspissated in the colon, mimicking meconium ileus. Slivers of glycerine suppositories administered twice daily for a few days will also encourage passage of bowel contents.

DUODENAL ATRESIA

The incidence is one in 10 000. In the majority of cases the atresia is distal to the opening of the bile duct. Bile-stained vomiting occurs with delayed passage of meconium or passage of only a small amount of stool. Abdominal distension will be absent or confined to the epigastrium. Visible gastric peristalsis may be apparent if the stomach is distended. An erect plain abdominal X-ray shows the classical "double bubble", a supine film demonstrates air outlining stomach and proximal duodenum only.

In a minority, the atresia occurs proximal to the opening of the bile duct. Vomiting is often copious and persistent but in the absence of bile its significance may not be appreciated. In addition, normal meconium is often passed. Abdominal distension is not present, so the three cardinal features of a bowel obstruction – bile-stained vomiting, distension and constipation – are absent. Not surprisingly delay in diagnosis is frequent, resulting in dehydration and gross electrolyte disturbance. Persistent vomiting in the neonate is as important as bile-stained vomiting and should prompt an abdominal X-ray.

Down syndrome is an associated finding in 30% of patients with duodenal atresia. A birth weight less than 2.5 kg is found in about 50% of cases, and of those with normal chromosomes at least 50% will have one or more additional congenital anomalies.

Pre-operatively the stomach must be kept empty with a size 6 or 8 FG tube on free drainage and hourly aspiration. If fluid and electrolyte disturbances have occurred these must be corrected, particular attention being paid to correcting the serum calcium. There is no urgency to operate on a duodenal atresia. At laparotomy the atresia is usually amenable to correction by anastomosing proximal duodenum to distal duodenum – a duodenoduodenostomy. Return of bowel function post-operatively may be delayed, and early intravenous feeding is advisable.

INCOMPLETE DUODENAL OBSTRUCTION, MALROTATION AND VOLVULUS

The onset of symptoms is often delayed for several days. The underlying cause may be an intrinsic duodenal stenosis, a mucosal web with a hole in it, an abnormality of intestinal rotation resulting in bands compressing the duodenum, or a volvulus of the midgut obstructing the duodenum. The intrinsic duodenal obstruction usually presents with persistent, often bile-stained, vomiting; meconium may have been passed, followed by changing stools if feeds have been tolerated for some days. The baby with a malrotation may tolerate feeds well but intermittently has bile-stained vomits – eventually the vomiting becoming persistent. Abdominal distention is unusual and meconium and normal stools will be passed.

Plain X-rays in a duodenal stenosis will show a dilated stomach and duodenum with a paucity of distal gas. In a malrotation, if the X-rays are taken when the baby is vomiting a distended stomach with little distal gas is seen; however, if the symptoms are intermittent the X-rays may appear entirely normal.

Where an incomplete duodenal obstruction is suspected a barium study should be done by an experienced radiologist. In duodenal stenosis the proximal duodenum is distended and peristalsis is vigorous, the contrast eventually passing into the distal duodenum which crosses the midline; the duodenojejunal flexure lies to the left of L1. In a malrotation, if the barium is administered when the baby is asymptomatic the contrast will flow freely, but it will demonstrate the duodenum failing to cross the midline and the first loops of jejunum lying to the right of the vertebral column. If the duodenum is obstructed at the time of the study the contrast may be seen "corkscrewing" through the upper jejunum, demonstrating a volvulus. A barium enema may demonstrate a centrally situated caecum in a malrotation, but a malrotation causing duodenal obstruction may occur in the presence of an apparently normally situated caecum; therefore a barium meal carefully performed and correctly interpreted is preferable to a barium enema if a malrotation is suspected.

If an intrinsic duodenal stenosis or web with normal rotation is diagnosed, surgical correction can be undertaken when the baby's fluid and electrolyte balance has been corrected.

If a malrotation/volvulus is present, or cannot be excluded, then urgent operation is essential because the vascular supply to the entire midgut (duodenum to transverse colon) runs through the narrow, possibly twisted pedicle of mesentery.

Less commonly a volvulus may present with abdominal distension, bile-stained vomiting and the passage of blood rectally. The baby is usually gravely ill and frequently anaemic. Resuscitation should commence, but the most urgent need is for laparotomy and untwisting of the volved bowel in the hope that a reasonable length of bowel can be salvaged, because this presentation indicates established intestinal vascular compromise.

SMALL BOWEL ATRESIA

The incidence is one in 5000. Bile-stained vomiting and abdominal distension are present within 48 hours of birth. Meconium may be passed. Distended loops of bowel are often visible and palpable through the abdominal wall. X-rays show loops of bowel of varying calibre with fluid levels. Intra-abdominal calcification suggests meconium peritonitis secondary to intrauterine bowel perforation.

A size 8 FG nasogastric tube should be left on free drainage and aspirated at least hourly. Delayed diagnosis will cause marked fluid and electrolyte deficits which require correction. A laparotomy will reveal the level of the atresia and confirm a solitary atresia or multiple atresias. It should be possible to resect most of the grossly dilated proximal bowel and perform an end-to-end anastomosis, but a period with enterostomies may be necessary. At laparotomy it is important to establish the length of bowel remaining, and whether it is jejunum or ileum.

While the surgery of the bowel atresias is relatively easy the postoperative problems associated with disordered gut motility and a short length of remaining bowel may present considerable problems. 15% of small bowel atresias are associated with meconium ileus. This may be apparent at laparotomy, but a sweat test should be performed routinely on all patients with jejunoileal atresia.

MECONIUM ILEUS

Between 10 and 20% of infants with cystic fibrosis present in the neonatal period with meconium ileus. The underlying problem is inspissated meconium packing the colon and ileum for a variable distance and producing an intraluminal obstruction – simple meconium ileus. Complications include bowel atresia, volvulus, and perforation with resulting meconium peritonitis producing calcification on the plain abdominal X-ray.

The clinical presentation is early abdominal distension, bile-stained vomiting and failure to pass meconium. Plain abdominal X-rays in simple meconium ileus show moderate small bowel distension, with few if any fluid levels. The presence of a coarsely granular appearance produced by bubbles of air within the meconium in obstructed bowel suggests the diagnosis, but this is also seen in other low bowel obstructions. The radiological appearances in complicated meconium ileus may be those of an atresia. An X-ray with a paucity of gas, calcification and a large gasless area may indicate a meconium cyst, usually a result of volvulus of loops of bowel with subsequent necrosis.

Initial management includes passage of a nasogastric tube and siting of an intravenous infusion. A gastrografin enema can be used to clear the distal bowel of inspissated meconium in simple meconium ileus, but should only be done by a suitably experienced radiologist with appropriate surgical support available. In complicated meconium ileus without radiological evidence of meconium peritonitis, a barium enema may be carried out for diagnostic purposes – demonstrating the microcolon containing pellets of inspissated meconium.

Laparotomy will be necessary in complicated meconium ileus, and in simple meconium ileus where the enema fails. An ileostomy may be fashioned after resection of grossly dilated bowel, relieving the obstruction and enabling washouts of the distal bowel to be undertaken through the mucus fistula. Alternatively the distal bowel may be washed out intra-operatively allowing a primary anastomosis to be performed.

The suspected diagnosis of cystic fibrosis is confirmed by a sweat test and the finding of one of the abnormal genes (ΔF508 is commonest) known to cause cystic fibrosis. Chest physiotherapy should be instituted early in any neonate with suspected cystic fibrosis. Start pancreatic supplements (0.25–0.5 g Pancrease powder per feed) once full oral feeds are established.

HIRSCHSPRUNG'S DISEASE

The incidence is one in 5000. Ganglion cells are absent from Auerbach's and Meissner's plexuses. In 70% of cases the absence of ganglion cells is confined to the sigmoid and the rectum, including the internal sphincter. Involvement of the entire colon and a variable length of small intestine occurs in 10% of cases. The typical infant is a full-term boy; associated anomalies are unusual apart from Down's syndrome. Any infant with Down syndrome with constipation must have Hirschsprung's disease excluded.

Failure to pass meconium within 48 hours is the cardinal symptom. Abdominal distension is progressive. Vomiting, particularly bile-stained vomiting, may not be a prominent early symptom, but poor feeding is frequently described. A rectal examination reveals an empty rectum which grips the finger, with often explosive passage of flatus and meconium following withdrawal of the finger. Reduction in the degree of abdominal distension following a PR may be dramatic, and passage of meconium may continue to the delight of the infant and onlookers. Beware!

DIAGNOSIS AND TREATMENT

If Hirschsprung's disease is suspected – and it should be in any full-term infant who has not passed meconium by 48 hours of age – a plain X-ray of the abdomen must be taken before a rectal examination is done. This will show dilated loops of bowel and some fluid levels. (In the neonate, distinguishing small from large bowel may be difficult.)

If a barium enema is performed it *must* precede any rectal examination or washout, or must be delayed for at least 12 hours after such manipulation. This is because the classical appearance of the narrow aganglionic bowel widening out at "the cone" to the distended ganglionic bowel will be altered by passive dilatation of the aganglionic segment and deflation of the obstructed bowel.

The definitive diagnosis is by rectal biopsy. This may be a full thickness biopsy or a suction biopsy.

Management depends on surgical preference. It is now common practice to keep the colon deflated by regular rectal washout or dilatation for a few weeks – performing the definitive pull through procedure to resect the aganglionic bowel and bring ganglionic bowel to the anal margin when the baby is feeding well and thriving. Formation of a colostomy and definitive surgery at 4–10 months is the alternative management strategy.

MECONIUM PLUG

A plug of inspissated meconium gives rise to signs of low intestinal obstruction. On rectal examination the rectum may be empty, but in a proportion of cases on withdrawing the finger the plug is expelled; following this there is dramatic relief of the obstruction. If a barium enema is carried out the diagnosis is obvious because the plug is outlined as a filling defect. The stimulus of the enema often results in passage of the plug.

The meconium plug may be the sole cause of the obstruction; but this can never be assumed until Hirschsprung's disease has been excluded by rectal biopsy, and cystic fibrosis by a sweat test, or gene probe.

IMPERFORATE ANUS

The incidence is one in 5000. The absence of an anal opening at the normal site will be apparent shortly after birth.

There are innumerable anatomical variations described. In the more serious "high" form, the normal calibre bowel ends above the levator ani – a fistula often communicating with the urethra in the male, or the vagina in the female. The majority of neonates with such an anomaly will require an initial colostomy.

In the "low" anomalies the bowel terminates either just under the perineal skin or at an ectopic site. A perineal procedure to open the bowel on to the surface or enlarge an ectopic opening is usually all that is necessary initially. However, if meconium is passed from the vagina the lesion is a high one, and perineal surgery in the neonatal period is not appropriate.

If there is no obvious opening on initial examination, no attempt to define the level with plain X-rays is likely to be successful within 12 hours of birth because the air in the bowel has to reach the lower colon. An inverted film is not necessary – placing the infant prone over a foam wedge with his bottom uppermost, waiting 10 minutes and then taking a shoot through lateral is much safer and gives equally accurate results. Early plain X-rays may be indicated if an oesophageal atresia or duodenal atresia is suspected. The sacrum should be scrutinized on the pelvic X-rays because of the association of sacral anomalies, particularly with the high anorectal lesions. Associated anomalies – genitourinary, cardiac, oesophageal and skeletal – are common, the baby with a high anomaly is at greatest risk.

It is often assumed, particularly in the female, that if stools are being passed through the ectopic, often stenotic, opening, referral for surgery is unnecessary for several weeks or even months. Delayed treatment leads to progressive rectal distension and usually a very sore, oedematous perineum. Rectal inertia then remains a chronic problem despite adequate surgery.

EXOMPHALOS

The incidence is one in 5000. There is a protrusion of abdominal contents through the umbilical ring covered with a transparent sac. The incidence of major associated anomalies – cardiac, genitourinary and gastrointestinal – is 40%. Features of the Beckwith-Wiedemann, trisomy 13 and trisomy 18 syndromes should be specifically sought. This anomaly is frequently diagnosed on an antenatal scan and major cardiac and chromosomal associations identified.

Unless the exomphalos ruptures emergency surgery is not essential. The abdomen should be wrapped in clingfilm and the sac carefully supported. A size 8 FG nasogastric tube should be aspirated frequently and left on free drainage. The blood sugar must be monitored frequently and appropriate amounts of dextrose infused if there is evidence of hypoglycaemia. The small and moderate sized exomphalos is readily closed. The large ones may require serial reduction using silastic or prolene (v.i.).

An entirely non-surgical approach can be used initially, painting the very large sac with an antiseptic drying agent and waiting for epithelialization to occur.

The associated anomalies and the size of the sac are the major factors contributing to an overall mortality of 25–30%.

GASTROSCHISIS

The incidence is one in 7500. The bowel protrudes through a defect in the anterior abdominal wall, either immediately adjacent to the umbilicus or separated from it by a strip of skin. There is no covering sac. The infant is frequently small-for-dates, but associated lethal abnormalities are rare. This anomaly can be readily diagnosed on prenatal ultrasound. Most evidence supports the view that *in utero* transfer to an appropriate unit is preferable to postnatal transfer. Very early surgery is then possible. Should *in utero* transfer not be possible then following delivery the infant should be kept warm, plasma and antibiotics should be started and urgent transfer arranged. Delay of even a few hours results in increasing thickening and oedema of the extruded bowel. Heat and fluid loss from the exposed bowel can be minimized by wrapping the entire abdomen in several layers of clingfilm, or by putting the lower half of the baby in a large polythene bag secured around the lower chest. A size 8 nasogastric tube should be left on free drainage and aspirated frequently – this is very important.

Hypoproteinaemia is a constant finding and an infusion of plasma 20 ml/kg will improve the infant's condition. Antibiotics should be commenced pre-operatively.

Replacement of the intestine into the peritoneal cavity with primary closure of the abdomen is possible in 80–90% of cases; but if it is not the intestine is enclosed in a silastic or prolene sac sutured to the edges of the abdominal wall defect, the contents of which are gradually reduced into the peritoneal cavity over a 1–2 week period with eventual closure of the abdomen.

Intestinal function may return surprisingly rapidly, but it is not unusual to have to support the infant with intravenous nutrition for weeks or even months before the absorptive capacity and motility of the bowel allow satisfactory oral nutrition.

DIAPHRAGMATIC HERNIA

The incidence is one in 2000–4000. The majority of neonates with this condition present with failure to respond to resuscitation following delivery, followed by considerable difficulty in establishing adequate oxygenation. Left-sided herniae through the foramen of Bochdalek occur in 90% of cases; the remainder are right-sided or herniae through the foramen of Morgagni or the oesophageal hiatus. Thus displacement of the heart sounds to the right chest, poor air entry into the left chest, and a scaphoid abdomen strongly suggest the clinical diagnosis. Confirmation is obtained by an X-ray of the chest and abdomen, showing the displaced mediastinum and loops of bowel in the chest in continuity with intra-abdominal bowel loops. Again the increasing use of prenatal ultrasound scanning allows the diagnosis of a diaphragmatic hernia to be made. Diagnosis in the second trimester is likely to be associated with significant pulmonary hypoplasia. As with gastroschisis *in utero* transfer to an appropriate unit has advantages. Prenatal diagnosis dictates the need to anticipate that the neonate is highly likely to require respiratory support immediately following delivery, and hopefully will prevent a period of mask ventilation which results in distension of the intrathoracic intestine.

Immediately the diagnosis is suspected a size 8 or 10 nasogastric tube should be passed and left on free drainage and aspirated frequently to prevent distension of the intrathoracic gut. Optimal respiratory support is essential using mechanical ventilation with high oxygen concentrations, paralysis with pancuronium, and infusions of base, aiming to achieve normal blood gases. Intravascular volume expansion with colloid or blood is often beneficial, an initial infusion of 20 ml/kg is given. Hypothermia is common unless efforts are made to prevent it during initial resuscitation.

Pulmonary hypertension with right-to-left shunting is a major problem pre and post operatively, and advice on management is given on p. 195. Operation is usually delayed for 24 hours or more to allow maximal reduction in pulmonary artery pressure to occur. Following operation ventilatory support may be required for a few days or several weeks because of pulmonary hypoplasia. Fast rates, high pressures, pharmacological agents and ECMO may all be required (pp. 191–194).

A degree of pulmonary hypoplasia is present in all babies with a diaphragmatic hernia presenting with early respiratory distress. The majority of babies surviving beyond the neonatal period can be expected to have good lung function but some have prolonged oxygen dependency. A significant proportion have such severe hypoplasia that despite intensive support, adequate oxygenation to maintain life is just not possible. The mortality of antenatally diagnosed CDH is still about 50% in most series, and this holds true in the North American ECMO experience.

A small proportion of babies with diaphragmatic herniae still present hours or days after birth, either with dyspnoea or evidence of bowel obstruction. A chest X-ray reveals the diagnosis. The prognosis following surgery is excellent.

POSTERIOR URETHRAL VALVES

The incidence is 1 in 4000.

This condition may present in the male neonate in a number of ways:

1. a palpable bladder with or without palpable kidneys;
2. ascites secondary to urinary extravasation, usually from a hydronephrotic kidney;
3. a poor urinary stream;
4. urinary tract infection, often with an associated septicaemia;
5. prenatal ultrasound diagnosis.

Impaired renal function may be reversible with adequate drainage, and correction of electrolyte and fluid imbalance; but frequently renal function remains abnormal because the obstruction has been present for many months during intrauterine life.

The diagnosis is confirmed by micturating cystourethrography.

Definitive treatment is disruption of the valves, usually endoscopically, and requires a skilled paediatric urologist. Temporary relief of the obstruction can be achieved by urethral catheterization.

If the diagnosis is suspected prenatally the advice of a paediatric urologist should be sought on the timing of the delivery and the immediate postnatal management.

HYPOSPADIAS

The incidence is one in 160. 70% are glandular or coronal, and in these the baby should be observed to make sure he passes urine in a good stream.

In the more severe forms – particularly if coexisting with bilateral undescended testes – an intersex problem must be excluded (pp. 275–277). Circumcision should not be carried out, the foreskin being essential to ensure an acceptable correction of the anomaly – usually at around 1.5–3 years of age.

BLADDER EXSTROPHY AND EPISPADIAS

The incidence is one in 30 000. There is a constellation of abnormalities, affecting boys more frequently than girls.

In epispadias in the male the urethra is represented as a strip of mucosa on the dorsum of the penis. In the female the urethra is split dorsally and is associated with a double clitoris.

In bladder exstrophy, in addition to a complete epispadias the bladder mucosa is exposed on the anterior abdominal wall, the symphisis pubis is widely splayed, the anus is anteriorly situated, and there may be an associated exomphalos. At the extreme end of the spectrum cloacal exstrophy may occur – the two halves of the exstrophic bladder being separated by the ileocaecal region of the bowel which is also exstrophic. The anus is imperforate, and upper urinary tract anomalies are common, as is sacral spina bifida in varying degrees of severity.

Early consultation with a specialist surgeon is essential because surgical intervention within the first 24–48 hours is now more widely advocated. In cloacal exstrophy fluid loss from the bowel may be considerable; urgent, expert assessment of this anomaly is essential.

TESTICULAR TORSION

This may occur pre- or postnatally. It appears to be painless and presents as an enlarged indurated mass with bluish-purple discolouration of the scrotum. If the diagnosis is made shortly after birth exploration is usually advised. Controversy exists on management if the testis is very ischaemic but not obviously necrotic. The majority view would be in favour of preserving the testis because interstitial cells may survive even severe ischaemia. The contralateral testis is usually fixed, although the likelihood of torsion of this testis is very small indeed. If the problem is noted but no action taken for 24–48 hours, exploration is not indicated and the testis will simply atrophy. Occasionally on exploring an apparent torsion, haemorrhagic infarction of the tunica vaginalis and testis is found without evidence of a torsion. This may represent idiopathic infarction, or possibly spontaneous correction of a torsion. Also found on occasions is blood clot either tracking from the peritoneal cavity or retroperitoneal tissues – presumed to be the result of birth trauma. An experienced ultrasonographer will distinguish testicular torsion from blood clot filling the tunica vaginalis.

UNDESCENDED TESTES

Three per cent of full-term and 30% of premature infants will have one or both testes undescended at birth. Bilateral undescended testes should prompt a search for other malformations. Spontaneous descent of the testes is possible during the first year of life, leaving one in a 100 requiring surgery. Follow-up is essential.

The timing of orchidopexy will depend on the individual surgeon. It may be as early as 1 year of age, but should certainly be no later than 4 years.

HYDROCELE

These are common, and require no treatment. They resolve spontaneously.

CIRCUMCISION

There is never any medical indication for this procedure in the neonatal period.

INGUINAL HERNIA

These are uncommon in the early days after birth. The premature infant, both male and female, is particularly prone to develop herniae. While the infant is in the NNU there is no need to operate but surgery is advisable before discharge home because of the high incidence of incarceration of herniae in the early months of life. If incarceration occurs, even if the hernia reduces with manipulation, surgery should be performed within a day or so and certainly before the infant is discharged.

SACROCOCCYGEAL TERATOMA

The incidence is one in 40 000. The infant is born with a cystic or solid mass overlying the sacrum and coccyx and frequently displacing the anus anteriorly. The majority occur in girls and are initially benign.

The mass may extend presacrally and even be palpable abdominally. The important differential diagnosis is from a sacral spina bifida. In the latter, X-rays will show a sacral abnormality, but at times interpretation in the newborn can be difficult.

Large sacrococcygeal teratomas require early referral for surgery. The significance of a small mass may not be appreciated. Early surgery for these is also essential, because the potential for malignant change rises very steeply with the passage of time.

POST-OPERATIVE CARE AFTER LAPAROTOMY

Post-operative management of all infants who have had a neonatal laparotomy is more or less identical and is based on the following.

1. Administration of appropriate IV fluids in general tending to use lower volumes (pp. 30–32).
2. Care of the nasogastric tube, ensuring its correct position and maintaining an empty stomach by appropriate aspiration.
3. Careful observation of vital signs, including ECG, BP and pulse oximetry. Ideally an arterial cannula should be *in situ* for BP and blood gas monitoring.
4. Daily estimation of electrolytes, serum albumin, bilirubin and calcium. A haemoglobin or PCV should be estimated as appropriate.
5. Antibiotics. Usually in combination to cover aerobic and anaerobic organisms.
6. Appropriate intensive care: some neonates will require IPPV post-operatively, for several days in those who are premature or have diaphragmatic hernia. (The treatment of the pulmonary hypoplasia of diaphragmatic hernia is given on p. 195.) The blood pressure must be maintained and renal failure avoided by attention to fluid balance, the BP, and the use of dopamine.
7. Analgesia (Chapter 9). Neonates do feel pain. Morphine is appropriate if the neonate is being ventilated but carries an appreciable risk of respiratory depression and if used the neonate will require very careful observation. The increasing use of local and regional analgesia will improve pain control and obviate the need for parenteral analgesia. Pain control is desirable but the unthinking use of opiates in a situation where adequate supervision of the neonate is not available may result in a respiratory arrest with permanent sequelae.

TOTAL PARENTERAL NUTRITION

(See also Chapter 4.)

In virtually all the conditions described here, oral feeding will not be possible for at least 3–4 days post-operatively. Some infants will not be able to take their full caloric requirements orally for several weeks. Intravenous feeding using the percutaneous long line technique (pp. 482–483), should, ideally, be started in virtually all these infants post-operatively.

FURTHER READING

Freeman, N.V., Burge, D.M., Griffiths, D.M. and Malone, P.S.J. (1994) *Surgery of the Newborn*. Churchill Livingstone, Edinburgh.

Jones, K.L. (1997) *Smith's Recognizable Patterns of Human Malformation*. W B Saunders, Philadelphia.

Stringer, M.D., Oldham, K.T., Mouriquand, P.D.E. and Howard, E.R. (1998) *Paediatric Surgery and Urology: Long Term Outcomes*. W B Saunders, Philadelphia.

26

NEONATAL TUMOURS

Malignant disease occurs in 2–4 per 100 000 live births; the main causes are listed in Table 26.1. The general management of neonates with malignant disease is beyond the scope of this book. These babies must be managed in the local paediatric oncology centre. Three common neonatal tumours, namely neuroblastoma, sacrococcygeal teratoma and mesoblastic nephroma, have an excellent prognosis and active assessment, investigation and treatment are always justified.

NEUROBLASTOMA

Perinatal and neonatal neuroblastoma is unique among malignancies because of its high spontaneous remission rate. As many as 1 in

Table 26.1 Causes of malignant disease in the neonate (<28 days)

Disease	Isaacs 1997* % of neonatal malignancy	Isaacs 1997* Incidence/ 100 000$^\phi$	Broadbent 1999[+] Incidence/ 100 000[++]
Neuroblastoma	27.5%	0.82	0.75
Teratoma	24.7%	0.74**	
Leukaemia	11.7%	0.35	0.45
Sarcoma	10.3%	0.31	0.33
Brain	9.3%	0.28	0.32
Renal	5.7%	0.15$^\$$	
Retinoblastoma	5.7%	0.15$^\sim$	0.13

* based on 795 cases from 11 published series.

[+] based on the UK children's cancer study group figures 1985–1992: overall incidence 2.27/1000.

$^\phi$ assuming an overall incidence of 3.0/100 000.

[++] precise figures based on an overall incidence of 2.7/100 000.

** this includes sacrococcygeal teratoma of which only 10–15% are malignant.

$^\$$ 80% of neonatal renal tumours are mesoblastic nephromas which are rarely malignant.

$^\sim$ the incidence of retinoblastoma will vary with local practice of screening family members of known cases of retinoblastoma.

40 neonates coming to autopsy have neuroblastomas found, which one must assume would have resolved if the baby had survived.

Neonatal neuroblastoma presents with an abdominal or thoracic mass, anaemia, and (in 30% of cases) with extensive cutaneous nodules – stage IV S disease. The masses may compromise respiration or compress the spinal cord. The diagnosis is confirmed by finding calcification on X-ray within the mass, neuroblastoma cells in a marrow biopsy, and a raised urinary vanillyl mandelic acid (VMA).

Aggressive early symptomatic treatment of anaemia or respiratory failure brought on by the mass is always justified because the prognosis is excellent. Around 91% of neonatal cases that survived in a recent UK series, including several cases of IV S disease, regressed without treatment (Moppett *et al.* 1999).

LEUKAEMIA

In the neonate, non-lymphoid acute leukaemia predominates. The neonate presents at birth with hepatosplenomegaly, anaemia, purpura and often widespread leukaemic infiltrates of other organ systems. There are classic findings of leukaemia on the blood film and marrow, usually with anaemia, a marked peripheral leucocytosis containing many primitive cells, and thrombocytopenia.

After confirming the diagnosis careful discussion with the parents is essential since the prognosis is dreadful, and the justification for treatment is thus borderline.

PROLIFERATIVE MYELOPROLIFERATIVE DISORDER

This condition is limited to babies with trisomy 21(Down syndrome). The clinical and haematological features are indistinguishable from acute leukaemia. The abnormal white cells are often megakaryocytes.

The condition resolves spontaneously in the first year just with supportive therapy, such as transfusion for anaemia.

TERATOMA

In some series teratoma has been found to be the commonest neonatal tumour, with an incidence as high as 1 in 25 000. The majority of teratomas are external tumours present at birth, most commonly in the sacrococcygeal area.

Active treatment of sacrococcygeal teratoma is always justified even when there are associated malformations of the rectum, bladder or genitalia, since in 90% of cases the tumour is benign and has an excellent prognosis.

All cases should have repeated alpha feto-protein measurement, as the plasma concentration of this protein remains grossly elevated long after its usual decline. Levels are normally high at birth but rapidly fall to <10 U/ml. If this does not happen in babies with teratoma it is a clue to the fact that the tumour has recurred or was malignant with some remaining.

The surgical management is discussed elsewhere (p. 408). Teratomas in other sites require careful clinical radiological, biochemical and surgical assessment. Extensive infiltration in the neck, for example, may preclude effective treatment.

RENAL TUMOURS

The commonest neonatal renal tumour is the mesoblastic nephroma which presents as an abdominal mass. These tumours should all be removed. The majority are benign and even local recurrence is rare.

REFERENCES

Broadbent, V. (1999) Malignancy in the neonate. In: *Textbook of Neonatology*, 3rd edn. Rennie, J.M. and Roberton, N.R.C. (eds), Churchill Livingstone, Edinburgh, pp. 1051–1061.

Isaacs, H. (1997) *Tumours of the fetus and newborn*. W.B. Saunders, Philadelphia.

Moppett, J., Haddalin, I. and Foot, A.B.M. for the UK CCSG (1999) Neonatal neuroblastoma. *Archives of Disease in Childhood* **81**: F134–F137.

FURTHER READING

Gallagher, P.G. and Lampkin, B.C. (1999) Neonatal tumours. *Seminars in Perinatology* 23, pp. 261–356.

27

NEONATAL JAUNDICE AND LIVER DISEASE

- *Two thirds of normal term babies develop visible jaundice in the first week of life.*
- *Jaundice which is present in the first 24 hours of life must be investigated and treated as an emergency.*
- *High bilirubin levels can cause encephalopathy, and once this develops the chance of permanent handicap is very high.*
- *Jaundice persisting after 14 days of age must be investigated. The minimum safe investigations are split bilirubin, PCV, thyroid function, urine for culture and a clinical examination.*

Jaundice is one of the most common clinical signs in neonatal medicine; two thirds of normal healthy term babies develop visible jaundice in the first week of life. Jaundice is the most frequent cause of admission after early discharge from the postnatal ward. In the vast majority of these babies the jaundice will be harmless, although healthy babies are not immune to the neurotoxic effects of bilirubin (*v.i.*). In a few babies with prolonged jaundice there is serious underlying disease such as biliary atresia, in which early diagnosis dramatically improves the chance of intact survival.

PHYSIOLOGY

The haem from 1 g of haemoglobin yields 600 μmol (35 mg) of unconjugated bilirubin, and the normal term baby breaks down about 0.5 g of haemoglobin every 24 hours. In the plasma, unconjugated bilirubin is mainly bound to albumin and less than 5 nanomol/l of free unconjugated bilirubin is normally present. Bound unconjugated bilirubin can be displaced by many drugs, although with the exception of sulphonamides and the Chinese herbal remedy Yin-chen it is doubtful whether this is of clinical importance (Wadsworth and Suh 1988; Ho 1996). Unconjugated

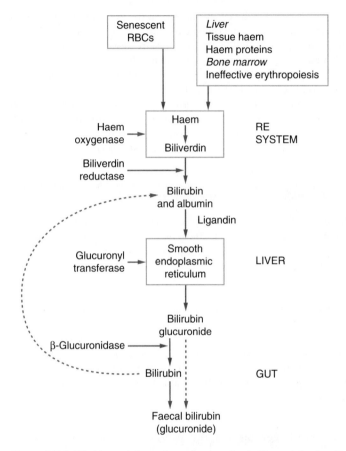

Figure 27.1 Bilirubin metabolism and excretion. Reproduced with permission from Tan 1995.

bilirubin is taken up in the liver by a cytoplasmic protein called ligandin, and is then combined with two molecules of glucuronic acid in the presence of the enzyme glucuronyl transferase to produce conjugated bilirubin (Fig. 27.1). This is actively transported out of the liver cell into bile and then travels into the gut where some passes out of the body in stool, being converted to urobilinogen by bacteria in the colon. Within the gut, if transit time is increased, conjugated bilirubin is deconjugated again by the glucuronidases produced by bacteria in the gut lumen and present in breast milk. The unconjugated bilirubin is absorbed into the enterohepatic circulation, and once more adds to the total pool of bilirubin which the liver has to metabolize. In the presence of obstruction to the biliary tree, conjugated bilirubin refluxes into the plasma and may be excreted in the urine.

All these hepatic functions are impaired in the preterm or ill term newborn compared to the normal healthy full-term baby and, in particular, defective conjugation cannot cope with a large post-natal bilirubin load from breakdown of red blood cells.

BILIRUBIN BIOCHEMISTRY

In most babies the majority of the bilirubin is present as the unconjugated form, with less than 20–40 micromol/l (approx = 1–2 mg%) of conjugated bilirubin. Unconjugated and conjugated bilirubin are also known as indirect-reacting and direct-reacting bilirubin, a name which reflects the chemical test for measuring bilirubin in the laboratory. If a "split" bilirubin test is asked for, the laboratory will do tests which measure both conjugated and unconjugated bilirubin. In routine neonatal practice bilirubin is measured in the nursery using a bilirubinometer. This equipment uses a colorimetric method and measures total bilirubin. The result obtained includes both unconjugated and conjugated bilirubin, together with the coloured photoisomers such as lumirubin (p. 428) which are non-toxic.

BILIRUBIN ENCEPHALOPATHY (KERNICTERUS)

Strictly speaking, kernicterus is a pathological diagnosis describing yellow staining of the basal ganglia. The term is also used to describe the clinical features of bilirubin encephalopathy, the underlying mechanism of which is still uncertain. The cells that are most prone to this type of damage, and which therefore become stained by the bilirubin to give kernicterus (literally "yellow nuclei"), are those which are metabolically active and receive the largest blood flow. In neonates these are the cells of the basal ganglia and the mid-brain. The damage is caused by free bilirubin in the extracellular fluid binding to neuronal cell membranes, with severe and complex biochemical sequelae for the cell (Ives 1999).

The likelihood of free bilirubin leaking out of the plasma and binding to cell membranes is increased by the acidaemia, hypoxia, hypercapnia and disruption of the blood-brain barrier seen in many ill neonates.

In early bilirubin encephalopathy the baby is hypotonic and lethargic, but later he becomes hypertonic and irritable and may seize. If left untreated the condition is fatal, or it may cause severe brain damage in survivors, who have athetoid cerebral palsy, deafness, upgaze palsy and intellectual retardation. Immediate treatment when early signs are present can prevent sequelae, but with late or long-standing signs, permanent CNS damage is inevitable.

The risk of kernicterus is increased by the following factors:

* short gestation;
* rapidly rising levels of serum bilirubin;
* low levels of plasma albumin for the bilirubin to bind to;
* the presence of hypoxia, acidaemia, hypoglycaemia, sepsis or some other serious illness that might disrupt the blood-brain barrier.

PREVENTING BILIRUBIN ENCEPHALOPATHY

We recommend the guidelines in Tables 27.1, 27.2 and 27.3. We would emphasize the lower values for both phototherapy and exchange transfusion in preterm babies. The rate of rise is important, and a bilirubin which is rising at more than 17 (micromol/h is likely to reach an exchange level. Our medico-legal and clinical experience suggests that the increased susceptibility of bigger preterm babies (33–36 weeks gestation) to bilirubin encephalopathy is often forgotten, perhaps because they are cared for on postnatal wards.

Table 27.1 Criteria for exchange transfusion[+] in low birth weight neonates (derived from Ahlfors 1994). Values are expressed in micromol/l

	<1250g	1250–1499g	1500–1999g	2000–2499g
Well baby, bilirubin	220	255	290	305
Well baby, bilirubin: albumin ratio	0.52	0.6	0.68	0.72
Sick baby*, bilirubin	170	220	255	290
Sick baby*, bilirubin: albumin ratio	0.4	0.52	0.6	0.68

*hypotensive, acidotic, hypoglycaemic, hypoxic, septic, with haemolysis of any kind, with GMH-IVH.
[+]we recommend that phototherapy is started at bilirubin levels 50 micromol/l below the exchange level.

Table 27.2 Management of jaundice in the healthy full term baby (from the American Academy of Pediatrics 1994)

Age in hours*	Bilirubin level in micromol/l	
	Phototherapy	**Exchange transfusion**
25–48	260	340
49–72	310	430
>72	340	430

*below 24 hours jaundice must always be investigated as it is usually due to a haemolytic process (*v.i.*). Whether to use phototherapy or to carry out an immediate exchange is a matter for clinical judgement and depends on the rate of rise, the absolute level, and the condition of the baby.

Table 27.3 Criteria for treatment of neonatal jaundice by gestational age. Values in micromol/l. Derived from various sources in the literature

	Phototherapy ill	**Phototherapy well Exchange ill, or rhesus disease**	**Mandatory exchange**
24–26 weeks	130	180	230
27–28 weeks	150	200	250
29–30 weeks	180	230	280
31–32 weeks	200	250	300
33–34 weeks	230	280	320
35–36 weeks	250	300	340

Clearly these data are not based on prospective studies in which the control group was allowed to develop bilirubin encephalopathy, but they are based on extensive clinical experience. Techniques for measuring free bilirubin or reserve albumin-binding capacity are not reliable enough for routine clinical application. The importance of the plasma albumin can be included in the assessment by measuring the bilirubin:albumin ratio (1g albumin = 15.15 micromol albumin, thus an albumin of 45 g/l = 680 micromol/l). An exchange transfusion should be carried out if either of the criteria shown in Table 27.1 is met. For term babies a bilirubin:albumin ratio of 0.8 is an indication for an exchange transfusion if they are well, and 0.72 if they are ill.

DIFFERENTIAL DIAGNOSIS OF NEONATAL JAUNDICE

The natural history and evolution of the jaundice often provides a clue (Fig. 27.2). It is important to remember that up to 66% of

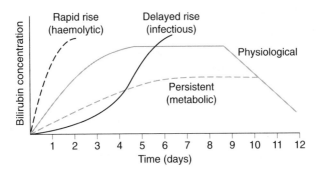

Figure 27.2 Patterns of neonatal jaundice.

entirely normal newborn babies become clinically jaundiced and it is unnecessary to submit them all to routine investigation. The scheme outlined in Table 27.4 will help to identify those conditions requiring treatment. The tests for common conditions should always be done. Tests for rare conditions should be done only if the first battery are negative or if there is a specific clinical lead.

PHYSIOLOGICAL JAUNDICE (UNCONJUGATED, INDIRECT REACTING HYPERBILIRUBINAEMIA)

AETIOLOGY

Whether a baby develops jaundice or not is determined by the balance between the load of haem that reaches the liver from RBC breakdown, and the liver's capacity to produce conjugated bilirubin.

The normal newborn, particularly if premature, is predisposed to jaundice because he has low levels of ligandin and glucuronyl transferase. Factors that increase the likelihood of a baby developing jaundice are listed below, and babies who become jaundiced for no other reasons than these are said to have "physiological jaundice". The factors include:

1. breast feeding;
2. neonatal red cells have a shortened life span, 60–70 days at term, about 40 days if premature;
3. polycythaemia increases the rate of RBC breakdown (p. 453). It

Table 27.4 Diagnostic tests in neonatal jaundice

	Diagnosis	Test
Rapidly developing jaundice on the first day		
Common	Rhesus, ABO, other blood group antibodies causing haemolytic disease	Haemoglobin
		Maternal and baby blood group Coombs' test
	Spherocytosis	Blood film, check family history
	Non spherocytic haemolytic anaemia e.g. G6PD deficiency (in some ethnic groups)	Appropriate enzyme test
Rare	Congenital infection	IgM, serology, platelet count, cultures
Rapid onset jaundice after the first 48 hours, or jaundice in a well baby which reaches treatment levels (Table 27.2 and 27.3)		
Common	Infection	WBC, culture urine, CSF, blood
Less common	Conditions listed above detected late, particularly G6PD deficiency	
Steady rise in jaundice still present at 5–7 days		
Common	Breast feeding	
Jaundice persisting beyond 14 days		
Common	Breast milk jaundice	Exclude conjugated hyperbilirubinaemia. Examine baby, check for UTI, consider G6PD if appropriate
Rare	Conditions in Tables 27.5 and 27.6 Must exclude hepatitis, galactosaemia hypothyroidism, biliary atresia	Appropriate blood and urine tests

is often the result of a large placental transfusion (p. 452). Delayed clamping of the cord increases the incidence of jaundice to over 30%;

4. breakdown of bruises or RBC extravasated into tissues. This may be marked, e.g. following breech presentation, forceps delivery or with large cephalhaematomata;

5. dehydration and a hypocaloric intake (usually breast fed babies (*v.i.*));

6. unconjugated bilirubin from the enterohepatic circulation (p. 415). The slower the intestinal transit time, the more bilirubin comes from this source;

7. "Shunt bilirubin" (20% of the total), from degradation of haem pigments made in the marrow but never incorporated into circulating red cells.

INVESTIGATION

When the bilirubin reaches treatment levels (Table 27.2 and 27.3) in a term baby the following investigations should be done as a minimum (see Table 27.4 for further, second line, investigations).

- Full blood count, PCV.
- Group, Coombs' test.
- Blood , urine and surface swab cultures.
- Thyroid function.
- Investigate for G6PD deficiency where appropriate.

BREAST FEEDING AND JAUNDICE

Breast fed babies develop higher levels of bilirubin than formula fed babies, and their jaundice persists for longer. The healthy term breast fed baby is not immune to kernicterus, although the condition is very rare in this group. In about 1 in 700 healthy term babies the serum bilirubin rises above 340 micromol/l, and most of these babies are breast fed. The cause of jaundice in breast fed babies is multifactorial. In the first week the main cause is probably a low calorie and fluid intake. The prolonged jaundice that is seen in thriving term babies after two weeks of age is due to agents in breast milk which inhibit bilirubin glucuronidation in the liver or deconjugate bilirubin glucuronide in the gut, enhancing the enterohepatic bilirubin circulation. The current combined, and justified, enthusiasm for breast feeding and early neonatal discharge means that babies are becoming markedly jaundiced in dimly lit bedrooms under the none too watchful eye of individuals hitherto lacking experience in assessing and managing neonatal jaundice. Disaster, in the form of kernicterus, can result. Neonatal units must ensure that those responsible for babies discharged early are trained to recognize significant jaundice and these professionals must have ready access to bilirubin estimations at all times.

In early onset breast feeding jaundice the small group of babies at high risk of developing potentially damaging levels of bilirubin can be predicted from an early estimation of the level (Bhutani *et al.*

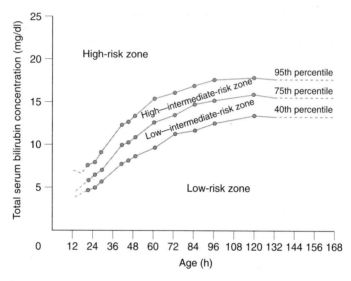

Figure 27.3 Hour specific bilirubin values from a group of over 13 000 healthy babies (from Bhutani *et al.* 1999 with permission). Note conversion of mg/dl to micromol/l requires multiplication by 17.1.

1999). A bilirubin level of 137 micromol/l at 24 hours is above the 95th centile for term babies (Fig. 27.3), and babies with breast feeding (physiological) jaundice "track" according to their bilirubin centile. Babies with haemolysis or another reason for jaundice do not track, and clearly two estimations are required before an entirely safe assumption can be made that this is the reason for jaundice in an individual baby. Repeat bilirubin estimation and careful clinical vigilance are essential for the group who reach the 95th centile early, because phototherapy is likely to be required. An adequate milk intake should be continued and if the criteria for phototherapy are met (Table 27.2), use it, continue breast feeding, and the bilirubin will fall and stay down.

The persisting late (>14 day) jaundice seen in thriving breast fed babies is an even rarer cause of kernicterus. Once the diagnosis is secure on the basis of the progression of the jaundice, a bilirubin consistently below 340 micromol/l and the exclusion of serious causes of prolonged jaundice (*v.i.*, Hannam *et al.* 2000), no treatment is required. Although stopping breast feeding for 24 hours will cause a rapid decline in the bilirubin level and establish the diagnosis, we consider that this practice should be abandoned as it will compromise the likelihood of successful long term lactation.

PATHOLOGICAL CAUSES OF JAUNDICE (UNCONJUGATED, INDIRECT REACTING HYPERBILIRUBINAEMIA)

HAEMOLYTIC DISEASE OF THE NEWBORN (HDN)

This is the commonest cause of severe jaundice which develops rapidly during the first 24 hours. Numerically ABO HDN is the commonest form, but Rh (D) is the most severe. Other blood group incompatibilities can, rarely, cause a similar picture. These conditions are considered in detail in Chapter 28.

HAEMOLYTIC ANAEMIA

Many intrinsic structural or biochemical disorders of the red cell present with early onset jaundice due to increased RBC breakdown, which may be severe enough to require phototherapy and exchange transfusion to prevent kernicterus. They include spherocytosis, glucose-6-phosphatase dehydrogenase deficiency, and the alpha thalassaemia syndromes (Chapter 28).

SEPTICAEMIA (see Chapter 14)

Bacterial infection causes increased RBC destruction, liberating more bilirubin, and impairs the ability of the liver to clear bilirubin from the plasma. Infection should always be suspected in any neonate with a sudden onset of jaundice not due to haemolytic disease or red cell abnormalities.

Jaundice with septicaemia may cause kernicterus. Phototherapy and exchange transfusion should be used as necessary.

PROLONGED NEONATAL JAUNDICE

There are various conditions in which neonatal jaundice is prolonged beyond the first week. These are summarized in Tables 27.5 and 27.6. The minimum investigations are a total bilirubin with conjugated and unconjugated bilirubin, PCV, urine for reducing

Table 27.5 Causes of prolonged jaundice

Group I	**Persistence of acute neonatal cause (unconjugated hyperbilirubinaemia)**
	Haemolytic anaemia (immune, spherocytic or non-spherocytic)
	Chronic low grade infection (bacterial or viral)
Group II	**Breast milk jaundice (unconjugated)**
Group III	**Rare causes of unconjugated hyperbilirubinaemia**
	Galactosaemia
	Hypothyroidism
	Aminoacidaemia (increased tyrosine, methionine)
	Pyloric stenosis
	Intestinal obstruction
	Drugs
	Fructosaemia
	Lucey-Driscoll syndrome (serum conjugation inhibition)
	Crigler-Najjar syndrome
	Gilbert's disease
	Cystic fibrosis
	Lipid storage disorders (e.g. Niemann-Pick, Gaucher's)
Group IV	**Conjugated hyperbilirubinaemia**
	Biliary atresia
	Other causes of obstructive jaundice (see Table 27.6)

substances and culture, thyroid function test and a clinical examination (Hannam *et al.* 2000).

PROLONGED UNCONJUGATED INDIRECT REACTING JAUNDICE

The conditions listed under Group I in Table 27.5 can usually be excluded quite easily by appropriate blood tests and cultures.

Of the conditions listed in Group III in Table 27.5 it is vital not to miss galactosaemia (p. 304) and hypothyroidism (p. 281), since these are preventable causes of mental subnormality. The possibility of cystic fibrosis can be investigated by a search for the commoner genetic deletions and by measurement of plasma immunoreactive trypsin. A sweat test can be carried out in older babies. The diagnosis and management of the other rare causes of jaundice are discussed by Mieli-Vergani and Mowat (1999).

Table 27.6 Causes of obstructive jaundice (which may be prolonged): often do not cause problems in the early neonatal period

Hepatitis
    A, B, C and others
    Congenital infection (e.g. rubella, CMV)
    Giant cell neonatal hepatitis
    Galactosaemia
    Other viral infection (e.g. Echovirus, reovirus)
Inspissated bile syndrome (can occur after rhesus disease)
Cystic fibrosis
Biliary atresia
Biliary hypoplasia
Endocrine disorders (hypothyroidism, hypopituitarism)
Inborn errors of metabolism (Tyrosinosis, Gaucher's, Neimann Pick, hypermethioninaemia)
Graft versus host disease
Alpha 1 antitrypsin deficiency
Inherited defects (Dubin-Johnson, Rotor)
Extrinsic biliary obstruction (bands, tumour, cholodochal cyst)
Gallstones; spontaneous perforation of the bile ducts
Prolonged TPN (p.59)
Lipid storage disease
Infantile polycystic disease
Neonatal haemochromatosis
Bile acid synthetic defects

PROLONGED CONJUGATED (DIRECT REACTING) HYPERBILIRUBINAEMIA (see Table 27.6)

It is surprising how rarely these conditions, particularly biliary atresia, present while the baby is still in the maternity hospital. When conjugated hyperbilirubinaemia is recognized, appropriate biochemical and serological tests should be carried out since accurate diagnosis is important on both prognostic and therapeutic grounds. Very pale stools and dark urine are not normal for babies, and this combination in a jaundiced baby should always lead to urgent investigation. Remember that many babies who develop obstructive jaundice will only have received oral vitamin K, and are at risk of late onset haemorrhagic disease of the newborn (p. 447–449). Giving an extra dose of IM vitamin K does no harm, and it can prevent devastating and damaging intracranial haemorrhage accompanying whatever is causing the jaundice. Bruising and bleeding are common presenting features in babies with obstructive liver disease.

TPN JAUNDICE

In routine neonatal practice by far and away the commonest cause of conjugated hyperbilirubinaemia is jaundice associated with TPN in the ill low birth weight neonate. Sepsis is undoubtedly a contributory factor. Other than stopping the TPN, no treatment is effective. Phenobarbitone, ursodeoxycholic acid and cholecystokinin have been found to reduce the level of bilirubin in some babies.

BILIARY ATRESIA

It is now clear that the earlier biliary atresia (incidence 1 in 14 000) is diagnosed, the better the results of surgery – usually a Kasai portoenterostomy. All babies still jaundiced at 14 days should have a urinalysis and split bilirubin measurement (*v.s.*). Those with marked bilirubinuria and/or a conjugated hyperbilirubinaemia should be referred at once to a paediatrician with special expertise in liver disease. Give vitamin K prior to transfer.

This is another reason for ensuring that all those seeing babies in the community are trained in the management of neonatal jaundice, including prolonged jaundice (see also breast milk jaundice, p. 421).

TREATMENT OF NEONATAL JAUNDICE

The underlying causes of the jaundice must always be sought and treated appropriately. In addition, specific therapy for the jaundice should be started if kernicterus is a threat.

TREATMENT OF PHYSIOLOGICAL JAUNDICE

Term babies

The vast majority of babies require no treatment. Dehydration and under-feeding may be present if the weight loss exceeds 10%. If the baby is being breast fed, increase the frequency of breast feeds to 2–3 hourly. We normally start phototherapy in term babies when the bilirubin has risen to 340 micromol/1, although there is no good evidence that this group are harmed by bilirubin levels below 425 micromol/1.

Preterm babies

In low birth weight babies who are already on the NNU, in whom kernicterus may develop at much lower bilirubin levels, give phototherapy when the total bilirubin reaches the appropriate level (Table 27.1, Table 27.3).

TREATMENT OF SEVERE JAUNDICE

Adequate hydration

In sick small babies under radiant heat sources, dehydration is an important contributor to jaundice. If there are no other constraints on the fluid balance, such babies should have their fluid intake increased to at least 150 ml/kg/24 h, if necessary by tube feeding or by giving intravenous fluid. Extra fluid should be given to preterm babies who require phototherapy.

Drugs

The enzymes of bilirubin glucuronidation can be induced by various drugs, in particular phenobarbitone. However, it takes 48 hours for phenobarbitone to have any effect, and this drug makes the baby sleepy and feed poorly. This therapy has no place in current neonatal practice except in the management of Type II Crigler-Najjar syndrome (Arias *et al.* 1969).

Although laxatives also lower neonatal serum bilirubin, their use is not justified even though it is often noted that the jaundice in preterm babies only starts to clear once they have had their bowels open. The metalloporphyrins reduce jaundice by inhibiting heme oxygenase and thus reducing the bilirubin load delivered to the liver. Trials are under way but these agents are not without side effects and they cannot be recommended in routine clinical practice.

Phototherapy

Phototherapy, with light of wave length 425–475 nm reduces the amount of unconjugated bilirubin in plasma by three methods (Ives 1999):

1. Geometrical isomerization of the bilirubin to produce water soluble isomers which are slowly excreted; they revert to toxic isomers in the dark or when phototherapy is discontinued.

2. Intramolecular photoconversion between adjacent pyrrole rings – this produces a stable isomer called lumirubin which is rapidly excreted.
3. Photo-oxidation to colourless pyrollic and dipyrollic compounds.

The isomers produced in reactions 1 and 2 are formed immediately phototherapy starts. They are yellow and indistinguishable from natural bilirubin in the bilirubinometer, but they are polar and non-toxic. Therefore as soon as phototherapy starts, although the measured bilirubin may not fall, some is present in a considerably less toxic form. By the time equilibrium is reached after twelve hours of phototherapy, about 20% of the total bilirubin measured by the bilirubinometer is in the form of non-toxic photoisomers.

Many phototherapy devices are now available. Not only are there overhead lamps, but fibreoptic pads and even "bili-blankets" which wrap the baby in a blue light source. These lights are powerful, generating spectral irradiance above 20 microW/cm^2 per nanometer of wavelength and combined use can reduce bilirubin in non haemolysing babies by more than 40% in 24 hours. Single phototherapy reduces bilirubin by about 20% of the initial value in 24 hours (Tan 1995). Combining light from a bilirubin blanket or pad with that from an overhead light source can avoid the need for an exchange transfusion if they are used together and immediately in term babies admitted from home with very high bilirubin levels (Maisels 1996).

The indications for phototherapy are as follows:

1. haemolytic disease – jaundiced babies with rhesus, ABO or other haemolytic disease of the newborn, or with RBC abnormalities, until it is clear that a permanent fall in bilirubin has occurred;
2. small sick babies, including those with sepsis, whose bilirubin levels rise above the phototherapy line (v.s.);
3. bilirubin levels >340 micromol/l (20 mg%) in mature healthy babies (v.s.).

Phototherapy should be used continuously until the bilirubin is falling consistently and is below the "safe" line for gestation (Tables 27.2 and 27.3). A small rebound is usual after stopping treatment, but if the bilirubin rises significantly once phototherapy is stopped, restart it and check that there is no new cause of hyperblirubinaemia. Do *not* give phototherapy for conjugated jaundice, because the baby is likely to turn a deep brown colour, probably due to photodegradation of porphyrins which are raised in the plasma of babies with conjugated hyperbilirubinaemia (Rubaltelli *et al.* 1983).

No serious long-term sequelae of phototherapy have been reported. However, phototherapy:

1. decreases gut transit time causing diarrhoea, probably owing to the irritant effect on the bowel of the photoisomers of bilirubin;
2. increases fluid loss through the skin and gut;
3. exposes the neonate to the risks of hypo- and hyperthermia, and powerful modern lights may cause superficial burns;
4. causes erythematous rashes.

Probably the most serious adverse effect of phototherapy is the anxiety it provokes in mothers who have their babies removed, blindfolded and laid naked under a bright light.

When giving phototherapy:

1. Give it in the postnatal ward beside the mother if the baby is otherwise well and weighs more than 2.0 kg.
2. Keep as much of the baby as unclothed as possible. Many babies are covered with nappies, hats, bootees, blindfolds and bits of sticky tape holding on various monitors, with the result that little light reaches the skin.
3. Take great care with the thermal environment. Naked babies in a cool room may become hypothermic, and preterm babies in incubators may overheat owing to the radiant heat output of the phototherapy unit.
4. Watch the baby's fluid balance. Phototherapy may double the fluid loss through a small baby's skin and gut, and appropriate increases in oral or intravenous fluid are necessary.
5. Blindfold the baby, but be careful that this does not cause conjunctivitis due to irritation from the bandaging; alternatively use a special plastic lightproof head box.
6. Check the irradiance of the lights after every 100–200 hours of use to ensure that they are still effective.
7. Make sure that the lamps are kept cool, and not used as dumping grounds for papers, towels, etc.

Exchange transfusion

This technique not only washes out bilirubin, but it also removes haemolytic antibody and corrects anaemia. It is therefore the treatment of choice in severe haemolytic jaundice. Furthermore, it is the only technique which can be used when the bilirubin must be lowered urgently because it has reached potentially toxic levels or the baby is showing early clinical evidence of kernicterus.

Exchange transfusion can also be used in the following situations:

1. severe non-haemolytic anaemia from any cause (p. 435);
2. sepsis (p. 237);
3. to remove drugs or accumulated toxic metabolites in depressed neonates;
4. in coagulopathies to remove factors that perpetuate the coagulation disturbance and replace coagulation factors (p. 450).

To achieve a 90–95% swap of the baby's blood, twice his blood volume (i.e. 2×85 ml/kg = 170 ml/kg) should be exchanged. Smaller volumes can be used when exchange transfusion is used in conditions other than HDN. Various techniques have been used but the following are the two most common approaches:

1. the serial withdrawal and injection of aliquots of blood through a central vein (usually the umbilical vein) until the required volume has been exchanged;
2. the continuous removal of blood from the umbilical or some other large artery, balanced by continuous infusion into a vein.

When using the push/pull technique, each cycle (withdrawing 5, 10 or 20 ml, and then injecting 5, 10 or 20 ml) should take 4–5 minutes, taking at least 2–3 minutes for the infusion. The smaller volumes should be used in low birth weight or sick babies. A full exchange by either technique should last about 1.5–2 hours.

Throughout the exchange the baby must have continuous ECG monitoring and be closely observed. In the very ill baby, the control of the exchange will be much better with continuous monitoring of BP, and frequent blood gas estimation.

Complications and hazards of exchange transfusion

Catheter induced complications   These include air emboli and aortic or portal vein thrombosis. Haemorrhage may occur from the umbilical stump or catheters. Exchange transfusion may cause NEC (p. 386). All these can usually be avoided by correct technique.

Haemodynamic complications   Unless great care is taken during the exchange transfusion, excess blood may be removed or injected, with disastrous consequences. In addition, too rapid an exchange by the push/pull technique can cause progressive cardiorespiratory deterioration (Aranda and Sweet 1977).

Hypoglycaemia   See p. 287, 291.

Hypocalcaemia The ECG should always be monitored during exchange transfusion to detect hypocalcaemia caused by the citrate in the bank blood. If cardiac arrhythmias occur give 1 ml of 10% calcium gluconate slowly IV and repeat it if necessary.

Hyperkalaemia In bank blood preserved in CPD-A, the "plasma" potassium increases steadily, by about 0.5 mmol per day. Hyperkalaemia may therefore develop if blood greater than 2–3 days old is used. Its treatment is outlined on p. 375.

Acidaemia Bank blood less than 24 hours old stored in CPD-A has a H^+ of 80 nmol/1 (pH 7.1). Therefore, during exchange transfusion in sick babies check the blood gases once or twice, and correct any metabolic acidaemia which develops.

Tissue hypoxia The 2:3 DPG levels are sustained reasonably well in CPD–A blood.

Age of blood

The quality of blood, even when stored in CPD-A deteriorates rapidly. The pH falls, the pCO_2 rises, the potassium concentration rises and the 2:3 DPG steadily falls. It is hyperosmolar, hypernatraemic, free of calcium and contains citrate which babies may find difficult to metabolize. For exchange transfusion in sick babies particularly those who are VLBW, blood less than 48 hours old should be used; blood older than this poses an unacceptable metabolic stress.

REFERENCES

Ahlfors, C.E. (1994) Criteria for exchange transfusion in jaundiced newborns. *Pediatrics* **93**: 488–494.

American Academy of Pediatrics (1994) Practice parameter: management of hyperbilirubinaemia in the healthy term newborn. *Pediatrics* **94**: 558–565.

Aranda, J.V. and Sweet, A.Y. (1977) Alterations in blood pressure during exchange transfusion. *Archives of Disease in Childhood* **52**: 545–548.

Arias, I.M., Gartner, L.M., Cohen, M., Ezzer, J.B. and Levi, A.J. (1969) Chronic nonhemolytic unconjugated hyperbilirubinemia with glucuronyl transferase deficiency. *American Journal of Medicine* **47**: 395–409.

Bhutani, V.K., Johnson, L. and Sivieri, M.S. (1999) Predictive ability of a predischarge hour specific serum bilirubin for subsequent significant hyperbilirubinemia in healthy term and near term newborns. *Pediatrics* **103**: 6–14.

Hannam, S., McDonnell, M. and Rennie, J.M. (2000) Investigation of prolonged neonatal jaundice. *Acta Paediatrica* **89**: 694–697.

Ho, N.K. (1996) Traditional Chinese medicine and treatment of neonatal jaundice. *Singapore Medical Journal* **37**: 645–651.

Ives, N.K. (1999) Jaundice. In: *Textbook of Neonatology*, 3rd edn. Rennie, J.M. and Roberton, N.R.C. (eds), Churchill Livingstone, Edinburgh, pp. 715–732.

Maisels, M.J. (1996) Why use homeopathic doses of phototherapy? *Pediatrics* **98**: 283–287.

Mieli-Vergani, G., Mowat, A. P. (1999). Disorders of the liver and biliary system. In: *Textbook of Neonatology*, 3rd edn. Rennie, J.M. and Roberton, N.R.C. (eds), Churchill Livingstone, Edinburgh, pp. 733–743.

Rubaltelli, F.F., Jori, G. and Reddi, E. (1983) Bronze baby syndrome: a new porphyrin-related disorder. *Pediatric Research* **17**: 327–330.

Tan, K.L. (1995) Phototherapy: Mechanism and clinical efficacy. In: *Physiological monitoring and instrumental diagnosis in perinatal and neonatal medicine*. Brans, Y.W. and Hay, W.W. (eds), Cambridge University Press, Cambridge pp 362–373.

Wadsworth, S.J. and Suh, B. (1988) In vitro displacement of bilirubin by antibiotics and 2-hydroxybenzoylglycine in newborns. *Antimicrobial Agents and Chemotherapy* **32**: 1571–1575.

28

NEONATAL HAEMATOLOGY

ANAEMIA IN THE NEONATE

- *Most anaemia in the non-jaundiced full term baby is due to perinatal blood loss.*
- *Perinatal blood loss may cause nothing more than mild pallor that requires treatment with iron and folate, but is occasionally responsible for a pale shocked baby with a haemoglobin of <4 g%.*
- *Anaemia of prematurity can be reduced by minimizing blood lost into the laboratory; routine use of haematinics is of no value and we do not currently use erythropoietin.*
- *Consider haemolytic disease in all jaundiced babies in the first 24 hours.*
- *Most cases of haemolytic disease of the newborn are now due to ABO incompatibility, but other incompatibilities and red cell disorders such as spherocytosis present in a similar way.*

DEFINITION

Anaemia is defined as a haemoglobin value of less than 12 g/dl in the first week or less than 10 g/dl later in infancy.

ANAEMIA PRESENT AT BIRTH

This may be due to haemorrhage, haemolysis or rarely to impaired red cell production.

Haemorrhage

This may be due to:

- twin-to-twin transfusion;
- fetal haemorrhage from normal or abnormal placental vessels, or from placental separation or injury (e.g. placental abruption,

placenta praevia, placental incision at caesarean section, velamentous insertion of the cord);
- fetal or neonatal internal haemorrhage (ruptured liver or spleen, subgaleal haemorrhage);
- fetomaternal haemorrhage.

Haemolysis

This may be due to:

- rhesus haemolytic disease (*v.i.*);
- other immune haemolytic processes e.g. anti-Kell, ABO incompatibility;
- congenital infection (e.g. parvovirus B19, cytomegalovirus).

Impaired red cell production

This may be due to:

- Blackfan Diamond syndrome and other disorders (see Brugnara and Platt, 1998);
- rarities such as α-thalassaemia (baby often hydropic) (see Orkin and Nathan 1998).

Marked pallor in the neonate may also be due to severe asphyxia (p. 83).

ASSESSMENT OF EARLY ANAEMIA

History and physical examination

- Was there unusual blood loss in labour? Examine the placenta for abnormal vessels, especially vasa praevia.
- Are there any findings in the baby to suggest bleeding (e.g. cephalhaematoma, boggy scalp swelling, rigid abdomen)? or haemolysis (hepatosplenomegaly, jaundice)?
- Was there a twin-to-twin transfusion? Compare haematocrits, discuss the obstetric history and antenatal ultrasound findings.
- Check the pulse and respiration. A steadily rising pulse rate, tachypnoea or air hunger are signs of massive haemorrhage.
- *Always* measure the baby's blood pressure.

Investigation

This should include the following:

- Haemoglobin and PCV measurement. Remember it takes 2–3 hours for these to fall after major acute haemorrhage.
- Serum bilirubin.
- Blood group and Coombs' test.
- pH. This is a good emergency test, since when the cardiac output falls, tissue perfusion deteriorates and an acidaemia develops.
- Check the mother's blood for feto-maternal haemorrhage by the Kleihauer test.

Treatment

In an emergency the baby will be pale and show signs of shock with weak pulses, shallow rapid respiration, hypotension and acidosis. In this life-threatening situation give an immediate transfusion (most easily through a UVC) of 15–20 ml/kg over 5–10 minutes using uncrossmatched O negative blood. Give oxygen if necessary, and then insert an umbilical artery catheter for regular monitoring of PaO_2, blood gases and haematocrit. Correct any acid–base abnormalities. Check that vitamin K was given.

If the baby is still pale and hypotensive repeat the transfusion over 15–20 minutes and if possible check the CVP through the UVC. Aim to achieve a normal blood pressure, normal pH and a haemoglobin above 12 g%.

If the baby with a haemoglobin level of 8–10 g is stable with no hypotension, tachycardia, acidaemia or respiratory distress, and in particular if no cause of acute blood loss can be found, he may be suffering from chronic, or acute on chronic haemorrhage such as a fetomaternal or twin-to-twin haemorrhage during late pregnancy. In such babies haemodilution is likely to have occurred, and they are unlikely to be hypotensive: if the anaemia is even more severe it may have caused fetal heart failure, or even hydrops (Chapter 29). In these situations, a single volume (80 ml/kg) exchange transfusion using packed cells is the safest way to raise the haemoglobin without exacerbating the heart failure.

With anaemia of 10–12 g% in an asymptomatic baby, a top-up transfusion of 20–30 ml/kg can be given over 2 hours with frusemide cover, and the need for further transfusions reassessed afterwards.

LATE-ONSET NEONATAL ANAEMIA (2–28 DAYS OF AGE)

The conditions listed in Table 28.1 may be responsible for anaemia of below 10 g% occurring later in the neonatal period in babies who

Table 28.1 Causes of chronic neonatal anaemia

Cause	Diagnosis
Haemorrhage	
Haemorrhage into the laboratory	Examine records of number of laboratory tests
Perinatal haemorrhage not recognized at the time of delivery	Check the history in more detail for such a problem
Chronic blood loss especially from the GI tract	Clinical examination, stool, urine analysis, iron-deficient picture on blood film
Haemolysis	
Mild haemolytic disease of the newborn – insufficient to cause jaundice	Maternal history, Coombs' test, antibody studies on the mother
Fragile red cells – e.g. spherocytosis	Blood film, family history
Enzyme deficiency (e.g. G6PD)	Enzyme assay, reticulocyte count
Chronic infection especially UTI and occasionally congenital infections	Clinical examination, stool, urine analysis, iron deficient picture on blood film
Impaired red cell/haemoglobin production	
Anaemia of prematurity (*v.i.*)	
Haemoglobinopathies	Haemoglobin electrophoresis, reticulocyte count, family studies
Drugs	History
Rare congenital bone marrow aplasias or congenital leukaemia	Physical examination for hepatosplenomegaly or skin infiltration; blood count, bone marrow

are otherwise well. The conditions fall into the same categories as before.

Investigation and treatment

In most cases, if no diagnosis is obvious, it is reasonable to assume that the baby received no placental transfusion, or had a small unrecognized perinatal bleed. If his haemoglobin is less than 10 g% transfuse him with 20 ml/kg packed red cells; but if it is above 10 g% give him iron and folic acid supplements in the expectation that he will develop a good reticulocytosis and his haemoglobin will rise.

Investigation for the last group of disorders in Table 28.1 should only be carried out if there are clinical clues, if the haemoglobin continues to fall, or there is other evidence of marrow disease (Brugnara and Platt 1998).

ANAEMIA OF PREMATURITY

The nadir in haemoglobin concentration in VLBW babies is 8 g/dl at the age of 4–8 weeks, and this section refers to babies who present at this time. In the critically ill neonate with RDS, sepsis, CLD, or GMH-IVH, it is essential to keep the haemoglobin above 14 g% (PCV >40) at all times (p. 142–143).

Erythropoietin deficiency This is almost certainly the single major cause of this disorder. EPO production switches off after birth in VLBW babies and increases only very slowly thereafter (Brown *et al.* 1983). There is a blunted EPO response to decreasing haemoglobin levels in preterm babies. In addition to EPO deficiency the *red cell survival* of premature babies is known to be short.

Folic acid deficiency Despite the fact that most premature babies, particularly those below 1.5 kg at birth, have low levels of serum folate by 6–8 weeks of age, megaloblastic change in the marrow is rare. However, we give babies of birth weight below 2.0 kg, and those with rhesus HDN, 0.1 mg of folic acid daily from 2 weeks of age while they are in the NNU.

Vitamin E deficiency We no longer give vitamin E supplements routinely. Vitamin E deficiency was a feature of feeding babies with the older milk formulas which were high in polyunsaturated fats.

Iron deficiency This is *not* important in the anaemia of prematurity. Premature babies do eventually become iron deficient, so start iron supplements when they weigh 2.0 kg and are ready for discharge. For the first 6 months we give 2.5 ml Sytron (equivalent to 13.75 mg Fe, 95 mg iron edetate) as a single daily dose.

Management

Check the haemoglobin and reticulocyte count of all the asymptomatic growing premature babies in the neonatal unit every week.

A small number of anaemic babies become lethargic, feed poorly and have mild tachycardia and tachypnoea with reduced weight gain and even apnoea. In those with a haemoglobin below 8 g% and more than $150 \times 10^9/l$ (about 4%) reticulocytes, the haemoglobin will rise slowly and transfusion is not required. If the reticulocyte count is below $50 \times 10^9/l$ (about 1–2%), and particularly if the baby is otherwise ready for discharge, a 20 ml/kg transfusion of packed cells should be considered.

Summaries of the results of randomized trials of recombinant human EPO show disappointing results, with only a small reduction in the numbers of untransfused babies, and this treatment is not currently widely used.

HAEMOLYTIC DISEASE OF THE NEWBORN

Pathophysiology

Throughout all pregnancies, very small amounts of blood leak from the fetal circulation into the mother. If it is rhesus positive (D positive) blood, about 5% of rhesus negative primiparae will develop a mild antibody response. However, in most women, major feto-maternal bleeding only occurs during labour, antepartum haemorrhage or spontaneous or therapeutic abortion. Although over 100 ml of blood may enter the mother's circulation in exceptional circumstances around the time of delivery, the usual volume is in the range 0.5–5.0 ml. However, this is enough to evoke a major antibody response, which will be most marked against the D antigen of the rhesus group.

The antibodies formed will be of the IgG class, which will cross the placenta and haemolyse fetal rhesus positive red cells.

In the 5% of first pregnancies in rhesus negative women where antibody is formed before delivery, the infant usually only suffers from mild rhesus HDN. In most first rhesus incompatible pregnancies, no antibody is formed until after the feto-maternal bleed at delivery, and so the infant has no neonatal problems. However, in subsequent pregnancies, if the fetus is again rhesus positive, the very small feto-maternal bleeds of 0.1–0.2 ml early in gestation will now evoke a major secondary antibody response in a sensitised woman. With each successive rhesus positive fetus, larger amounts of anti-D will be made, and the disease in the fetus will become more severe.

Not all rhesus positive babies inside rhesus negative women provoke an antibody response. The presence of ABO incompatibility between the mother and her fetus protects against rhesus HDN, since if A positive fetal cells cross into an O negative woman, her natural isoimmune anti-A will destroy the fetal RBC before they evoke an antibody response to the rhesus antigen.

Antenatal care

There are three stages in the antenatal care of these women:

1. Detect all rhesus negative women and screen them for the presence of antibody by appropriate blood tests in the booking antenatal clinics. Also check whether their partner is homozygous or heterozygous for D.
2. Assess how severely affected the baby is.
3. Plan the optimal time to deliver the baby.

Assessment of severity

This is done in three ways (Table 28.2). First, the level of maternal antibodies is measured. If this is high, either amniocentesis or fetal blood sampling should be carried out. At amniocentesis the colour of the liquor is assessed by measuring the change in optical density of the fluid (compared to a standard) at a wavelength of 450 mμ. This is plotted on the chart shown in Fig. 28.1. Those in zone 1 have no or mild disease, those in zone 2 have disease that needs watching, and those in zone 3 require urgent therapy. Serial examinations should be repeated every 2–3 weeks.

For babies below 28 weeks gestation, and for those who reach upper zone 2 or are in zone 3 fetal blood sampling should be done to measure the haemoglobin in the fetus (Table 17.1). If the level is normal, or just below normal (fetal haemoglobin rises from 11 g% at 28 weeks to 15 g% at term) no treatment is required, but if it is more than 2 g/l below the mean the fetus should be transfused always aiming to keep the fetal haemoglobin above 7–8 g/l. Severity is also assessed by serial ultrasound measurements looking for fetal ascites, pleural effusions or hydrops.

Timing of delivery

If the amniocentesis results approach the action line under 33 weeks, fetal transfusion is indicated. After 33 weeks, fetal delivery should be considered.

If fetal transfusions are being used, the aim should be to continue these until the baby is at least 33–34 weeks gestation and

Table 28.2 Antenatal management of Rh affected women

Maternal anti-D level (iu/ml)	Repeat sample (weeks)	Fetal blood sampling	Rh D typing of fetus^	PCV level	Intrauterine transfusion	Time at which delivery is recommended (weeks)
<0.5	4	Not required	No	No	No	40
0.5–3.9	2	Not required	No	No	No	40
4.0–9.9	2	Not required	No	No	No	36–38
10–20	2	28 weeks*	Yes	Yes	Probably no~	33–38~
>20	2	20 weeks	Yes	Yes	Probably yes+	33–38+

* if after 28 weeks, within one week of the maternal anti-D level first being >10 iu/ml.

~ precise timing determined from PCV levels (see text), the objective being to reach at least 34 weeks of gestation.

+ in many units for babies >28 weeks this would be preceded by amniocentesis, referring the baby for blood sampling if he was in upper zone 2 or zone 3 on the chart (Fig. 28.1).

^ if fetus is Rh negative no further action is required.

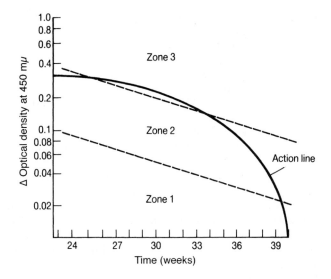

Figure 28.1 Chart for interpreting amniocentesis results with Whitfield's action line superimposed (Whitfield 1970).

has a mature L:S ratio, and so is no longer at risk from RDS after delivery. If fetal demise is imminent for any reason, the baby should be delivered regardless of gestation.

Whenever possible the baby should be delivered at a time that is convenient for both the paediatrician and the transfusion service. Friday is therefore not a good day! Always ensure that at least 2 units of suitable fresh whole blood are available before delivery.

Postnatal care

Resuscitation In severely affected infants efficient resuscitation is paramount. If the infant is very anaemic it is easy to underestimate the severity of coexisting RDS, since an anaemic baby cannot become cyanosed. Therefore, in severe rhesus HDN an arterial catheter should be inserted as quickly as possible for assessment and control of PaO_2 and pH. All the tenets in Chapter 7 on first-hour care are particularly important to this group of infants.

In cases that are predicted to be in zone 1 or lower zone 2 (Fig. 28.1), particularly where the infant is more than 36 weeks gestation, difficulties with resuscitation are rare. Nevertheless, a paediatrician must attend all such deliveries in case the baby is unexpectedly severely affected, and also to get the initial investigations under way.

Laboratory investigation The cord blood of babies born to all affected mothers must be analysed for blood group, direct Coombs' test, serum bilirubin and haemoglobin. The first two confirm the diagnosis, while the second two give an indication of the severity of the disease. Haemoglobin values from blood collected later (during the first 4–6 hours of life) are often 10–25% higher than the cord blood values.

Anaemia The timing of the first exchange transfusion is decided on the basis of the *cord* haemoglobin results. Levels less than 10 g% are an indication for an immediate exchange transfusion, and the further below 10 g% the greater the urgency. With haemoglobin values in the range 10–12 g%, an exchange transfusion will be needed within the next few hours. With cord haemoglobin values above 12 g% it is safe to wait, and base the decision to do an exchange transfusion on the serum bilirubin values.

Jaundice In all affected infants, estimate the bilirubin on capillary blood at least 6 hourly, and record the results on a graph. This will allow an estimate of the time at which a serum bilirubin of 340 micromol/1 (20 mg%) might be reached. Carry out the exchange transfusion before that time. Infants with cord bilirubin values exceeding 100–135 micromol (6–8 mg%), or who have a bilirubin rising at 17 micromol (1 mg) per hour or faster at any age, will almost certainly need an exchange transfusion. In premature infants who often have other problems increasing the risk of kernicterus (p. 417), exchange transfusion should be carried out at lower bilirubin levels (Table 27.3).

A bilirubin estimation should always be done at the beginning and the end of an exchange transfusion, which should lower the plasma bilirubin by 50–60%. Immediately after the exchange there is usually a rapid rise in bilirubin as the tissue levels equilibrate with the plasma levels. Bilirubin levels should continue to be measured 4–6 hourly as before, and repeated until the levels fall consistently or a further exchange is needed.

All infants with rhesus HDN should be placed under phototherapy (p. 427–429) until it is apparent that no further exchange transfusions will be required. Drug therapy for jaundice should not be used.

Other haematological problems The infants may have a low platelet count, but bleeding problems are rare unless DIC develops in a severely affected infant. If DIC does develop it should be treated as outlined on p.449–450, and platelet transfusion should be given if the infant is bleeding and has a platelet count below $50 \times 10^9/1$ (50 000/mm^3), or below $30 \times 10^9/1$ if not bleeding.

Infants with severe rhesus HDN have many circulating nucleated red cells. These nucleated cells may cause confusion in white cell counts measured in Coulter counters and in the examination of blood stained CSF (p. 246).

Prevention of infection Prophylactic antibodies are not indicated in rhesus HDN or following insertion of an umbilical venous catheter for exchange transfusion.

Cardiovascular status Hepatosplenomegaly in the presence of extramedullary haematopoiesis, cardiomegaly in the presence of anaemia, and hydrops in the presence of anaemia and hypoalbuminaemia are poor indicators of whether or not severely affected babies are in heart failure. On the contrary many are markedly hypovolaemic and hypotensive.

Blood pressure must therefore always be measured, as well as CVP if possible, although it is often difficult to get a UVC through the ductus venosus, and the value of CVP measurements from a UVC wedged in the liver is uncertain. Hypotension should be treated vigorously, and 20–30 ml/kg of saline may need to be given combined with dopamine or dobutamine. After the first exchange transfusion it is often wise to leave the baby with a surplus of 20–30 ml depending on his BP.

Hypoglycaemia Rhesus babies are prone to hypoglycaemia, especially after exchange transfusion (p. 287, 291). In infants with cord haemoglobin values below 10 g%, hypoglycaemia may arise at any time, and such babies should have regular glucose estimations for at least 48–72 hours after delivery. All babies need glucose measurements 1, 2 and 4 hours after exchange transfusions (Table 17.1).

Chronic liver disease (p. 425) Following severe HDN, infants may develop obstructive jaundice (inspissated bile syndrome) which clears by 3–4 weeks of age. It is now very rare.

Late anaemia In Coombs' positive infants who do not require exchange transfusion, anaemia of less than 6 g% may develop by

2–3 weeks of age. Similar but milder degrees of anaemia may also be seen in infants who have had an exchange transfusion. All survivors of HDN should be checked regularly during the first month of life and top up transfusions given if the haemoglobin falls to less than 7 g%, particularly if the reticulocyte count remains low.

Folate deficiency Survivors of HDN have low serum folate levels, and although they rarely develop megaloblastic anaemia their growth during the first year may be improved by giving them supplementary oral folate.

Treatment following intra-uterine transfusion

Irrespective of whether transfusions were given intraperitoneally or intravenously at cordocentesis, since rhesus negative blood is given, the cord blood results will be peculiar – even suggesting that the baby is not affected because the haemoglobin can be normal and the Coombs' test negative. However, management of such babies is no different to that outlined above. Not infrequently though, because most of their circulating red cells are rhesus negative, they do not require exchange transfusion.

Prevention of rhesus haemolytic disease

The antibody response following feto–maternal haemorrhage can be prevented by giving the mother 500 international units of anti-D immunoglobin. This is routinely given intramuscularly to all rhesus negative women who deliver rhesus positive babies within 72 hours (ideally within 24 hours) of delivery. A maternal Kleihauer test (for fetal RBC) should always be done and a further 125 units (1 ml) of anti-D immunoglobulin given for each 4 ml by which the feto-maternal transfusion is calculated to exceed 4 ml.

Anti-D immunoglobulin should always be given to all rhesus negative women in pregnancy after any of the following complications. The dose is 250 units at less than 20 weeks of pregnancy and 500 units thereafter.

1. Spontaneous miscarriage;
2. Ectopic pregnancy;
3. Chorionic villus sampling;
4. Amniocentesis;
5. Termination of pregnancy;

6. Antepartum haemorrhage;
7. Road traffic accidents, falls and abdominal trauma;
8. External cephalic version.

These routines will prevent rhesus sensitization in 95% of women. There is an unresolved debate about whether all rhesus negative women should receive a dose of anti-D at 28 weeks of gestation in order to protect the 5% of women who develop rhesus antibodies in response to the small feto-maternal haemorrhages which occur throughout pregnancy. Such treatment is currently not offered in all regions of the UK.

ABO incompatibility

Group A, B and most group O women have IgM isoagglutinins which do not cross the placenta, but about 10% of these women have an IgG anti-A haemolysin in their plasma (and rarely anti-B) which can cross the placenta and haemolyse the RBC of a group A (or group B) infant.

The antibody is present before pregnancy, so first babies may be affected. Furthermore, it is very unusual for the titres of these antibodies to rise as a result of feto-maternal bleeding at any stage of pregnancy, and successive pregnancies are therefore rarely more severely affected than the first one.

In terms of absolute numbers ABO HDN is 5 to 10 times more common than rhesus HDN. Fortunately, because the anti-A and anti-B haemolysins are comparatively weak antibodies, and much of the antibody which crosses the placenta is absorbed by A and B antigens in body tissues other than the RBC, ABO HDN rarely causes severe problems.

ABO HDN usually presents in the first 24 hours of life in an otherwise healthy full-term infant who rapidly becomes jaundiced. Jaundice recognized on the third or fourth day of life may also occasionally be due to ABO HDN. The haemoglobin is usually normal, and the direct Coombs' test is either negative or weakly positive. The mother and baby are ABO incompatible. Proof of the diagnosis depends on identifying the haemolytic anti-A in maternal plasma or in the infant's plasma, after eluting it from his RBCs.

Treatment If phototherapy is given from the time of diagnosis, the bilirubin rarely rises to dangerous levels. However, if it does exceed

350–400 micromol/l (20–24 mgm%) an exchange transfusion is required in term babies, starting at lower levels in babies under 37 weeks gestation (Chapter 27).

The other problems of rhesus HDN – such as hypoglycaemia, heart failure or chronic liver disease – are rarely seen, but babies who do not require exchange transfusion should be followed up carefully to ensure that anaemia does not develop.

Other blood group incompatibilities

The other rhesus groups C,E,c,e, and other groups such as Kell and Duffy, have all been responsible for HDN of varying severity, including rare cases of hydrops. The management is no different to that already described for rhesus disease. Anti-Kell may cause severe neonatal anaemia without jaundice.

CONGENITAL SPHEROCYTOSIS

This can present within the first 48–72 hours with jaundice which may become severe enough to require exchange transfusion.

The diagnosis can be made from the family history and the infant's blood film which shows many spherocytes, although less than in later life. The infant usually has a normal haemoglobin; but once spherocytosis is diagnosed, whether or not exchange transfusion is carried out, he should receive 1 mg of folic acid per day.

NON-SPHEROCYTIC HAEMOLYTIC ANAEMIAS

These are due to inherited red cell metabolic defects. Although they usually present later in life with a haemolytic anaemia, they occasionally present neonatally with severe jaundice that requires phototherapy or exchange transfusion.

BLEEDING AND BRUISING

- *All babies should receive vitamin K to prevent VKDB. The most effective prophylaxis is obtained with 1 mg IM given shortly after birth.*
- *Late VKDB is virtually confined to breast fed infants and those with liver disease, and is not reliably prevented by oral vitamin K prophylaxis.*
- *Thrombocytopenia and DIC are common in sick babies with many diagnoses.*

- *Platelet transfusion in the absence of overt bleeding is indicated if the platelet count is below $30 \times 10^9/l$: if bleeding is a clinical problem give platelets if there is any thrombocytopenia.*
- *With DIC, treating the precipitating cause is the priority; use fresh frozen plasma, cryoprecipitate, platelets and exchange transfusion to control bleeding in severe cases.*

The neonate, particularly if born prematurely, is deficient in all the factors involved in the intrinsic clotting mechanism with the exception of fibrinogen, factors V and VIII (Appendix G). The levels rise to adult values within a few weeks.

The levels of the natural anticoagulants antithrombin III and proteins C and S are low in neonatal plasma, as are the levels of plasminogen. Although in theory this might make neonates hypercoagulable this has not been found to be the case in practice.

Coagulation in the neonate is usually evaluated by a platelet count together with the prothrombin time, thrombin time, fibrin degradation products and activated partial thromboplastin time (Fig. 28.2). Beware of heparin in the sample, which can give rise to a very prolonged PTT and a minor prolongation of the PT. The D-dimer test is the most sensitive indicator of intravascular formation of fibrin and the presence of D-dimers usually indicates DIC in the newborn. The prothrombin time in the normal term newborn is 13–16 seconds, being prolonged to about 13–20 seconds in preterm babies. This result is increasingly reported as an International Normalized Ratio (INR) which takes account of laboratory variation; this result centres around 1.0 with a range of 0.5–1.5 in term babies. The APTT also varies between laboratories, but is prolonged in babies compared to adults. Absolute values of 40–70 seconds at term and 40–100 seconds in preterm babies are usually reported. Interpretation of common patterns of abnormal test results is shown in Table 28.3.

HAEMORRHAGIC DISEASE OF THE NEWBORN (VITAMIN K DEFICIENCY BLEEDING)

This is due to a deficiency of the vitamin K dependent clotting factors II, VII, IX and X and can be prevented by routine administration of 1 mg of the natural analogues of vitamin K (e.g. Konakion) IM at birth. This preventive treatment is recommended for all newborn babies. The incidence of the disorder if vitamin K

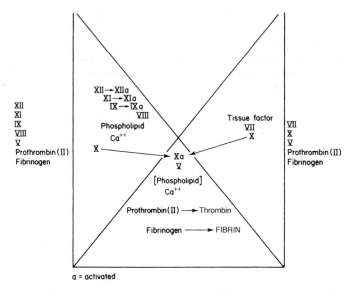

a = activated

Figure 28.2 Activated partial thromboplastin time (APTT) and prothrombin time (PT). Those portions of the coagulation mechanism measured by the APTT are in the triangle on the left; those measured by the PT in the triangle on the right. Listed on the left are those factors which influence the APTT and on the right those which influence the PT (from Abildgaard 1981).

Table 28.3 Interpretation of coagulation tests in neonatal bleeding: derived from Gross and Stuart 1977

Coagulation test	VKDB	DIC	Liver disease
PT	very prolonged	prolonged	prolonged
APTT	prolonged	prolonged	prolonged
TT	normal	prolonged	prolonged
FDPs	normal	increased	normal or ↑
Fibrinogen	normal	reduced	reduced
Platelet count	normal	reduced	normal or ↓
Response to vitamin K	dramatic	no response	diminished response

prophylaxis is not used at all is about 1 in 10 000, whereas a single intramuscular dose of vitamin K prevents virtually all cases. Oral vitamin K regimens are not totally effective but have become popular since the publication of evidence which linked vitamin K with later childhood leukaemia. There are three forms of the disorder;

early, classical and late. The early form is limited to babies of mothers who have taken drugs such as anticonvulsants during pregnancy and should be prevented by giving extra folate to these women.

The classical form of VKDB presents on the second to fourth day of life with umbilical stump haemorrhage, haematemesis and/or melaena, ecchymoses, epistaxis or scalp haemorrhage. The baby may also bleed from puncture sites and circumcision. The prothrombin time and APTT are very prolonged, but the thrombin time and fibrinogen level are normal (Appendix G, Table G.4).

Once haemorrhage has occurred, the baby should be managed as described on page 435. An immediate replacement transfusion is indicated if the baby is shocked, but more gradual correction by exchange transfusion should be used if the baby has had time to haemodilute. Always give 1 mg of vitamin K intravenously (to avoid a haematoma) irrespective of what was thought to have been given at delivery. Fresh frozen plasma should be given at the same time because vitamin K takes several hours to correct the coagulation deficit.

Late VKDB is largely a disease of breast fed babies. Intracranial haemorrhage is a devastating complication, which is seen in about one third of cases. There are often small warning bleeds from the gum or rectum. The time of onset tends to be later (30–60 days) now that almost all babies receive at least a single oral dose of vitamin K as prophylaxis. It is now clear that more than one oral dose is required to prevent this disorder. The optimal oral regimen has not yet been devised, but the manufacturers of Konakion MM recommend 2 mg orally on days 0, 28 and 56. Remember that VKDB is often the presenting condition in babies with liver disease.

DISSEMINATED INTRAVASCULAR COAGULATION

This is seen in neonates with severe birth asphyxia, septicaemia, intracranial haemorrhage, hypothermia, hypotension, hypoxia and acidaemia. It usually presents as petechial bleeding into the skin, or oozing from skin puncture sites and the umbilicus, but haemorrhage may occur anywhere.

Thrombin formation, triggered *in vivo* by microbial endotoxin or by thromboplastin released from damaged tissues and endothelial cells, results in intravascular coagulation which consumes platelets, factors II, VIII, XIII and fibrinogen, and leaves the baby with a bleeding diathesis. The fibrinolytic system is activated, and the fibrin degradation products so produced, further aggravate the bleeding tendency by interfering with fibrin polymerization.

Diagnosis

The PT, APTT and thrombin time are all prolonged, confirming consumption of intrinsic coagulation factors and fibrinogen. Fibrin degradation products will be increased in the blood. The platelet count is usually below $100 \times 10^9/l$ (<100 000/mm³) and blood films show distorted RBC. The D-dimer test may be available and levels are raised. The minimum criteria for the diagnosis of DIC are as follows:

- compatible clinical signs;
- abnormal clotting studies, including a prolonged PT and APTT;
- some other laboratory evidence (e.g. fibrinogen consumption, low platelets, elevated FDP, elevated D-dimers).

Treatment

1. Remedy the underlying disease (e.g. correct hypotension or acidaemia).
2. Replace clotting factors by transfusing fresh frozen plasma (10–15 ml/kg). If the underlying condition is being adequately treated, FFP transfusion should not provide the fuel for further DIC.
3. In severely affected babies, or those with continuing DIC despite intravenous FFP, exchange transfusion with blood <48 hours old not only provides the missing clotting factors, but also washes out the various toxins that are perpetuating the DIC. Cryoprecipitate can be used, and provides fibrinogen, factor VIII and von Willebrand factor.
4. In a bleeding neonate, heparinization is unjustified and is not used.
5. Give an extra dose of intravenous vitamin K.

CONGENITAL DEFICIENCIES OF COAGULATION FACTORS

(Barnard 1984)

These may all present in the neonatal period, usually with bleeding from surgical incisions such as circumcision, but rarely from other sites. If bleeding in a neonate does not respond to vitamin K, and DIC is not present, specific assays for these conditions should be arranged. Haemophilia (factor VIII deficiency) is present in 90% of such cases.

NEONATAL THROMBOCYTOPENIA

The normal neonatal platelet count is the same as that in the adult, namely $150–450 \times 10^9/l$. Thrombocytopenia is a common finding in the NNU, occurring in 20–30% of all admissions. The condition is rare (about 1%) in the general neonatal population, and in a well term baby the most likely cause is neonatal alloimmune thrombocytopenia (NAITP) or maternal ITP. Thrombocytopenia usually presents with purpura, ecchymoses or large cephalhaematomata. Bleeding at other sites (including the gut, umbilicus, skin and CNS) can occur but is comparatively rare. Differential diagnosis is usually possible on the basis of a history, clinical examination, coagulation studies, platelet count (mother and baby), platelet antibody studies and occasionally bone marrow examination.

Causes include the following:

1. DIC, and hence all the conditions that may cause DIC, especially sepsis (*v.s.*), hypoxic ischaemic encephalopathy, necrotizing enterocolitis;
2. Neonatal alloimune thrombocytopenia – usually a mother who is human platelet antigen (HPA) 1a negative with a HPA 1a positive fetus but other platelet alloantigens can be involved such as 5 and 3;
3. Giant haemangiomas (Kasabach-Merritt syndrome);
4. congenital infection including HIV (p. 261–262);
5. maternal idiopathic thrombocytopenia or SLE with transplacental passage of antiplatelet IgG;
6. in association with Rh HDN (p. 443);
7. marrow abnormalities (leukaemia, hypoplasia);
8. drugs (administered to mother or baby – quinidine, thiazides);
9. inherited abnormalities (e.g. Wiskott-Aldrich, thrombocytopenia – absent radius syndrome);
10. maternal disease such as PET;
11. organic acidaemias (p. 297).

Treatment

One major source of anxiety is whether the thrombocytopenia will lead to an intracranial haemorrhage, and for all the conditions listed above this seems to be exceptionally rare except in babies with alloimmune thrombocytopenia. In neonatal alloimmune thrombocytopenia the risk of *in utero* haemorrhage justifies the risk of antenatal platelet transfusion. In this and in the other conditions specific therapy for thrombocytopenia is not indicated unless platelet counts are $<30 \times 10^9/l$ ($<50 \times 10^9/l$ if sick or very preterm in the first few days of life) *or* there are clinical problems with haemorrhage and any degree of thrombocytopenia.

Treatment of alloimmune thrombocytopenic purpura should be with transfusion of platelets from donors who are CMV negative and HPA-1a negative. In the UK this product has replaced washed maternal platelets, which carry a risk of graft-versus-host disease. Steroids and immunoglobulin (1 g per kg daily for 3 days) may prolong survival of the transfused platelets. In the non-immune thrombocytopenias such as DIC, platelet transfusion will usually control the bleeding.

Most cases of neonatal thrombocytopenia resolve quickly, either because the underlying infection is treated, or because the antibody responsible for the thrombocytopenia disappears. Only if thrombocytopenia is persistent should some of the rarer conditions listed above be sought. Persistent thrombocytopenia may be the only clue to congenital HIV infection.

NEONATAL POLYCYTHAEMIA

The viscosity of blood increases linearly up to a PCV of 65%. Above this there is a progressively larger increase in viscosity per unit change in PCV. Furthermore, at a given PCV and shear rate *in vitro*, neonatal blood is more viscous than adult blood (Mackintosh and Walker 1973).

Newborn babies become polycythaemic in the following situations:

1. recipients in twin-to-twin transfusion;
2. recipients of large placental transfusions (delayed cord clamping);
3. small-for-dates babies;
4. babies of diabetic mothers;
5. rarities (e.g. neonatal thyrotoxicosis, Beckwith-Wiedemann syndrome).

Diagnosis

Polycythaemia should only be diagnosed if the venous haematocrit is greater than 65–70% since capillary haematocrits are inaccurate, and may be 15% greater than the true central haematocrit.

The following symptoms are attributed to hyperviscosity and polycythaemia:

1. CNS depression, fits and cortical venous thrombosis;
2. heart failure;
3. respiratory distress, cyanosis and persistent fetal circulation;
4. jaundice;
5. hypoglycaemia;
6. hypocalcaemia;
7. renal vein thrombosis;
8. NEC.

Treatment

Some authorities recommend therapy for all babies with a venous haematocrit of 65–70%. However, we believe that therapy is only needed for polycythaemia when the central haematocrit exceeds 80%, or if one of the symptoms listed above occurs at haematocrits of 70–80% in the absence of other causes. The PCV can be lowered by carrying out an exchange transfusion using saline, and exchanging 20–30 ml/kg depending on the severity of the polycythaemia.

NEONATAL THROMBOSIS

Increasing use of central lines and arterial catheters, sometimes combined with a genetic predisposition to thrombosis, has resulted in increasing problems with thrombotic disease in the newborn. It is important to make the diagnosis, as timely action can save a limb. Prevention should be attempted, and all infusions into an aterial catheter should be heparinized.

Inherited disorders which increase thrombotic risk include the following:

- Factor V Leiden deficiency;
- Protein C deficiency;
- Protein S deficiency;
- Homocystinuria due to cystathionine β-synthase deficiency;
- Antithrombin III deficiency;
- Increased lipoprotein A.

DIAGNOSIS

Clinical signs of venous obstruction include oedema and cyanosis of a limb, head and neck or chest with increased collateral vessel circulation. There may be an abdominal mass and haematuria if the renal vein is thrombosed.

Clinical signs of arterial thrombosis include a pale, cold limb with absent pulses which may be obviously painful, seizures, or increased ventilatory requirements due to pulmonary emboli. Hypertension can be a clue to renal artery obstruction. Damping of a transduced arterial trace may be an early sign of thrombus formation.

The diagnoses can be confirmed with real time and Doppler ultrasound or venography, but may have to rest on clinical suspicion. MR angiography is available in a few centres. Protein C deficiency may present as purpura fulminans, haemorrhagic necrosis of the skin with DIC.

TREATMENT

For arterial obstruction which is threatening a limb, surgical embolectomy should be seriously considered. If an arterial catheter is *in situ*, consider infusing streptokinase or tissue plasminogen activator (tPA) down the catheter on to the clot before removing it. Whole body heparinization can be tried in babies who are not at high risk of intracranial haemorrhage. If amputation looks inevitable, a time delay may allow the line of demarcation to move proximally (p. 473).

Venous lines which are blocked can sometimes be restored to patency by flushing with urokinase or tPA. The role of thrombolytic therapy in other cases of venous obstruction and renal vein thrombosis is unclear.

BLOOD COMPONENT THERAPY

A plethora of different blood component products is now available, and Table 28.4 gives a summary of the indications for their use.

Any blood component which is to be given to newborns must be CMV negative. For an exchange transfusion blood must be fresh, and preserved in CPD, not SAG-M. Potassium levels reach concentrations of up to 30 mmol/l in 5 week old blood. For top up transfusions older blood is suitable, and the use of satellite (octopus) packs reduces donor exposure. SAG-M is acceptable as a preservative in

Table 28.4 Blood component therapy

Blood component	Indication
Whole blood (plasma reduced)	Exchange transfusion, haemorrhage, hypotension with anaemia
Packed cells	Top up transfusion
Fresh frozen plasma	DIC, VKDB
Cryoprecipitate	Bleeding, severe DIC
Platelets	Thrombocytopenia

this situation. Guidelines regarding the irradiation of blood products for the newborn vary (Voak *et al.* 1994), but there is a risk of graft-versus-host disease so many units irradiate all blood products which are to be given to newborns. Directed donations from relatives are a particular problem in this respect.

REFERENCES

Abildgaard, C.F. (1981) Diseases of coagulation. In: *Hematology of Infancy and Childhood*, 2nd edn. Nathan, D.G. and Oski, F.A. (eds), W. B. Saunders, Philadelphia.

Barnard, D.R. (1984) Inherited bleeding disorders in the newborn infant. *Clinics in Perinatology* 11: 309–337.

Brown, M.S., Phibbs, R.H., Garcia, J.F. and Dallman, P.R. (1983) Postnatal changes in erythropoietin levels in untransfused premature infants. *Journal of Pediatrics* 103: 612–617.

Brugnara, C. and Platt, O.S. (1998) The neonatal erythrocyte and its disorders. In: *Hematologic Problems in the Newborn*, 5th edn. Oski, F.A. and Naiman, J.L. (eds), W. B. Saunders, Philadelphia, pp. 19–52.

Gross, S.J. and Stuart, M.J. (1977) Hemostasis in the premature infant. *Clinics in Perinatology* 4: 259–304.

Mackintosh, T.F. and Walker, C.H.M. (1973) Blood viscosity in the newborn. *Archives of Disease in Childhood* 48: 547–553.

Orkin S.H. and Nathan, D.G. (1998) The thalassemias. In: *Hematologic Problems in the Newborn*, 5th edn. Oski, F.A. and Naiman, J.L. (eds), W.B. Saunders, Philadelphia, pp. 811–886.

Voak, D., Cann, R., Finney, R.D. *et al.* (1994) Guidelines for administration of blood products: transfusion of infants and neonates. *Transfusion Medicine* 4: 63–69.

Whitfield, C.R. (1970) A three year assessment of an action line method of timing intervention tests in rhesus isoimmunization. *American Journal of Obstetrics and Gynecology* 108: 1239–1244.

29

HYDROPS FETALIS

- *All hydropic babies should be vigorously resuscitated until the underlying diagnosis is established.*
- *Resuscitation includes IPPV from birth plus continuous BP and ideally CVP measurement. Consider thoracocentesis, paracentesis and peritoneal dialysis.*
- *Many causes of hydrops are fatal, and after establishing the diagnosis it is appropriate to offer to withdraw intensive care.*

There are many causes of hydrops, in which the baby is born with gross oedema and serous effusions (Table 29.1). Non-immune hydrops has an incidence of approximately 1 in 2000 births.

An attempt should be made to resuscitate all hydropic babies since some, including those with severe rhesus disease, have conditions which are compatible with neurologically intact survival, and in others it is important to keep the baby alive long enough to establish a diagnosis to assist with genetic counselling, or the management of subsequent pregnancies. With the falling incidence of rhesus haemolytic disease of the newborn, 80–90% of cases now have a non-immune aetiology.

PATHOPHYSIOLOGY

Physiologically, hydrops is usually due to one or more of the following four interrelated factors:

1. anaemia – at times profound;
2. hypoalbuminaemia and a low colloid osmotic pressure – this is often due to liver damage caused by massive extramedullary haemopoiesis or liver infection;
3. heart failure – due to anaemia, cardiac abnormality, or high output state;
4. fetal illness with leaky capillaries and fluid transudation.

Table 29.1 Causes of hydrops fetalis

Haemolytic disease of the newborn
  Rhesus, ABO incompatability, Kell, Duffy
Fetal anaemia (10–27%)
  Haemorrhage into mother or twin
  αThalassaemia, G6PD deficiency
Fetal cardiac disease (19–26%)
  Congenital heart disease
  Arrhythmias
  A/V malformations e.g. vein of Galen malformations, and heart failure
Congenital infection (1–8%)
  Parvovirus B19, CMV, toxoplasmosis, syphilis, leptospirosis, Chagas disease
Placental anomalies (2–6%)
  Chorionic, umbilical vein thrombosis
  Chorioangioma
Fetal lung malformation (8–10%)
  Lymphangiectasia
  Cystic adenomatoid malformation
Fetal renal disorders (2–3%)
  Congenital nephrotic syndrome
  Renal dysplasia
Fetal GI tract abnormalities (2%)
  Atresia, hepatitis
Twinning (4–8%)
  Monozygotic twins with twin-twin transfusion
Maternal diabetes, toxaemia, anaemia
Achondroplasia and short-limbed dwarfs (4%)
Fetal malignancy e.g. neuroblastoma (rare)
Malformations, chromosomal disorders and metabolic errors (40–45%)
Idiopathic (20%)

From Etches et al. 1999. Figures in parentheses show the percentage of non-immune hydrops due to the individual conditions.

TREATMENT

The following steps should be taken irrespective of aetiology:

1. Get help immediately in the labour ward. More than one person is needed to manage these babies.
2. Unless the baby is in very good condition, intubate him and give IPPV from the moment of delivery, in order to try to control the pulmonary oedema and severe hypoxaemia which virtually always accompany hydrops. IPPV should be continued until the

hydrops is under control, which usually means at least 24–48 hours. The babies are often premature with surfactant-deficient RDS as well as pulmonary oedema and pleural effusions. The initial ventilator settings should therefore be those for severe RDS, namely 80% O_2, 25/5 cm H_2O, 80 breaths/min and an inspiratory time of 0.3–0.35 s.

3. Examine the baby (including measuring his blood pressure), looking for stigmata of conditions listed in Table 29.1.
4. Insert umbilical venous and arterial catheters as soon as possible after delivery to monitor BP and CVP (if possible) and to obtain blood for analysis.
5. Organize the investigations in Table 29.2 in all cases as soon as possible.

Table 29.2 Investigation of the hydropic neonate

I. Samples, procedures to be requested on admission
   blood gas*
   FBC including reticulocyte count and examination of the film*
   Group, Coombs, cross match*
   Blood glucose*
   Bilirubin*
   Albumin and liver function tests
   Full coagulation screen
   Haemoglobin electrophoresis
   Immunoglobulin levels
   TORCH, syphilis, parvovirus serology
   Routine cultures, blood culture, CRP
   Urinalysis for protein*
   CXR*
   Skeletal survey*
   ECG*
   Ultrasound scan of brain*
   Photograph*

2. Subsequent tests
   Examination of pleural/ascitic fluid
   Echocardiogram
   CT/MR scan for lung malformations
   Blood, urine, WBC for enzyme assays for IEMs
   Skin, liver biopsy for IEM
   Genetic studies for inherited conditions

* Results of these tests should be available by 60–90 minutes of age.

6. Cultures of the usual sites should be sent, including a blood culture (p. 232–233).
7. Aspirate the peritoneal and pleural effusions, taking care to avoid puncturing an underlying viscus. Save the fluid for analysis. This step should precede arterial catheterization if the baby does not respond to resuscitation at delivery.

These initial procedures should be completed within 30–60 minutes of delivery, and the results of routine investigations should be available shortly after that. If the PCV is less than 25%, carry out an exchange transfusion at once, using fresh uncrossmatched rhesus negative blood from the labour ward. A hydropic baby's blood volume is usually less than normal due to the low plasma albumin and colloid osmotic pressure, and it is therefore dangerous to start the exchange transfusion by removing 30–40 ml of blood.

Carefully monitor the ECG, blood pressure and CVP during the exchange transfusion. At the end of the exchange the aim is to achieve a BP of at least 40 mmHg systolic, a PCV of 40% and a CVP of between 0 and + 5 mmHg.

After the exchange transfusion, or if no exchange transfusion is needed, take stock of the situation. Ensure that the BP is normal by giving more plasma expanders or by using dopamine. Perform any other diagnostic tests that seem to be indicated. If the baby has not passed urine by this stage give 5–10 mg of frusemide IV. Continue routine intensive care, and maintain normal blood gases, blood glucose, electrolytes and PCV.

If everything else is under control, and the baby is not suffering from some lethal abnormality, but he still does not pass urine, give more frusemide, and consider peritoneal dialysis or haemoperfusion to remove the excess fluid.

Specific problems should be treated. Arrhythmias should be controlled (p. 368–369), correctable malformations should be operated on (e.g. excision of sacrococcygeal teratoma) and babies with potentially treatable infections (toxoplasma, syphilis) given appropriate antibiotics. Full intensive care with IPPV, blood pressure support and control of blood gas, biochemical and haematological abnormalities should be maintained until the diagnosis is established or it is clear that the baby has a fatal condition. Sadly the latter conclusion is common in non-immune hydrops which has a mortality of 80–90%.

FURTHER READING

Etches, P., Demianczuk, N.N., Okun, N.B. and Chari, R. (1999) Hydrops fetalis. In: *Textbook of Neonatology*, 3rd edn. Rennie, J.M. and Roberton, N.R.C. (eds), Churchill Livingstone, Edinburgh, pp. 845–857.

30

GENETIC DISEASE

In any odd-looking baby:

- *Compare his appearance with his next of kin.*
- *Carefully list his dysmorphic features and consult the computerized databases.*
- *Send blood for cytogenetic analysis.*
- *Consult an expert in dysmorphology if the suspicion remains high.*

About 2–3% of babies are born with a malformation, and malformation sequences are still a common cause of neonatal death. The diagnosis of genetic disease requires a high index of suspicion in the neonatal period, although some disorders, such as Down syndrome, are well known and easily recognized. Fetal medicine has changed the pattern of malformations which present in the neonatal period; for example Patau syndrome (Trisomy 13) and Edward syndrome (Trisomy 18) are now very rare because cases are diagnosed early in pregnancy and most parents choose termination. Some conditions are known to result from sub-microscopic deletions of the genome, so that a specific request is required before the laboratory can help, by using fluorescent *in-situ* hybridisation. If one of these conditions is suspected (e.g. a microdeletion of chromosome 22 in a child with congenital heart disease and an absent thymus – Di George syndrome or "catch-22") it is always worth repeating a chromosome test which was thought to be normal antenatally. FISH-ing generally for microdeletions is not possible, and a specific request is required.

The first clue to possible genetic disease is usually the appearance of the infant, who does not "look right" – in other words he is dysmorphic. This instant recognition, which is based partly on the examiner's past experience, is often called "Gestalt" recognition, from the German word meaning shape or form. Infants appear dysmorphic for any of the following three reasons:

- Malformation. A malformation is present when there is an anomaly in an organ, or part of an organ. Examples include polydactyly, craniosynostosis, cleft lip, congenital heart disease or microcephaly. More subtle, but equally important malformations are findings such as micropenis, hypertelorism, accessory nipples and misshapen digits. Multiple minor malformations are always suspicious.
- Deformation. Deformation exists when the anatomy is normal, but has been distorted by intra-uterine forces. The most common example is talipes secondary to oligohydramios.
- Disruption. This is rare, but it occurs when there is an alteration of the normal process of development, such as from an amniotic band. Disruptions are non-genetic in nature.

When examining a baby with a possible malformation, always remember that any mention of a deviation from normal will be devastating to the parents. Sensitive handling is obviously essential, as is the provision of accurate information. Parent support groups are often excellent sources of information and support once a specific diagnosis has been made. The world-wide web is another source (see the list of useful websites at the end of this chapter).

Experienced help from a clinical geneticist is required when considering the diagnosis of a malformed baby who may have a genetic disorder. Once the baby has been examined thoroughly and carefully, and a detailed family history has been prepared, the combination of malformations can be entered into a computer programme or looked up in a book with the appropriate tables to see whether a specific "syndrome" diagnosis can be made. The number of "hits" can be optimised by using a small number of the best "handles". This means choosing the abnormal features which are not common, such as imperforate anus, rather than those which are common in the general population (e.g. clinodactyly). Measurements, cranial imaging and X-rays may all contribute to a diagnosis. Ophthalmological examination can be invaluable. One or two genetic diseases can be diagnosed with serum biochemical tests, perhaps the best known example being Smith-Lemli-Opitz syndrome in which there is an elevated 7-dehydrocholesterol concentration. Some genetic disorders only ever occur as mosaics (e.g. Pallister-Killian syndrome), so that a skin biopsy has to be done to make the diagnosis because white cell chromosomes will be normal.

Malformations can result from fetal exposure to teratogens, (e.g.

fetal alcohol syndrome, rubella) and the cause of many malformations remains unknown. Photographs should be taken as a record, because in many cases it is just not possible to reach a diagnosis in the nursery and follow up and discussion with experts will be required.

GOOD "HANDLES" FOR GENETIC DIAGNOSIS

Microcephaly
Macrocephaly
Polydactyly
Syndactyly
Cataract
Hypertelorism
Cleft lip and/or palate
Small mandible
Very short limbs
Absent radius
Anal atresia
Skin abnormalities

FURTHER READING

BOOKS

Baraitser, M. and Winter, R.M. (1996) *Colour Atlas of Congenital Malformation Syndromes*. Mosby-Wolfe, London.

Jones, K.L. (1997) *Smith's Recognizable Patterns of Human Malformation*, 5th edn. WB Saunders, Philadelphia.

Wiedemann, H-R., Kunze, J. and Dibbern, H. (1992) *An Atlas of Clinical Syndromes*. Wolfe, London.

USEFUL WEBSITES

http://www.ncbi.nlm.nih.gov/Omim/
OMIM: a completely free resource which is a mine of information. Fully referenced, up to date information and a gene map.

http://rarediseases.info.nih.gov/
Office of Rare Diseases: good but a payment is required for detailed information.

http://www.medinfo.cam.ac.uk/
Public Health Genetics Unit in Cambridge: useful site.

http://www.rarediseases.org/lof/lof.html
Rare diseases database.

http://bisance.citi2.fr/GENATLAS/
Genatlas.

http://www.bham.ac.uk/BSHG/
British Society for Human Genetics. No specific disease information.

http://www.hgmp.mrc.ac.uk
UK medical research council resource centre; links to other sites.

http://www.cafamily.org.uk/
A very useful site containing information and pictures of many conditions, with addresses and websites of parent support groups in the UK. Well designed and easy to use.

31

PROGNOSIS

Uncertainty and worry about the outcome for their child preoccupy the thoughts of all parents whose baby requires any sort of special care. Counselling about prognosis is an everyday task for neonatologists, and it takes knowledge and experience to pitch the information at the right level, to include enough detail to explain but not confuse, and to be "honest but not cruel". Trainee paediatricians are often asked about a baby's prognosis, partly because they are present on the neonatal unit at all hours of the day and night and partly because parents like to canvass a second opinion. The aim of this chapter is to help trainees to give an accurate answer, but it cannot be over-emphasized that much damage can be done by inaccurate and ill-timed advice. As in any other area of neonatology, if in doubt, ask! Encourage your consultant to document what he or she has already told the parents and to let you sit in on the counselling consultations for "your" babies. Always remember that there is a huge spectrum of disability, that there are always exceptions, and that quality of life is a value judgement. The following list represents situations in which, in our combined experience, wrong information is often given and/or errors of judgement made. Conflicting advice gives rise to anger and bitter resentment in parents, and litigation often ensues.

- Never, ever give a poor prognosis based on 1–10 minute Apgar scores alone (p. 68).
- Do not withdraw (or fail to initiate) intensive care without senior input.
- If it has been decided not to offer full cardiopulmonary resuscitation to a very premature baby, do not leave the baby uncovered and unattended on the resuscitaire after you have made an assessment at delivery. Always treat the baby's body with respect.
- Do not base a prognosis solely on the appearance of the baby – bronzing, oedema, peeling flaky skin and bruising will all clear in time.

- A single, unilateral parenchymal haemorrhage is not necessarily associated with a poor prognosis (p. 324–329).
- The cysts of periventricular leukomalacia (p.330–331) normally disappear after a few months, but this does not mean that the condition is cured.
- Treating retinopathy of prematurity does not guarantee intact vision, nor does a "normal" eye screen.

MORTALITY

MORTALITY BY BIRTH WEIGHT, SEX AND GESTATIONAL AGE

Many datasets exist, but useful look-up tables are provided in the recent review of survival for the years 1994–7 in Trent, UK (Draper *et al.* 1999) and are reproduced as Figs 31.1 and 31.2. Outcome is reported to be better in Australia and the USA.

NEURODEVELOPMENTAL OUTCOME

Preterm babies have a higher incidence of neurodevelopmental disability than full-term babies. Fig. 31.3 shows the outcome by gestational age. However, it is important to remember that the burden of disability in the general population is surprisingly high. Around 2–3% of all children have a major neurological disability, including cerebral palsy and/or mental retardation, a further 2–3% have hearing impairment or impaired vision and 10–20% have language delay, clumsiness or learning difficulty. The best follow up studies are geographically based, include controls, have a low dropout rate and continue to assess the enrolled cohort of children until they are well into school age. However, not many of the multitude of published studies meet these criteria.

PRETERM BRAIN INJURY

There are serious limitations in using ultrasound evidence of brain injury as a proxy for neurodevelopmental outcome, and brain imaging will never replace follow up studies. The significance of transient parenchymal abnormalities has yet to be defined. Nevertheless, this method provides a rapid early result which is undoubtedly useful to parents and doctors alike. The efforts of many groups, such as those in New Jersey, Liverpool and London (Pinto-Martin *et al.* 1995,

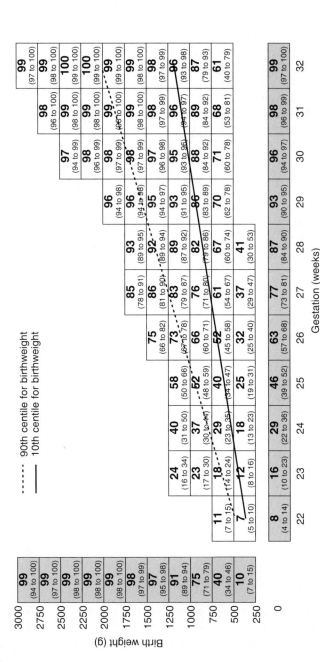

Figure 31.1 Median (95% confidence interval) predicted percentage survival for European female infants admitted alive to NNU in Trent 1994–7. Reproduced from Draper *et al.* (1999) with permission.

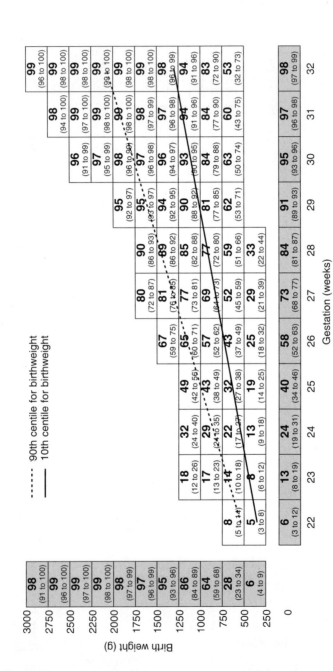

Figure 31.2 Median (95% confidence interval) predicted percentage survival for European male infants admitted alive to NNU in Trent 1994–7. Reproduced from Draper *et al.* (1999) with permission.

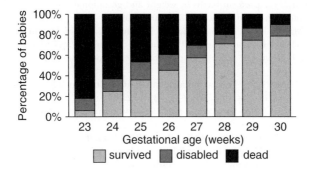

Figure 31.3 Survival by gestational age. Modified from Rennie 1996.

Cooke 1987, Stewart *et al.* 1987), who have imaged large cohorts of preterm neonates and carefully followed them up have led to the following broad conclusions (see also Rennie 1997).

- A preterm baby who is discharged from a neonatal unit with a consistently normal cranial ultrasound scan is at low risk (approximately 5%) of subsequent neurodevelopmental problems.
- This risk is not substantially increased in the presence of an uncomplicated GMH or IVH which is not followed by ventricular enlargement.
- Bilateral cystic change in the occipital cortex, corresponding to the pathological lesion of periventricular leukomalacia, is associated with a very high probability (more than 90%) of cerebral palsy.
- Unilateral parenchymal haemorrhagic lesions (haemorrhagic parenchymal infarction) usually evolve into a porencephalic cyst, and the prognosis can be surprisingly good if there is no other lesion. Children often have good intelligence with a monoplegia which is not unduly disabling.
- Not all VLBW survivors with neurodevelopmental problems, or later MRI evidence of PVL, have early ultrasound abnormalities.

REFERENCES

Cooke, R.W.I. (1987) Early and late cranial ultrasonographic appearances and outcome in very low birthweight infants. *Archives of Disease in Childhood* **62**: 931–937.

Draper, E.S., Manktelow, B., Field, D.J. and James, D. (1999) Prediction of survival for preterm births by weight and gestational age: retrospective population based study. *BMJ* **319**: 1093–1097.

Pinto-Martin, J.A., Riolo, S., Cnaan, A., Holzman, C., Susser, M. and Paneth, N. (1995) Cranial ultrasound prediction of disabling and nondisabling cerebral palsy at age two in a low birthweight population. *Pediatrics* **95**: 249–254.

Rennie, J.M. (1996) Perinatal management at the lower margin of viability. *Archives of Disease in Childhood* **74**: F214–F218.

Rennie, J.M. (1997) *Neonatal Cranial Ultrasound*. Cambridge University Press, Cambridge.

Stewart, A.L., Reynolds, E.O.R., Hope, P.L., Hamilton, P.A., Baudin, J., Costello, A.M de L., Bradford, B.C. and Wyatt, J.S. (1987) Probability of neurodevelopmental disorders estimated from the ultrasound appearance of brains of very preterm infants. *Developmental Medicine and Child Neurology* **29**: 3–11.

FURTHER READING

Stewart, A.L. and Roth, S.C. (1999) Neurodevelopmental outcome. In: *Textbook of Neonatology*, 3rd edn. Rennie, J.M. and Roberton, N.R.C. (eds), Churchill Livingstone, Edinburgh, pp. 79–100.

32

IATROGENIC DISEASE

- *Iatrogenic disorders are an unavoidable complication of intensive care of the critically ill neonate.*
- *Complications from arterial lines can be minimized by correct insertion technique, heparinizing the infusate, and removing the lines when there is clear evidence of vascular compromise.*
- *The commonest complication of long lines used for TPN is CONS sepsis. Bizarre findings or collapse in babies with long lines in place may be due to extravascular accumulation of the infusate in unexpected sites.*
- *Most peripheral neonatal IV infusions end their life by extravasation. Tissue damage must be prevented by detecting "tissuing" early. Alarms are not enough and regular inspection of the site is mandatory.*
- *Subcutaneous irrigation of the site of an extravasation injury remains controversial, but may be of value if the infusate contained calcium or TPN.*

Many complications of the techniques and drugs used in NNUs have been described (Brain *et al.* 1999). In this chapter we shall only consider problems that are relatively common and require urgent treatment.

HAEMORRHAGE FROM ARTERIAL LINES – UMBILICAL OR PERIPHERAL

This should not happen (p. 98), but sometimes does! Never cover the umbilicus with a sheet when a UAC is *in situ*. If bleeding does occur then do not compound the mistake by under-estimating the volume of blood lost. Although 10 ml of blood makes only a small stain on the blanket, in a 1 kg baby it represents a 10–15% of his blood volume, equivalent to a pint in an adult. Always transfuse babies in this situation, starting with 10ml/kg, giving saline whilst waiting for blood if there is clear evidence of cardiovascular decompensation. Signs of decompensation are an increasing pulse rate, peripheral under perfusion, acidaemia and hypotension (p. 434) (although the latter may take time to develop).

PERIPHERAL ISCHAEMIA FROM ARTERIAL LINES — PERIPHERAL AND UMBILICAL

This may be due to spasm caused by irritation of the artery which can lead to thrombosis, primary thrombosis of the artery, or emboli. The basic rule is remove the catheter if there are signs suggesting peripheral ischaemia or peripheral emboli. These signs include pallor, reduced pulses, blue tips to fingers or toes, or major organ involvement such as NEC or haematuria.

If in doubt, take it out

It may be acceptable to leave the catheter in place with continued careful observation and heparinization of the infusate if there is only transient (less than 5–10 minutes) pallor after using the line for sampling. The benefit may outweigh the risk in very ill ELBW neonates in whom vascular access to monitor PaO_2 to prevent ROP is crucial.

If the pallor occurs shortly after insertion in a very ill hypotensive baby, it is justified to see whether the perfusion rapidly improves after volume infusion to raise the blood pressure. However if the pallor does not improve within 15 to 30 minutes or it recurs, the line must be removed. In the vast majority of cases this results in return of the peripheral perfusion to normal within a few minutes. If normal colour does not return within 60 minutes, consider local application of nitroglycerine ointment or the infusion of a bolus of tolazoline (0.5 mg/kg) for their peripheral arteriolar dilating capacity (Heath 1986, Wong *et al.* 1992). If this fails there is a significant risk of peripheral gangrene and tissue loss. Urgent investigation with ultrasound to assess arterial flow should be carried out, backed up if possible by arteriography. Renal ultrasound and Doppler scans should be done in babies with suspected renal artery thrombosis.

The alternatives if arterial thrombosis is identified are thrombolysis or surgical exploration of the artery, proceeding to embolectomy if possible. For thrombolysis we and others have had success with tissue plasminogen activator 0.5 mg/kg administered over 10 minutes followed by 0.5 mg/kg/h until the signs resolve.

If gangrene does develop wait until there is a clear line of demarcation between viable and non-viable tissue. This may result in considerable peripheral recovery and a lower level of amputation (Brain *et al.* 1999). The complications reported to occur with umbilical artery catheters include the following:

- aortic thrombosis, aneurysm
- renal thrombosis
- gut artery thrombosis
- hypoglycaemia (p. 291)
- hypertension
- haemorrhage (p. 98)
- paraplegia from spinal artery damage
- ischaemia of legs, buttocks, toes

LONG LINES

The four major complications are:

- sepsis;
- thrombosis;
- ectopic placement and/or extravasation;
- retention.

Sepsis, especially that caused by slime producing CONS is a common complication (Freeman *et al.* 1990). If continuing TPN is essential, consider leaving the line *in situ* and administering antibiotics through the line; adding urokinase may be beneficial (p. 60). If the infection persists, or the line thromboses with propagation of the thrombus into the vascular tree, there is no alternative but to remove the line.

Extravascular accumulation of TPN has been recorded in many sites (Table 32.1). An X-ray to check the position following insertion or manipulation is mandatory, and our preferred site is in the vena cava, not the right atrium. The only treatment for extravasation is to remove the line and treat the tissue injury which results from the local accumulation of the irritant fluid. The accumulating reports should

Table 32.1 Reported sites of extravasation from silastic long lines

Pericardial	
Pleural	direct
	secondary to SVC obstruction
	with phrenic nerve injury
Intrapulmonary	
Intra-abdominal	
Intraspinal	
Intracranial	

be a warning to all neonatologists that any bizarre and unexpected complication in a baby on TPN could be due to extravasation.

Silastic long lines are fragile and can rupture if too much pressure (>900 mmHg) is applied. If they block, *gentle* flushing can be used, and remember that a large syringe produces a lower pressure than a small syringe in this context, and the manufacturers recommend using a 10 cc syringe. Do not push hard on the syringe. Once these lines have clotted, their small size makes them difficult to rescue and in general we remove them. However, if the line is particularly precious it may be worth trying urokinase. Flush the urokinase solution (1 ml of 5000 units/ml) into the line, leave it to dwell for 10 minutes, and try to aspirate the clot. Do not try to swill the clot into the circulation. If this fails, it can be repeated once or twice over a maximum period of an hour.

Silastic lines have been known to break on removal, with embolization of the remaining fragment into the circulation, so check that the whole length is removed from the baby, and pull gently.

TISSUE DAMAGE FROM SUBCUTANEOUS INFUSIONS

This is the commonest iatrogenic injury in neonates. Most peripheral drips end because they "tissue", rather than just stop because the vessel has thrombosed. It is surprising that there is not more tissue injury from this cause, but it is only if infusions contain TPN or calcium that serious damage is likely to occur.

Some consider that the risk of permanent tissue damage and scarring can be reduced by flushing the tissues with hyaluronidase and saline, although this has never been subjected to a controlled trial. If irrigation is chosen, inject 500–1000 units of hyaluronidase into the damaged subcutaneous tissues, make two small skin incisions on each end of the affected area and open the tissue planes with artery forceps. The area should then be irrigated with up to 500 ml of normal saline (Davies *et al.* 1994).

COMPLICATIONS OF IPPV

A wide range of different types of damage to the nose, lips, gums and palate has been reported secondary to prolonged endotracheal intubation. These scars should be prevented by appropriate immobilization. Once tissue damage has occurred, it is too late. Plastic surgery may be required for correction.

The management of laryngeal and tracheal complications of IPPV are described on p. 176.

CHEST DRAINS

The cannula may penetrate the lung at insertion. This complication should be suspected in cases where placing the chest drain does not successfully control the pneumothorax. The remedy is to remove the drain and start again – carefully!

AIRWAY AND GASTRO-INTESTINAL TRACT RUPTURE

Perforation of the pharynx, larynx, trachea, oesophagus and stomach has been described secondary to endotracheal tubes, pharyngeal suctioning, or placing nasogastric tubes. This need not have been an overtly traumatic procedure.

The clue that suggests airway damage is pneumomediastinum or pneumothorax, coupled with difficulties in re-intubation or re-insertion. Oesophageal injury presents like TOF with pooling of secretions (p. 395–396). Occasionally, perforation of either organ will result in mediastinal infection which can spread to the pleura.

Treatment of airway rupture is usually conservative. The injury should be bypassed with an ETT until the lesion is likely to have healed. The same also applies to oesophageal perforation, although a gastrostomy may be necessary.

REFERENCES

Brain, J.L., Roberton, N.R.C. and Rennie, J.M. (1999) Iatrogenic disorders. In: *Textbook of Neonatology*, 3rd edn. Rennie, J.M. and Roberton, N.R.C. (eds), Churchill Livingstone, Edinburgh, pp. 917–938.

Davies, J., Gault, D. and Buchdahl, R. (1994) Preventing the scars of neonatal intensive care. *Archives of Disease in Childhood* **70**: F50–51.

Freeman, J., Goldman, D.A., Smith, N.E., Sidebottam, D.E., Epstein, M.F. and Platt, R. (1990) Association of intravenous lipid emulsion and coagulase negative staphylococcal bacteraemia in neonatal intensive care units. *New England Journal of Medicine* **323**: 301–308.

Heath, R.E. (1986) Vasospasm in the neonate: response to tolazoline. *Pediatrics* **77**: 405–408.

Wong, A.F., McCulloch, L.M. and Sola, A. (1992) Treatment of peripheral tissue ischaemia with topical nitroglycerine ointment in neonates. *Journal of Pediatrics* **121**: 980–983.

33

PROCEDURES

ANALGESIA FOR PROCEDURES

Babies who are ventilated should be receiving sedation and probably some background analgesia (Chapter 9). If this is the case, the morphine infusion should be increased, if there is time, before a painful procedure is carried out. Babies who are not receiving analgesia already should be given it wherever possible. Local anaesthetic should be used for procedures involving skin incisions, such as chest drains or paracentesis. EMLA cream can be used for suprapubic aspiration or long line insertion, but does not appear to work on the heel – perhaps because the skin is too thick. Umbilical catheterization should be a painless procedure, and lumbar puncture is usually quick and easy; use of local anaesthetic does not improve the success rate of these procedures and is not generally warranted.

BLOOD SAMPLING

CAPILLARY SAMPLES

Tissue atrophy, painful inclusion dermoids and osteomyelitis of the os calcis can follow excessively deep and frequent heel pricks on the plantar part of the heel pad. The area to be used is shown in Fig. 33.1; Jain and Rutter have recently recommended a wider field based on ultrasound studies of the soft tissue of the heel (Jain and Rutter 1999, Blumenfeld, Turi and Blanc 1979).

If the heel is not well perfused, rub it, or warm it in water at 40°C. Sterilize the skin with one of the standard skin antiseptics, but do not apply vaseline. Use a spring-loaded device such as an Autolet which inserts a sharp disposable stilette to a predetermined depth, and has been shown to be less painful.

Capillary samples can be used for most haematological and

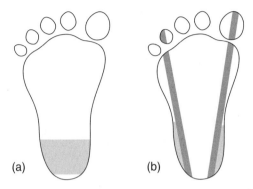

Figure 33.1 Alternative sites for capillary sampling from the heel. From Jain and Rutter 1999 (a), and Blumenfeld *et al.* 1979 (b).

biochemical tests, but they are unreliable for blood gases, haemoglobin and PCV on the first day or two of life and for blood cultures. After 48–72 hours acid–base and haematological data can be satisfactorily obtained from capillary samples, but capillary PO_2 values are unreliable and bear no relationship to PaO_2 (p. 101).

VENOUS BLOOD

Open-ended needle technique

A special open-ended FG21 or FG23 needle with a fixed plastic wing for gripping can be inserted (without a syringe attached) into a peripheral vein which has been distended in the usual way in either the hand, the foot or some more proximal site in the arm or leg. If the venous occlusion is gently continued blood will drip out of the end of the needle (Fig. 33.2) and can be collected in an appropriate bottle.

Although the broken needle technique was a very efficient and minimally traumatic way of obtaining blood for most investigations it is no longer recommended. Concerns have been raised about this method because in one or two cases the needle has been left in the crib rather than being appropriately disposed of, and later worked its way into the baby's body. This danger can be avoided by leaving the hub on the needle and allowing the blood to drip from the plastic luer lock fitting, or using a similar gauge butterfly with the plastic

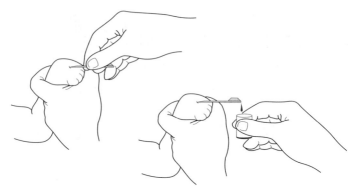

Figure 33.2 Collecting blood by the open-ended needle method. Modified from Wilkinson and Calvert 1992.

tubing cut off very short. The new device illustrated, which is specifically designed for neonatal venepuncture, appears equally effective. Needles must always be disposed of properly.

Venepuncture

The site which is safest and most likely to be successful in the neonate is the antecubital fossa. Two points should be remembered when taking blood from this site:

1. Do not use too great an occluding pressure around the upper arm, as this obstructs arterial flow.
2. Use a big needle (FG21 or FG23) to minimize the problems caused by excessive suction through a narrow needle.

Avoid using the femoral vein for venepuncture if at all possible, since there is the risk that the hip joint may be entered and infected. If this vein has to be used because there is no alternative, lie the baby on his back with his legs partially flexed and fully abducted at the hip. Palpate the femoral artery in the midpoint of the groin just below the inguinal ligament. The femoral vein lies just medial to it. Hold the needle and syringe vertically, and advance through the skin towards the vein while applying constant gentle suction so that blood flows back as soon as the vein is entered. In our experience it is very rarely necessary to resort to femoral venepuncture.

ARTERIAL PUNCTURE

Eight sites can be used: radial, ulnar, posterior tibial, dorsalis pedis, brachial, temporal, axillary and femoral. The drawbacks of any type of arterial puncture are listed on p. 100.

RADIAL ARTERY PUNCTURE

The artery should be entered just proximal to the transverse wrist creases after confirming that there is an ulnar artery either by palpation or by showing that the hand is perfused when the radial artery is occluded.

A very useful technique is to place a fibre-optic light source behind the baby's wrist; this makes the artery clearly visible, especially in low birth weight babies.

Local anaesthetic is not routinely used (v.s.). However, it can be used if accurate PaO_2 measurement is critical, since it minimizes the crying and struggling which causes PaO_2 to fall.

The wrist is held slightly extended (Fig. 33.3). The artery should be approached at an angle of 25–30° to the skin – particularly if you hope to cannulate it. Either an FG23 or FG25 needle attached directly to a 1–2 ml heparinized syringe, or a FG23 or

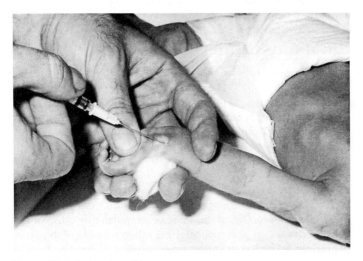

Figure 33.3 Position for radial artery puncture.

FG25 butterfly needle with its attached plastic tubing can be used for puncture (for details of cannulation, *v.i.*). The options are to attempt to enter the lumen of the artery directly, or you can deliberately transfix the artery, and then gradually withdraw the needle while sucking gently on the syringe, which will rapidly fill as soon as the artery is entered.

ULNAR ARTERY PUNCTURE

The technique is identical to that for radial puncture.

POSTERIOR TIBIAL ARTERY PUNCTURE

The baby's foot is held partly plantar flexed, and using either of the above techniques the needle is inserted at an angle of 30–40° to the skin midway between the posterior margin of the medial malleolus and the back of the Achilles tendon. Sampling is then carried out as described above.

DORSALIS PEDIS ARTERY PUNCTURE

The baby's foot is held partially plantar flexed and the artery entered in the midpoint of the foot where it lies between the first and second metatarsals. Sampling is then carried out as described above.

BRACHIAL ARTERY PUNCTURE

The baby's arm is fully extended at the elbow and slightly externally rotated at the shoulder. The artery is entered proximal to the antecubital fossa as it lies on the brachialis muscle on the medial side of the arm just before it turns laterally under the bicipital aponeurosis. It should not be cannulated, as it is an end artery.

TEMPORAL ARTERY PUNCTURE

The temporal artery and its branches over the lateral part of the skull can be entered at any point, usually using a heparinized FG23 scalp vein needle. They should not be cannulated because of the risk of reflex spasm or emboli affecting other branches of the external carotid, including the middle meningeal.

FEMORAL ARTERY PUNCTURE

The contraindications to femoral arterial puncture are identical to those for femoral venepuncture. The artery is entered by a vertical approach about 0.5–1.0 cm distal to the inguinal ligament.

PERCUTANEOUS ARTERIAL CANNULATION

An FG23 or FG24 intravenous cannula can be inserted percutaneously into the radial, ulnar, posterior tibial or dorsalis pedis arteries, but should not be inserted into the brachial or temporal arteries. The technique for puncturing the artery is described above. Once the artery is entered, the Teflon cannula is advanced over the needle, usually 2–3 mm along the artery. The cannula is connected to an infusion of heparinized saline with a luer lock extension tubing, and then the cannula and the limb are carefully immobilized. Femoral artery cannulation using a catheter inserted over a guide wire is increasingly being used, especially in term babies. It appears to be very successful and safe, but as the artery is an end artery the toes should be watched carefully for signs of arterial obstruction. All indwelling arterial cannulae should be perfused with heparinized saline (1 unit/ml) at a rate of 0.5–1.0 ml/h. They can be left *in situ* for as long as they stay patent, but they must never be used for anything other than sampling and BP monitoring.

To remove these cannulae, simply pull them out of the artery and apply firm manual pressure over the puncture site for at least 5 minutes. Apply a tight dressing and keep a close watch for haemorrhage developing.

INTRAVENOUS INFUSION

SITES

The preferred sites are the veins on the back of the hand, the top of the foot, the long saphenous vein at the ankle, veins in the antecubital fossa and the scalp veins, but in practice any superficial vein can be used.

FG22–FG25 cannulae or butterfly needles can be used. The latter are easier to insert into very fine scalp veins, whereas Teflon cannulae are less irritant to vessels and last longer. At least an FG24 needle or cannula must be used if blood is to be transfused.

TECHNIQUES

The veins in low birth weight babies lie in lax subcutaneous tissue. Hold them steady during insertion by asking an assistant to hold the subcutaneous tissue sufficiently taut on each side of the vein to prevent it from moving, but not taut enough to occlude it. Leave the cap off the end of the cannulae, or off the scalp vein needle tubing during the procedure, since this allows blood to flash back rapidly into the device as soon as the vein is entered, by a combination of the venous pressure and capillarity.

Good immobilization is essential, and this is a very individual activity among neonatologists. Small splints are commercially available. The practice of using "home-made" splints is now rare, since a batch of the wooden tongue depressors that were used as the basis for making them was found to be contaminated with a rare fungus. Because of the dangers of tissue damage resulting in permanent scarring from extravasated infusion fluid (p. 474) it is important to leave the site as exposed as possible. This maximizes the chance of recognizing tissued infusions quickly, and minimizes the consequences.

VENOUS CUT-DOWN FOR INTRAVENOUS INFUSIONS

There is nothing special about this in the neonate, except that everything is smaller! The usual veins to try are those in the antecubital fossa, and the long saphenous vein either at the ankle or more proximally in the leg. In general if it is necessary to resort to a cut-down, this should be done by a surgeon with the appropriate skills, in the operating theatre with full anaesthesia and aseptic precautions. In these circumstances a long-term multi-lumen catheter such as a Hickman is inserted, usually into the subclavian vein with a subcutaneous tunnel in the chest wall, with the intention that this will last longer than the baby's illness.

INSERTION OF A LONG LINE

This technique is valuable when long-term intravenous fluids are to be given, especially intravenous feeding with high concentrations of dextrose. The procedure must be carried out with full sterile precautions. Vygon manufacture a set containing a 19-gauge scalp vein needle and 23-gauge silicone tubing with a special connecting set. The length of the line to be inserted must be estimated by using

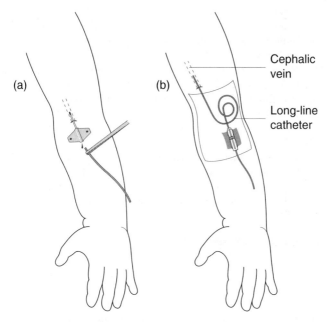

Figure 33.4 (a) and (b) Insertion of long line. From Kelsall (1999) with permission.

a tape measure to measure the distance from the point of insertion to the expected end-point of the line. The butterfly needle is inserted into a suitable vein such as one of the larger veins at the elbow (the medial antecubital vein is better than the lateral one), the long saphenous vein at the ankle or the external jugular vein. Once the needle is inserted, a 0.025 inch outside-diameter silastic catheter is threaded through the needle and fed up the vein (Fig. 33.4(a)). The butterfly needle is then removed, by withdrawing it carefully over the whole length of the catheter. The compression hub of the catheter is then secured, making sure that the black mark on the catheter is completely hidden. The catheter is taped in place with a loop to take up any strain (Fig. 33.4(b)). This procedure is fiddly and takes some practice; always use non-toothed forceps to avoid damaging the fragile material of the catheter. Failing to fit the end of the catheter back into the compression hub correctly is a common cause of leakage. A training video is available which demonstrates the correct technique. For advice on flushing and unblocking these catheters see p. 474. Remember that a small syringe generates more pressure than a large syringe. Never use a syringe smaller than 2 ml, and do not use force when attempting to unblock catheters.

The position of the cannula, irrespective of how it is inserted, is confirmed radiographically by injecting a small amount of radio-opaque dye into it. In our experience opacification is required, although the manufacturers of the silastic line claim that the line is radio-opaque. The aim is always to have the catheter in the vena cava, but more proximal positioning is acceptable if the catheter cannot be pushed in further. We prefer not to aim for the right atrium, because we consider that the incidence of complications, particularly extravasation causing a pericardial tamponade or cardiac arrhythmias, is higher with the line in this position (p. 473).

UMBILICAL CATHETERIZATION

Both the umbilical vein and artery can be catheterized up to 7–10 days after delivery. Catheterization is easiest just after birth, and whether or not it can be done later depends on the condition of the umbilical stump. If this has remained clean and sterile, when the dried Wharton's jelly is cut off, the distal ends of the umbilical arteries and umbilical vein can usually be identified easily and then catheterized.

Umbilical vein catheterization is very easy to do, so it should always be left until *after* arterial catheterization.

UMBILICAL ARTERY CATHETERIZATION

When inserting a catheter within 6–12 hours of delivery, there is a risk of haemorrhage from the arteries when the cord is cut. For this reason a ligature should always be loosely in place around the base of the cord before it is cut. The cord is cut about 5 mm distal to the junction between the skin and the Wharton's jelly. A common mistake is to cut further away (1.0–1.5 cm). This leaves a long, curly, badly supported stretch of artery within the Wharton's jelly and markedly increases the risk of creating a false passage. The vein is a large patulous opening lying superiorly. The arteries often protrude from the Wharton's jelly as tortuous white structures 2–3 mm in diameter (Fig. 33.5(a)).

One of the arteries should be cut flush with the Wharton's jelly

(a)   (b)

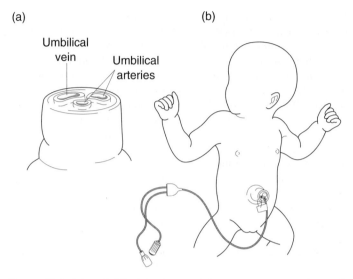

Umbilical
vein   Umbilical
              arteries

Figure 33.5 (a) and (b) The appearance of the cut surface of the umbilicus, and a method of positioning an inserted umbilical catheter using a "flag" of tape. From Kelsall (1999) with permission.

and the orifice gently teased open to a depth of 5–10 mm with a pair of fine forceps. Hold the edge of the artery and surrounding Wharton's jelly with a pair of fine-toothed forceps, and introduce an FG4.5–5.0 PVC catheter full of heparinized saline (1 unit/ml). This is used to continue the arterial dilatation. The cord stump should be pulled up towards the baby's head to straighten out the artery as it turns caudally in the anterior abdominal wall just below the umbilicus. Most cases of failed catheterization are due to the creation of a false passage into the vessel wall at this level. Once this has been passed it is rare not to be able to pass the catheter up into the aorta. The length to be inserted can be looked up on a graph, or calculated by Shukla's formula. This formula states that the correct catheter length (in cm) to be inserted to reach a level between T6 and T10 (diaphragm) is 2.5 × the weight of the baby (in kg) plus 9.7 (Shukla and Ferrara 1986).

Once inserted, the catheter should be immobilized. There are several methods of achieving this. One approach involves inserting a suture with the first "bite" made into the junction of the Wharton's

jelly and the skin and the second into a flag of tape stuck firmly to
the catheter higher up (Fig. 33.5(b)). This method has the advantage that it is not too cumbersome, and it remains possible to move
the catheter if an X-ray shows that it is wrongly positioned. The
anchoring suture has to take a small bite of skin, because over time
the Wharton's jelly will dry out and a suture into the jelly alone will
not hold. If this method is chosen, haemostasis needs to be achieved
via another method, either by suturing through the unused vessels
or by leaving the umbilical tape in place around the base of the
umbilical stump. Another method involves the use of an H-bridge
of tape across the abdomen and the catheter.

Finally, the stump is sprayed with antibiotic powder. A dressing is
not needed. The position of the catheter tip must be checked radiologically and the position altered if necessary (p. 98–99). The
abdomen should be included on the X-ray. The problems with
UACs are listed on p. 473. The correct position of the catheter is at
the level of T10–T12 or L5. It is important to avoid leaving the tip
of the catheter in the aorta between these levels, because the renal
and superior mesenteric arteries arise here and complications can
ensue. The hallmark of an arterial catheter on an X-ray is that it
takes an apparent downturn before heading off into the descending
aorta. This is the reason for requesting that the chest and abdomen
are included on the X-ray; if the catheter travels straight towards the
thorax then it is venous and not arterial.

UMBILICAL VEIN CATHETERIZATION

An FG-6 PVC catheter filled with heparinized saline is used, and it
is usually extremely easy to insert into the umbilical vein after lifting
out any small thrombi that may be lying in the vessel. At a depth of
about 5–7 cm, with the tip of the UVC in the portal sinus, blood is
easily withdrawn. Within 24 hours of birth it is usually possible to
pass the catheter from the portal sinus through the ductus venosus
into the inferior vena cava, right atrium and left atrium. The
catheter should be secured *in situ* in the same way as a UAC.

Umbilical venous catheters passing through the ductus venosus
into the thorax pose the constant threat of an air embolus (p. 105).
Great care should be used when they are in this position and the
end must never be disconnected. If the catheter cannot pass
through the ductus venosus, its tip lies in a vessel with comparatively
sluggish blood flow with the attendant risk of thrombotic complications. Hypertonic solutions should not be infused into these

catheters because if the endothelium is damaged the risk of a clot increases.

REMOVING CATHETERS

There is a risk of haemorrhage when removing a UAC. To prevent this, the ligatures around the catheter should be divided, all the dried and caked Wharton's jelly removed, and the umbilical stump freshened. A black silk suture is then inserted around the stump *before* the catheter is removed. When the catheter has been removed, the sutures can be pulled tight. In addition, it is important to withdraw the catheter slowly and wait a minute or two before removing it the final centimetre to allow the vessel to go into spasm proximally.

The tip of the catheter should always be put in transport medium and sent for culture.

INTUBATION

Intubation is an essential skill which can only be perfected with practice. Training with mannequins can help. Essential equipment consists of an appropriate sized laryngoscope with a straight blade, suction, oxygen, an appropriate sized ETT and a fixation system. An assistant who understands the procedure is invaluable. Before starting, check the equipment and if the intubation is elective consider premedication (p. 151). Position the baby with his head in the midline and his neck slightly extended. Clear any secretions with suction. Insert the laryngoscope into one side of the mouth (usually the right for right-handed operators), and apply gentle vertical traction. This, together with a little cricoid pressure, will bring the vocal cords into view.

Pass the ETT through the cords when they are open. Do not push against closed cords because this can cause damage. If you encounter spasm of the vocal cords, send for help and bag the baby for a while before trying again. Nasal intubation at resuscitation should only be attempted by experienced operators, and involves passing a lubricated ETT into the nostril in a vertical direction, through the choanae into the oropharynx where the tip can be grasped with a Magill's forceps and the tube placed between the cords.

NEUROLOGICAL PROCEDURES

LUMBAR PUNCTURE

This can be carried out with the baby lying down or sitting up. His lumbar spine should be flexed, but since many babies who require LP are very ill, and doubling them up obstructs their airway and compromises tidal breathing, the degree of flexion that is used has to be a compromise. Contraindications to LP include severe respiratory disease, thrombocytopenia and coagulation disturbances.

In general, babies tolerate LP best in the *upright* position. Use the L3/4 space and a proper stiletted spinal needle. Advance the needle slowly, as the subarachnoid space is only 5–7 mm from the surface in the premature baby and 1 cm from it in full-term babies, and there is often no "give" as the subarachnoid space is entered. For this reason it is extremely easy to go in too far, and hit the anterior vertebral venous plexus. One ml of CSF is adequate for all purposes.

When the needle has been removed, the hole in the skin is best sealed with a plastic spray dressing.

VENTRICULAR PUNCTURE

This may be required for the insertion of intraventricular antibiotics in neonatal coliform meningitis, or for measurement of pressure and CSF examination in posthaemorrhagic ventriculomegaly. Always assess ventricular size ultrasonically before attempting a ventricular puncture, and do not attempt the procedure if the ventricles are very small.

Lie the baby on his back with the top of his head facing towards you, and position yourself comfortably in a seated position so that you are at the same level as him. Ask an assistant to hold the baby's head still. Choose an entry point in the lateral angle of the fontanelle as far away from the midline (and the dural sinus!) as you can get, and clean the skin thoroughly with a suitable antiseptic. Use full sterile procedure.

The ventricles are entered by passing a fine 4–5 cm spinal needle through the chosen spot in the lateral margin of the anterior fontanelle and aiming forward and slightly inwards towards the inner canthus of the opposite eye. Usually, if a ventricular tap is being performed, the ventricles are large and are easily entered at a shallow depth of around 1 cm. Ultrasound guidance can help.

Always insert and withdraw along the same track. If you are

aiming in a different direction after a dry tap, always withdraw the needle to just below the calvarium before taking a fresh aim.

SUBDURAL PUNCTURE

These are rarely indicated (p. 323). A spinal (LP) needle with a flat bevel and stilette should be used. The subdural space is entered at the same point as described above for ventricular puncture. As soon as any "give" is felt, the stilette should be withdrawn. If nothing drips out, do not advance the needle any further, and do not point the needle in different directions seeking fluid. If subdural taps are indicated, they should be done bilaterally.

If fluid is encountered it should be allowed to drain away completely, and subdural taps repeated on subsequent days, as these effusions have a habit of re-accumulating.

SUPRAPUBIC BLADDER PUNCTURE

This should be the method of choice for obtaining clean urine samples if bag urine gives equivocal evidence of UTI (p. 232–233).

At least one hour after the last wet nappy, a 21-gauge needle attached to a 10 ml syringe should be inserted in the midline 1 cm above the symphysis pubis, and angled slightly down into the pelvis. At a depth of 1–2 cm the bladder is entered and the urine aspirated. Do not deviate from the midline or enter more than 2 cm.

The needle is then withdrawn and the wound on the abdominal wall closed with nobecutaine and a small adhesive dressing.

BLADDER CATHETERIZATION

This is sometimes required in order to assess urine output or where neurological problems prevent bladder emptying. Use a fine 5 or 6 gauge feeding tube and sterile KY jelly.

THORACENTESIS

PLEURAL EFFUSION

The baby is usually supine, and an FG17 or 19 Jelco or Medicut attached via a 3-way tap to a 20 ml syringe should be inserted into the fourth intercostal space in the midaxillary line. Large quantities of fluid can then be slowly and safely aspirated without disconnecting the syringe, which would allow air or infection to enter the pleural cavity.

PNEUMOTHORAX

In an emergency situation with a tension pneumothorax, the chest should be tapped in the third intercostal space in the anterior axillary line using the above technique. The alternative is just to use a butterfly needle with a 3-way tap. The 3-way tap allows repeated aspiration of the air without disconnecting the syringe from the needle or the cannula.

This emergency procedure should always be followed by insertion of a thoracentesis tube. Either an FG10 or 12 tube should be used even in very small babies. Appropriate tubes mounted on a disposable trocar are commercially available. We remove the trocar altogether and use the following technique. If time allows, a small amount of local anaesthetic should be inserted. A nick is then made in the skin with a scalpel blade, and a track made for the cannula through the intercostal muscles with a pair of fine forceps. The cannula is inserted by holding it with the forceps, a distance of 2–3 cm aiming to get the tip lying under the sternum (since air rises!). The drain should then be connected to an underwater seal drain with 10–20 cm H_2O suction pressure. Great care must be taken not to transfix the lung as the cannula is inserted. In all cases the drain must be held in place with a suture, and the skin incision made airtight with a dressing.

When the drain is removed care should be taken to prevent air from entering along its track during or following removal. We try not to use purse-string sutures because the scar they produce is cosmetically disfiguring, and usually close the wound with steri-strips. Occasionally there is no alternative but to insert a suture, usually because the drain has been in a long time.

PERICARDIAL PUNCTURE

This is occasionally indicated in cardiac tamponade due to a pneumopericardium, or for aspiration of TPN from the pericardial cavity. The procedure is made easier and safer if it is done under ultrasound control. An FG21 cannula connected via a 3-way tap to a 10 ml syringe is inserted under the rib cage to the left of the xiphis-

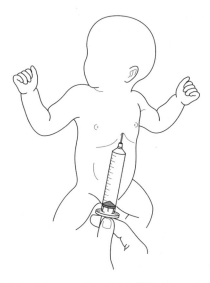

Figure 33.6 Pericardial puncture (from Kelsall 1999 with permission).

ternum (Fig. 33.6). It is then advanced upwards and to the left at 45° from the vertical and 45° from the midline while applying gentle suction. At a depth of about 1 cm the pericardium will be entered and air withdrawn. If necessary, the cannula can be left *in situ* and connected to underwater seal drainage.

PARACENTESIS ABDOMINIS

The conditions in which ascites develops are commonly associated with organ enlargement (e.g. hepatosplenomegaly in severe rhesus HDN). For this reason blind needle aspiration should not be carried out because of the risk of entering a major viscus.

Under local anaesthetic a small nick should be made through the skin and linea alba at the junction of the upper and middle third of the line joining the umbilicus to the symphysis pubis. When the peritoneum is entered and fluid gushes out, an FG8 nasogastric feeding tube with extra holes cut in the side can be inserted and pushed to the paracolic gutters. Alternatively, the puncture can be made in the right or left iliac fossae. When all the ascites has been drained or aspirated, the tube is removed and the incision closed with a single suture. A similar procedure can be used in the occasional baby with a pneumoperitoneum. Tubes inserted in either position can be left for long-term drainage of fluid or air or for peritoneal dialysis (p. 376).

REFERENCES

Blumenfeld, T.A., Turi, G.B. and Blanc, W.A. (1979) Recommended site and depth of newborn heel skin punctures based on anatomical measurements and histopathology. *Lancet* i: 230–233.

Jain, A. and Rutter, N. (1999) Ultrasound study of heel to calcaneum depth in neonates. *Archives of Disease in Childhood* 80: F243–F245.

Kelsall, A.W.R. (1999) Procedures. In: *Textbook of Neonatology*, 3rd edn. Rennie, J.M. and Roberton, N.R.C. (eds), Churchill Livingstone, Edinburgh, pp. 1369–1384.

Shukla, H. and Ferrara, A. (1986) Rapid estimation of insertional length of umbilical catheters in newborns. *American Journal of Disease in Childhood* 140: 786.

Wilkinson, A. and Calvert, S.A. (1992) Procedures. In: *Textbook of Neonatology*, 3rd edn. Rennie, J.M. and Roberton, N.R.C. (eds), Churchill Livingstone, Edinburgh, pp. 1167–1191.

34

THE DEATH OF A BABY

Helping the parents after the death of a baby is often a neglected part of the service provided by a neonatal unit.

Parents always grieve for a stillbirth or a neonatal death regardless of the circumstances. The grief may last for a year or more, and must be allowed to run its course. The grief reaction after the death of a baby is no different to that after bereavement at any other time, and involves the following stages:

- numbness, shock and disbelief;
- intense bouts of tearfulness;
- feelings of guilt, despair and anger (the "pangs of grief");
- searching for a cause of death;
- insomnia, anxiety and social withdrawal;
- stage of resolution, with a return to society.

The duration of the individual stages vary enormously, and some parents get "stuck" at one stage. Parents can be helped to pass through the normal stages of grief with sensitive handling and good communication.

CARE OF THE DYING BABY

Always keep parents fully informed about the medical progress of their baby, and if the prognosis is hopeless this should be explained fully to them. When death has become inevitable because of, for example, brain death following severe intrapartum asphyxia, the baby should be disconnected from the paraphernalia of intensive care and the parents should be encouraged to hold and cuddle their dying or dead baby. Appropriate religious ceremonies should always be arranged if requested in such cases.

KEEPSAKES

These serve to emphasize the reality of the event, and include photographs, locks of hair, footprints and even the cot cards. Parents treasure these and find them helpful in the grieving process. Keepsakes should therefore always be offered. Photographs can be filed in the notes in an envelope if the parents do not want them at the time, as they often appreciate receiving them later on. Parents should be encouraged to name their baby.

POSTMORTEMS

The aim should be to get a postmortem on every neonatal death and stillbirth. The appropriate time to ask permission is usually 12–24 hours after the death of the baby, or when the parents are given the death certificate or the stillbirth certificate.

Parents who are averse to the idea of a postmortem often have bizarre notions of what it involves. When told that it does not affect burial or funeral arrangements, and can be conducted in a way that does not interfere with the baby's appearance, they may well often agree to it. Limited postmortems can often yield vital information, if, for example, parents do not want the head or face of their baby interfered with.

It is important to explain to parents that an autopsy can check that nothing unsuspected was present which might influence the outcome of subsequent pregnancies, and also to reassure them and the neonatologist that nothing that should have been done was left undone. Many parents who refuse consent for a postmortem subsequently regret that this type of information is forever denied to them. Furthermore, postmortem is one of the most important components of audit in neonatal intensive care.

DOCUMENTATION

BIRTH CERTIFICATE

All live births, irrespective of birth weight and gestation, have by law to be registered within 42 days of the birth. The mother or her husband can do this at any registry office. Currently, a father who is not married to the baby's mother cannot register a birth or a stillbirth.

DEATH CERTIFICATE

This must be issued for all neonatal deaths irrespective of their birth weight and gestation. It is usually given to the parents the day after the baby's death, and, if relevant, the certificate should be appropriately marked if postmortem data will be available later. It is not usually justifiable to delay issuing the death certificate until after the postmortem has been carried out.

The death must be registered within 5 days. It must be done in the town (registration district) in which the baby died – not his place of birth or home address – and this can be done by the mother or father irrespective of whether they are married. The registrar will issue the parents with a certificate for the undertaker to allow funeral arrangements to take place.

BURIAL

The hospital can arrange the burial of neonatal deaths and stillbirths, usually in a numbered, but unmarked, grave in the local cemetery. However, parents can and should be encouraged to have a normal funeral irrespective of the baby's gestation.

STILLBIRTHS

The definition of a stillbirth was changed in 1992 to include all

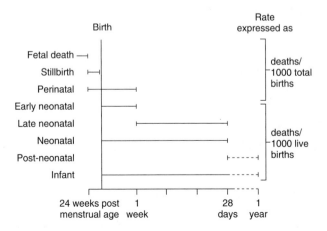

Figure 34.1 Definitions of stillbirth and infant mortality rates.

babies born dead after 24 weeks of gestation (Fig. 34.1). Parents should be actively encouraged to see and hold their dead baby. This also applies to those whose stillborn child is malformed. Even babies with anencephaly can be wrapped up in a blanket so that the face can be seen and the shock of seeing the whole malformation minimized. The baby can be given a first name, which is included in the stillbirth certificate.

Although, in many hospitals, stillborn babies are buried at the hospital's expense in an unmarked plot in the local cemetery, the baby can have a normal funeral and the parents should always be asked if they wish to arrange this in the normal way with an undertaker. The registrar will give the parents a certificate for the undertaker to enable him to arrange the funeral. Funerals of stillbirths are, however, not eligible for the death grant. For stillbirths of less than 24 weeks gestation a funeral can also be arranged in the absence of a stillbirth certificate, so long as a doctor provides the undertaker with a letter explaining the situation.

Parents of stillborn babies should also be offered a full post-mortem examination which should include a chromosome analysis.

APPENDIX A

ASSESSMENT OF GESTATIONAL AGE

It is our belief that this has become an unnecessarily complex endeavour. In most cases the aim is to achieve an assessment of whether the mother's estimated gestational age from the first day of her last menstrual period is correct or whether she or her obstetrician are one menstrual cycle out in their calculations.

The following scheme is based on the work of Robinson (1966) and Parkin *et al.* (1976). The Robinson score, based on serial assessment to determine when various reflexes first become elicitable, performed better than scores based on physical characteristics in a comparative study (Wariyar *et al.* 1997). None of the scores were nearly as accurate as an estimate based on early antenatal ultrasound.

NEUROLOGICAL ASSESSMENT

This is best for infants less than 36 weeks gestation (Table A.1).

Beyond this period one is dependent on cutaneous and soft tissue assessment, and the following is that described by Parkin *et al.* in 1976.

Table A.1 Assessment of gestational age. Source: Robinson 1966

| Reflex | Stimulus | Positive response | Gestation in weeks if reflex is: | |
			Absent	Present
Pupil reaction	Light	Pupil constriction	≤31	≥29
Glabellar tap	Tap on glabella	Blink	≤34	≥32
Traction response	Pull up by wrists from supine	Flexion of neck or arm	≤36	≥33
Neck righting	Rotation of head	Trunk follows	≤37	≥34

CUTANEOUS AND SOFT TISSUE ASSESSMENT

SKIN TEXTURE

This is tested by picking up a fold of abdominal skin between finger and thumb and by inspection:

0: very thin with gelatinous feel
1: thin and smooth
2: smooth and of medium thickness, irritation rash and superficial peeling may be present
3: slight thickening and stiff feeling with superficial cracking and peeling especially evident in the hands and feet
4: thick and parchment-like with superficial or deep cracking.

SKIN COLOUR

This should be estimated by inspection when the baby is quiet:

0: dark red
1: uniformly pink
2: pale pink, though the colour may vary over different parts of the body; some parts may be very pale
3: pale, nowhere really pink except on the ears, lips palms and soles.

BREAST SIZE

This is measured by picking up the breast tissue between finger and thumb:

0: no breast tissue palpable
1: breast tissue palpable on one or both sides, neither being more than 0.5 cm diameter
2: breast tissue palpable on both sides, one or both being 0.5–1.0 cm diameter
3: breast tissue palpable on both sides, one or both being more than 1 cm diameter.

EAR FIRMNESS

This can be tested by palpation and folding of the upper pinna:

0: pinna feels soft and is easily folded into bizarre positions without springing back into position spontaneously

Table A.2 Calculation of the Parkin score (Parkin *et al.* 1976)

Score	Gestational age in weeks
4	34.5
5	36
6	37
7	38.5
8	39.5
9	40
10	41
11–12	>41

1: pinna feels soft along the edge and is easily folded, but returns slowly to the correct position spontaneously
2: cartilage can be felt to the edge of the pinna, although it is thin in places and the pinna springs back readily after being folded
3: pinna is firm with definite cartilage extending peripherally, and springs back immediately into position after being folded.

Add up the total scores, and the mean gestation for that score can be read off Table A.2.

Two other pieces of assessment which are useful are:

1. Infants with fused eyelids are usually 26 weeks of gestation or less;
2. In the first hour or two after birth, assess the plantar skin creases. After this time all babies tend to get wrinkly as they dry out. In infants of 36 weeks or less there are one or two transverse plantar creases at the level of the metatarsal heads. By 38 weeks these creases have migrated to the midpoint of the sole, and by full term they have reached the heel.

REFERENCES

Parkin, J.M., Hey, E.N. and Clowes, J.S. (1976) Rapid assessment of gestational age at birth. *Archives of Disease in Childhood* **51**: 259–263.

Robinson, R. J. (1966) Assessment of gestational age by neurological examination. *Archives of Disease in Childhood* **41**: 437–447.

Wariyar, U., Tin, W. and Hey, E. (1997) Gestational assessment assessed. *Archives of Disease in Childhood* **77**: F216–F220.

APPENDIX B

ASSESSING THE ILL NEONATE

Many attempts have been made to develop scoring systems which can be applied to neonates in the first few hours of life. These can help both in discussion of the prognosis with parents and in identification of babies with a very high mortality risk, in whom new therapies can justifiably be evaluated. In the past very simple clinical markers such as the inability to achieve a PaO_2 of 13.3 kPa (100 mmHg) in 100% oxygen or the need for IPPV in the first few hours identified babies who had a mortality rate of $> 75\%$.

Several relatively simple techniques are available:

SCORES BASED ON OXYGENATION

These can be used at any time during the neonatal period and they only require measurement of blood gases and F_IO_2.

a) A-aDO$_2$ (alveolar-arterial oxygen difference)
    This requires a calculation of the alveolar oxygen tension (PAO_2) using the alveolar air equation:

$$PAO_2 = P_IO_2 - \frac{PACO_2}{R} + \{PACO_2 \times F_IO_2 \times \frac{1-R}{R}\}$$

Where:

P_IO_2 is the partial pressure of inspired O_2 in mmHg and equals

(F_IO_2 [as as fraction] $\times$ 760 [atmospheric pressure] – 47 [water vapour pressure])

$PACO_2$ is the alveolar CO_2 partial pressure – assumed to be the same as $PaCO_2$, in mmHg

R is the respiratory quotient – assumed to be 0.8

Thus in 100% oxygen PAO_2 is 678 mmHg if the $PaCO_2$ is 35 mmHg (example a, v.i.)

In air (21% oxygen) PAO_2 is 108 mmHg if the $PaCO_2$ is 35 mmHg (example b, v.i.)

The A-aDO$_2$ is then the arterial PaO_2 subtracted from the

PAO_2. A normal adult breathing air with a PaO_2 of 100 mmHg has an A-aDO_2 of 8 mmHg (example a, *v.i.* and *v.s.*), whereas a baby with a PaO_2 of 50 mmHg in 100% oxygen has an A-a DO_2 of 628 mmHg (example b, *v.i.* and *v.s.*). Babies with an A-a DO_2 of more than 610 mmHg are in serious trouble.

b) aAO_2 ratio (arterial-alveolar oxygen ratio)

This also requires a calculation of the P_AO_2 as above. The ratio of PaO_2 and PAO_2 is then expressed numerically. Using the above examples the ratios are:

Example a) $100/108 = 0.93$
Example b) $50/678 = 0.07$

In general babies with aAO_2 ratios < 0.1 are seriously ill.

c) Oxygenation index

$$OI = \frac{\text{mean airways pressure (cmH}_2\text{O)} \times F_IO_2 \times 100}{PaO_2(\text{postductal) mmHg}}$$

The units are the same as for calculating A-aDO_2.

An OI >40 identifies a baby with a severe oxygenation deficit, though some workers find that it is not until OI is > 60 that it is a good predictor of mortality (Ortega *et al.* 1988).

CRIB SCORE (CLINICAL RISK INDEX FOR BABIES)

This score, developed in Dundee (International Neonatal Network 1993), is based on clinical and laboratory variables collected in the first 12 hours of life (Table B.1). It is easy to use and provides a useful separation beween groups with markedly different outcomes (Fig. B.1).

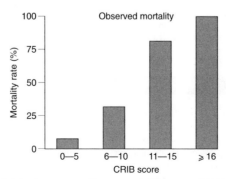

Figure B.I Relation between ascending ranges of CRIB score and hospital mortality.

Table B.1 Items used for the CRIB score

Factor	Score
Birth weight	
>1350 g	0
851–1350 g	1
701–850 g	4
< 700 g	7
Gestation (weeks)	
>24	0
≤24	1
Congenital malformations*	
None	0
Not acutely life-threatening	1
Acutely life-threatening	3
Maximum base excess in first 12 hours (mmol/l)	
>−7.0	0
−7.0 to −9.9	1
−10.0 to −14.0	2
>−15.0	3
Minimum appropriate F_iO_2 in first 12 hours	
< 0.39	0
0.41 to 0.60	2
0.61 to 0.90	3
0.91 to 1.0	4
Maximum appropriate F_iO_2 in first 12 hours	
<0.39	0
0.41 to 0.8	1
0.81 to 0.9	3
0.91 to 1.0	5

* excluding inevitably lethal malformations.

^ for example −3.0 mmol/l scores 0; −16 mmol/l scores 3.

REFERENCES

International Neonatal Network (1993) The CRIB (clinical risk index for babies) score: a tool for assessing initial neonatal risk and comparing performance of neonatal intensive care units. *Lancet* **342**: 193–198.

Ortega, M., Ramos, A.D., Pltzaker, A.G. *et al.* (1988) Early prediction of ultimate outcome in newborn infants with severe respiratory failure. *Journal of Pediatrics* **113**: 744–747.

APPENDIX C

BLOOD PRESSURE VALUES

Various reports of normal blood pressures in the first few days of life have been published. We find the data of Bada *et al.* (1990) and the Northern Neonatal Nursing Initiative (1999) the most useful (Fig. C.1, Fig. C.2(a) and C.2 (b)).

The figures produced by Tan (1988) (Table C.1) are also a useful guide for normality up to 2 months of age. Intensive care support

Table C.1 Normal blood pressures in the first 2 months of life (Tan 1988)

	Days				Weeks			
	1	3	5	7	2	3	4	8
Systolic	68	74	74	76	76	76	78	86
Diastolic	44	49	49	48	46	49	49	52
Mean	58	64	62	64	58	60	65	69

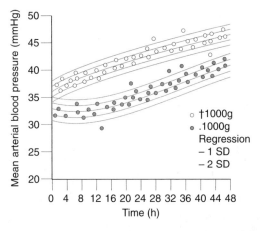

Figure C.1 MAP during the first 48 hours of life (from *Bada et al.* 1990 with permission).

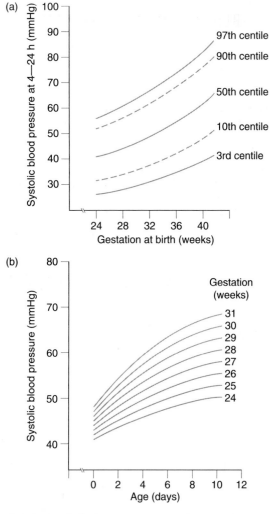

Figure C.2 (a) Systolic blood pressure in the first 24 hours of life related to gestational age at birth, (b) Systolic blood pressure during the first 10 days of life related to gestational age at birth from the Northern Neonatal Nursing Initiative 1999.

should aim to provide a blood pressure which gives adequate oxygenation for the metabolic demands of all the body's organs. Assessing the adequacy of blood pressure can be difficult in ill preterm babies, in whom the usual methods of assessing perfusion may not be accurate. Although there is no proof that the commonly used rule of thumb which states that the mean blood pressure is roughly equivalent to the gestational age in weeks is completely accurate, it has the merit of simplicity and is easily recalled.

REFERENCES

Bada, H.S., Korones, S.B., Perry, E.H. *et al.* (1990) Mean arterial blood pressure changes in premature infants and those at risk for intraventricular haemorrhage. *Journal of Pediatrics* **117**: 607–614.

Northern Neonatal Nursing Initiative (1999) Systolic blood pressure in babies of less than 32 weeks gestation in the first year of life. *Archives of Disease in Childhood* **80**: F38–F42.

Tan, K.L. (1988) Blood pressure in very low birthweight infants in the first 70 days of life. *Journal of Pediatrics* **112**: 266–270.

FURTHER READING

Cunningham, S. (1999) What is an adequate blood pressure in the newborn? In: *Current Topics in Neonatology 3*. Hansen, T.N. and McIntosh, N. (eds), Saunders, London, pp. 62–92.

APPENDIX D

THE NEONATAL ECG

The ECG remains essential to the study of cardiac arrhythmias (p. 368) and it can aid in the assessement of chamber enlargement, hypertrophy and strain.

A systematic approach to the ECG enables the maximum information to be extracted from it, and should include an assessment of rate, rhythm, axis, atrial and ventricular information.

RATE AND RHYTHM

The normal heart rate for babies varies according to age. On the first day the range is 95 to 145 beats/min with a mean of 120 beats/min. By the end of the first month the mean heart rate is 150 beats/min with a range of 115 to 185. Extrasystoles of supraventricular or ventricular origin are not rare, but in the absence of CHD they subside spontaneously over the first week. In sinus rhythm every QRS complex is accompanied by a P wave; the distance between the two is the PR interval. The P waves should be upright in leads 1 and V_6. If they are not, either the atria are not normally sited, or there is a supraventricular rhythm.

THE PR INTERVAL

The PR interval is measured in lead II from the beginning of the P wave to the beginning of the QRS complex. It increases slightly with age and is normally of no more than 0.12 seconds duration in neonates. The PR interval is reduced to less than 0.07 seconds in nodal rhythm and in WPW syndrome. A long PR interval indicates first degree block. This can be familial or due to structural disease e.g. ASD.

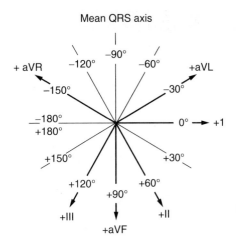

Mean QRS axis

Figure D.1 Hexaxial reference system for calculating frontal plane axis of QRS complex. To obtain the QRS axis:

1. Identify the lead in which R and S waves are mostly nearly of equal size.
2. Look at right angles to the lead identified in step 1.
3. One of the leads identified in step 2 will be predominantly positive, and the other predominantly negative.
4. The predominantly positive lead identified by step 3 is approximately the QRS axis.
5. The approximate QRS axis obtained from step 4 can be made more accurate by estimating the equiphasic lead (step 1) more accurate by "imaging" it between actual leads.

If all leads appear equiphasic the QRS axis is described as "indeterminate"; this is rarely normal.

THE AXIS

THE MEAN FRONTAL QRS AXIS

Use the compass diagram shown in Fig. D.1.

The mean neonatal frontal QRS axis is + 135° with a normal range between + 110° and + 180°. There is a rapid change to the left (i.e. a less positive or more negative axis) in the first month, to a mean axis of + 75°, and then a further and more gradual change to the left until adult life is reached. Left axis deviation (sometimes called a superior axis) is seen in tricuspid atresia, atrioventricular septal defects, and in babies with pulmonary stenosis and Noonan syndrome.

INFORMATION ABOUT THE ATRIA

THE P WAVE

A peaked P wave more than 3 mm tall, best seen in lead II and V_1, indicates right atrial enlargement. This is seen in anomalies with a high right atrial pressure, tricuspid and pulmonary atresia, or a very dilated right atrium, as in Ebstein's anomaly. The normal P wave is not more than 2.5 mm high and lasts for less than 120 ms. A bifid P wave lasting more than 120 ms, or late inversion of the P wave greater than 1 mm in V_1, suggests left atrial enlargement.

INFORMATION ABOUT THE VENTRICLES (see Table D.I)

THE QRS COMPLEX

QRS voltages may be very low in the first week, particularly in preterm babies. At birth the R wave should be dominant in V_1, and in V_6 the S wave is commonly, but not invariably, dominant. However, by one month the R wave should be dominant in V_6 too. The RS complex represents depolarization of the ventricles and rarely exceeds 0.08 seconds in duration. Complexes that exceed 0.08 seconds indicate prolongation of intraventricular conduction, but partial right bundle branch block is the normal pattern in 20% of neonates. The QRS complexes evolve across the chest leads from a dominant R in V_1 to more S in V_6.

Table D.I Criteria for diagnosing ventricular hypertrophy on neonatal ECGs

Right ventricular hypertrophy
1. R in V_1 20 mm or more
2. S in V_6 0–7 days 14 mm or more, 8–30 days 10 mm or more
3. R/S ratio in V_1 0–3 months 6.5:1 or more
4. T upright in V_1 after 4 days
5. Q wave in V_1

Left ventricular hypertrophy
1. S in V_1 more than 20 mm
2. R in V_6 more than 20 mm
3. Q in V_5, V_6 more than 4 mm

THE Q WAVE

The Q wave represents septal depolarization. Absent (40%) or small Q waves may be seen in the left chest leads in the perinatal period, but deflections of more than 4 mm are abnormal and indicate septal hypertrophy (Table D.2). A Q wave in V_1 is abnormal and indicates right ventricular hypertrophy, or may be seen in congenitally corrected transposition. An rsR pattern is normal but may easily be confused with a qR pattern, if the primary r wave is very small.

THE ST SEGMENT

Normally this begins from a point within 2 mm of the isoelectric line (the TP segment). Elevation of the ST segment is seen with myocardial injury, in myocarditis or in acute ischaemia. ST segment depression may occur with electrolyte disturbances, digoxin therapy, ischaemia, "strain" – pressure overload of either ventricle and endocardial fibroelastosis.

THE QT INTERVAL

The QT interval is measured from the beginning of the QRS complex to the end of the T wave. It varies with heart rate and should not exceed 0.28 seconds at a heart rate of 160 beats/min, and 0.31 seconds at a heart rate of 120. The QT interval corrected for heart rate, or QTc, is the QT interval divided by the square root of the RR interval. The RR interval measured is the one immediately preceding the QRS complex whose QT interval has been measured. There is disagreement about the upper limit of the normal QTc interval in neonates, with no published data on the values in preterm babies. Certainly a value of more than 0.5 seconds is prolonged, and some authors suggest an upper limit of normal of 0.45 seconds in the newborn (Schwartz *et al.* 1982). A prolonged QTc is seen with hypocalcaemia, and marked prolongation is seen with the rare QT prolongation syndrome which is associated with potentially lethal ventricular arrhythmias. Cisapride treatment should not be given to preterm babies with a QTc of above 0.5 and the interval must be measured before this treatment is considered at all in this group.

Table D.2 Normal ranges for rate, axis and voltages in the neonatal ECG

ECG standards (neonatal period)

Age in days	Centile	Rate	QRS axis	PR (ms)	PII (mV)	R V$_1$ (mV)	R V$_5$ (mV)	R V$_6$ (mV)	S V$_1$ (mV)	S V$_6$ (mV)	R/S ratio V$_1$
0–1	95%	150	+185	140	0.25	2.35	1.8	1.0	1.8	0.8	7.0
	50%	120	+135	105	0.16	1.3	1.0	0.4	0.8	0.3	2.5
	5%	100	+90	82	0.07	0.7	0.3	0.1	0.1	0.0	0.4
1–3	95%	150	+185	132	0.25	2.4	1.9	1.0	1.8	0.75	6.0
	50%	120	+135	105	0.16	1.5	1.1	0.4	0.8	0.3	2.5
	5%	100	+90	85	0.05	0.7	0.4	0.1	0.1	0.0	0.4
3–7	95%	160	+180	130	0.27	2.1	1.9	1.1	1.5	0.8	7.0
	50%	125	+135	103	0.17	1.25	1.3	0.5	0.7	0.3	2.9
	5%	100	+90	80	0.08	0.5	0.5	0.15	0.1	0.0	0.5
7–30	95%	175	+150	128	0.28	1.7	2.1	1.3	1.0	0.8	6.3
	50%	145	+110	100	0.18	1.0	1.4	0.5	0.4	0.3	3.7
	5%	110	+75	75	0.08	0.4	0.6	0.25	0.1	0.0	1.0

Values relate to term neonates. From: Daignon et al. (1979/80) Normal ECG standards for infants and children. Pediatric Cardiology I: 123–133 and 133–152.

At a paper speed of 25 mm/s 1 mm = 0.04 s = a small square.

5 mm = 0.2 seconds = 1 large square: rate count the number of divisions between 2 RR complexes and divide into 300.

REFERENCE

Schwartz, P.J., Montemerlo, M., Facchini, M *et al.* (1982) The QT interval throughout the first 6 months of life: a prospective study. *Circulation* **66**: 496–501.

TRANSPORTATION OF THE SICK NEONATE

There will always be a need to transport infants, either postnatally or *in utero*. A survey in 1991 revealed about 2000 of each type of transport in the UK. The number of transfers appears to be increasing as the pressure on neonatal intensive care cots mounts. A recent survey of the 37 tertiary centres in the UK showed that these units alone were transferring about 1500 babies a year (1991 data; *in utero* and postnatal figures included). The most frequent reasons for transport are because the referring hospital does not provide long-term ventilation, or that it lacks a staffed intensive care space. Other babies need specialized surgical or cardiology services. Transport teams are usually sent from the accepting unit, ideally the nearest hospital that provides neonatal intensive care. The team consists of a neonatologist and a neonatal nurse equipped with a portable incubator and appropriate equipment for the care of the sick infant during transfer back to their own hospital. In a few regions of the UK, and in the US and Australia, transport teams are provided from a specialized central unit. This system has several advantages; the personnel are additional and the accepting unit is not denuded of staff during the retrieval, the team can build up special expertise and evaluate equipment; a dedicated ambulance and crew can be justified because of the number of trips per day; and formal training and experience can be arranged. In future it seems likely that UK neonatal transport will be centralized in this way but in the short term local *ad hoc* arrangements continue. This chapter aims to provide practical advice on how to go about arranging a retrieval. Transport is always a hazardous business and practice makes perfect.

COMMUNICATION

When accepting a request for retrieval the following information should be collected (structured forms can be helpful):

- the baby's name, the mother's name and the exact location for the retrieval;
- the working diagnosis and reason for request;
- the baby's current condition and level of intensive care support;
- the latest laboratory results.

Basic advice about ventilator settings, blood pressure support, drainage of air leaks etc. can be given before the team departs from the accepting unit. Always be polite; remember how difficult it can be to organize blood gases and chest X-rays in some hospitals.

EQUIPMENT

Most transfers in the UK take place by road, but the equipment is the same whether the journey is made by road, rail, sea ferry or aircraft.

The portable incubator and associated monitoring equipment should aim to replicate the intensive care setting and must be versatile enough to:

1. run off mains electricity or various batteries;
2. sustain an ambient temperature of at least 36°C within the (preferably double-glazed) canopy, despite very cold environmental temperatures;
3. allow access to the infant through portholes without allowing dissipation of heat or ambient oxygen from within;
4. have adequate ports to allow drip tubing, oxygen tubing etc. into the incubator without leaving the portholes open;
5. have at least two IV infusion pumps for maintaining intravenous and arterial lines during the journey;
6. give and sustain any concentration of oxygen from 21% to 100% throughout the journey, and to carry enough oxygen to allow for this with plenty to spare;
7. ventilate the infant, or give CPAP during the journey;
8. monitor ECG and PaO_2 (or SpO_2) continuously during the journey;
9. have a portable blood pressure monitoring device;
10. provide adequate illumination of the infant.

No commercially available portable incubator fulfils all these criteria, with the result that most referral units build their own transport trolley by incorporating a transport incubator on to a standard

Table E.1

Equipment	Drugs (1 or 2 ampoules of each)
Baby notes and consent forms	10% calcium gluconate
Syringes 1 ml, 2 ml, 5 ml, 10 ml, 20 ml	1: 1000 and 1:10000 adrenaline
Blood bottles	Atropine
Cannulae FG 22, 24	Pancuronium
Scalp vein needles FG 21, 23, 25	Frusemide
Needles FG 21, 23, 25	Surfactant
LP needle	Naloxone
3-way taps	Hydrocortisone
Cord clamps	8.4% sodium bicarbonate (5 ampoules)
Cord ligatures × 2	Tolazoline
Splints	7% THAM (5 ampoules)
Thermometer	Konakion
Glucometer and BM stix	Diazepam
Blue litmus	Glucagon
Lancets	Dopamine
Razor	1% Isoprenaline
Black silk sutures	Phenobarbitone
Scalpel and blades	Paraldehyde
Stitch cutters	Water for injection
Safety pins	1000 units/ml heparin
Sterile toothed and non-toothed forceps	Normal (0.9%) saline (5 ampoules)
Artery forceps × 2 (1 sterile)	Dextrose saline (500 ml bag)
Scissors × 2 (1 sterile)	10% Dextrose (500 ml bag)
Arterial dilator	50% Dextrose (1 × 50 ml)
Micropore 0.5 inches	
Plasters	
Bandages	
Sterets and Steristrips	
ET tubes 2.5 mm, 3.0 mm, 3.5 mm	
(oral and nasal)	
KY jelly (one tube)	
ECG electrodes	
BP cuffs — neonatal sizes	
Connector for Ambu bag and ventilator	
Magills forceps	
Laryngoscope (and spare blades, bulbs and batteries)	
Heimlich valves	
FG 10 trocars	
Self inflating bag	
Stethoscope	
Plastic tube connections (various sizes)	
Suction tubes 5, 6, 8 and 10 FG	
UAC FG 3.5 and 4 including continuously recording ones	

Table E.1 (contd)

Equipment	Drugs (1 or 2 ampoules of each)
Tape measure	
Name bands	
Oxygen analyser	
ECG	
BP monitor (oscillometric)	
UAC catheter read out box for PO_2	
Oximeter	

ambulance trolley and attaching the various monitoring devices and infusion pumps.

In addition to the incubator, the transport team should take sufficient drugs, catheters, endotracheal tubes and other equipment to resuscitate the infant at the referring hospital, and to establish all the components of care necessary. The equipment listed in Table E.1 is a suggested list.

The drugs should include an orally active anti-emetic for the medical personnel, since the back of an NHS ambulance is the most efficient motion-sickness provoking environment yet invented! The personnel must be warmly clothed and prepared to remain at the referring hospital for several hours.

On arrival at the referring hospital it is important not to be in too much of a rush to get back to base. There is no place for the "swoop and scoop" retrieval in neonatal medicine. Assess the infant, and be prepared to work on him for some time using the facilities available in the local hospital together with the transport equipment. Insert catheters, start CPAP or IPPV and drain pneumothoraces. Check blood gases, correct metabolic abnormalities, remedy hypotension with plasma expanders or dopamine and control infusions. Consider whether surfactant should be given and, if so, be prepared to stay longer in order to monitor the baby during the time of rapid changes in ventilatory requirements that usually occur. Collect a sample of maternal blood and consent forms for surgery if necessary. Only when the infant's condition is satisfactory should you wrap him warmly, place him in the transport incubator, and start the journey back. If in doubt, ventilate the unventilated baby. The back of an ambulance in cold weather is no place to start trying to intubate.

Check the following as a bare minimum before leaving:

- Are the blood gases reasonable?
- Chest X-ray (is there a pneumothorax? – if so drain it and attach a flutter valve for transfer);
- Is the blood pressure satisfactory?
- Is the temperature within the normal range?
- Is the blood glucose normal and is there a secure intravenous line?
- Is sedation (or paralysis) adequate?
- Is there a patent nasogastric tube in place to empty the stomach?

Never forget to talk to the parents of the baby, let them see (and if possible hold) their baby, and explain what is happening. If feasible arrange for the mother to be transferred to the hospital housing the intensive care unit later. Take a photograph of the baby and give it to the mother before leaving.

Although there is much to be said for getting to the referring hospital as quickly as possible with blue lights flashing and police escorts, on the journey back, small sick infants (and indeed the transport team) do not benefit from being bounced around in the back of an ambulance. A more sedate rate of progress is often in order, using the blue light, siren and police escort only to get through congested traffic.

Keep the ambulance heater full on. Despite swaddling and a warm incubator, infants cool very rapidly if the ambulance is cold. If you are unhappy about the infant during the journey stop the ambulance while you sort him out. Many teams now carry mobile phones in order to call the consultant for advice during transport, and to give an ETA to their own unit.

SPECIAL PROBLEMS

Babies with surgical conditions often need transporting. Wrap gastroschisis or exomphalos in clingfilm to avoid heat loss, and make sure that the fluid balance is reasonable before setting off. Transport babies with suspected TOF head up with a large bore nasogastric tube in the pouch, and aspirate this very frequently to avoid spill-over into the lung. Babies with diagphragmatic hernia, or persistent pulmonary hypertension must be paralysed and sedated before transfer and any necessary adjustments made to the ventilation before leaving. Nitric oxide can be given in transfer but requires special equipment to monitor delivery and waste gases.

APPENDIX F

NORMAL BIOCHEMICAL VALUES IN THE NEWBORN

The values here have been derived from many sources in the literature and appendices to major textbooks of neonatology. For simplicity in many cases we have rounded up or down some numbers.

Alanine aminotransferase	9–44 IU/l
Albumin	24–44 g/l
Alkaline phosphatase	125–373 iu/l Up to 500 u/l in preterm babies
Alpha-1-antitrypsin	1.0–2.2 g/l (values <1.0 suggest deficiency)
Alpha fetoprotein	<55 000 U/ml at term. Levels decline rapidly after birth, and are higher still in preterm babies.*
Ammonia	10–160 micromol/l
Aspartate aminotransferase	20–100 IU/l
Bicarbonate	18–22 mmol/l
Bilirubin	Up to 200 micromol/l in the first 10 days, see p. 418 Conjugated bilirubin <20 micromol/l
Cholesterol	0.6–3.2 mmol/l (prem) 1.9–4.3 mmol/l (term)
Copper	1.4–11.0 micromol/l (9–70 µg/dl)
Cortisol	330–1700 nmol/l (at birth), 1st week 200–770 nmol/l
Creatinine kinase	<500 IU/l (may be higher at <100 hours of age)
Ferritin	150–900 microg/l (prem)
Folic acid	5–21 ng/ml

(erythrocytes)	>160 ng/ml
Gamma-glutamyl transpeptidase	<250 IU/l in the first two weeks, <150 IU/l 2–4 weeks
Growth hormone (1st week)	15–404 ng/ml
17-hydroxyprogesterone	<30 nmol/l (2–7 days), <14 nmol/l (>6 days)
IgA	<0.1 g/l
IgG	5–17 g/l
IgM	<0.2 g/l
Immunoreactive trypsin	up to 120 microg/l
Insulin	Usually <20 mu/l; should suppress with hyperglycaemia
Iron	10–33 micromol/l (higher at birth)
Lactate	0.8–1.2 mmol/l after 24 hours
LDH	325–1825 U/l
Osmolality	275–300 mosmol/kgH$_2$0
Proteins – Total	55–75 g/l (5.0–7.5 g%)
– Albumin	25–45 g/l (2.5–4.5 g%)
Pyruvate	up to 120 micromol/l
Testosterone	<10 nmol/l (male) <2 nmol/l (female)
TSH	<10 mU/l after 3 days
T4	75–300 nmol/l (<200 in prems, >100 at term)
T3	0.8–4.0 nmol/l
Triglycerides	0.06–1.60 mmol/l (5–140 mg%)
Uric acid	0.15–0.5 mmol/l
Vitamin A	15–50 microg/dl
Vitamin D (25-OHD$_2$)	7–19 microgm/dl
Vitamin E	1.0–3.5 microg/dl
Zinc	8–20 micromol/l

*Reference: Blair, J.I., Carachi, R., Gupta, R. *et al.* (1987) Plasma, alphafetoprotein references ranges in infancy: the effect of prematurity. *Archives of Disease in Childhood* **62**: 362–365.

Table F.1 Normal blood electrolyte and urea values

	Na (mmol/l)	K (mmol/l)	Cl (mmol/l)	Ca (mmol/l)	PO$_4$ (mmol/l)	Mg (mmol/l)	Urea (mmol/l)	Creatinine micromol/l
Premature newborn	130–145	4.5–7.2	95–117	1.75–2.80	1.00–2.60	0.62–1.25	0.5–6.7	55–150
Full term	130–145	3.6–5.7	92–109	2.10–2.70	1.8–3.0	0.7–1.0	1.6–10.0	35–115
One week	–	4.0–6.0	92–109	2.20–2.70	1.4–3.0	0.85–1.05	1.6–5.0	14–86
One month	–	4.0–6.0	92–109	2.15–2.65	1.7–3.0	0.65–1.0	1.9–5.2	12–48
Child	136–145	3.3–4.6	95–108	2.2–2.5	–	0.7–0.95	3.3–6.6	–

NORMAL URINE BIOCHEMISTRY

Ca	0.2–1.6 mmol/l	0.05–0.21 mmol/kg/24 h
Phosphate	<10 mmol/l	5–25 micromol/kg/24 h
Na	1–15 mmol/l	0.8–2.2 mmol/kg/24 h*
K	2–28 mmol/l	0.2–5.0 mmol/kg/24 h
Cl	5–30 mmol/l	1.3–3.3 mmol/kg/24 h
Creatinine clearance	0.5 ml/kg/min in preterms <1 week 1.5 ml/kg/min in term babies	
Urea	1–9 mmol/l	1.3–5.9 mmol/kg/24 h
7 Ketosteroids	< 2.5 mg/24 h	
Pregnanetriol	< 0.2 mg/24 h	

* Much higher in preterm infants (see Chapter 3)

APPENDIX G

HAEMATOLOGICAL VALUES IN THE NEWBORN

The normal haemoglobin at birth is about 14 g% in babies at 28 weeks gestation, and about 17.0 g% at term (Table G.1). The haematocrit is about 55% at term; the capillary haematocrit is always about 15% higher than arterial or venous haematocrit. Up to 0.5×10^9/l nucleated red cells (500/mm³) may be present in the blood of the normal term neonate, and up to 1.5×10^9/l (1500/mm³) in the premature baby. Very high levels of nucleated red cells, up to 10 000/mm³, have been recorded after fetal stress and haemorrhage. These usually disappear within 48 hours of delivery.

Following the rise in $Pa\mathrm{O}_2$ after delivery, the level of erythropoietin falls, and it is undetectable in the plasma for 1–2 months. This is associated with a dramatic decrease in red cell production, which is very high in fetal life. In both full-term and premature babies the haemoglobin falls as a consequence, and in premature babies it reaches a nadir of 7–8 g by the end of the second month. After the

Table G.1 Haematological values during the first weeks of life in term babies (95% intervals in brackets) (adapted from Brugnara and Platt 1998)

Value	Cord blood	Day 1	Day 3	Day 7	Day 14
Haemoglobin (g/dl)	16.8	18.4	17.8	17.0	16.8
	(13.7–20.1)	(14–22)	(13.8–21.8)	(14–20)	(13.8–19.8)
Venous Hct (%)	53	58	55	54	52
Red cells × 10¹²/l	5.25	5.8	5.6	5.2	5.1
MCV (fl)	107	108	99	98	96
MCH (pg)	34	35	33	32.5	31.5
MCHC (%)	31.7	32.5	33	33	33
Reticulocytes (%)	3–7	3–7	1–3	0–1	0–1
Nucleated RBC (per mm³)	500	200	0–5	0	0

Table G.2 Neutrophil and lymphocyte count x 10^9/l (mean and range) in full-term and premature babies (derived from various sources in the literature)

Age	Neutrophil		Lymphocyte	
	Full-term	**Premature**	**Full-term**	**Premature**
0	11 (5–26)	5 (2–9)	5.5 (2–11)	4 (2.5–6)
24 hours	11 (5–21)	7.5 (3–9)	5 (2–9)	3.5 (1.5–3)
72 hours	5.5 (2–7)	4.5 (3–7)	3.5 (2–5)	3 (1.5–4)
1 week	5 (2–8)	3.5 (2–7)	5 (3–6)	4.3 (2.5–7.5)
1 month	3.8 (1–9)	2.5 (1–9)	6 (3–15)	6.5 (2–15)

Table G.3 White cell counts in full-term and premature babies*

Cell type	Cell count
Metamyelocytes	
≤ 3 days (term and preterm)	Up to 2.0×10^9/l (2000/mm³)
> 3 days (term and preterm)	Rarely >0.5×10^9/l (500/mm³)
Myelocytes	
≤ 3 days (term)	Up to 0.75×10^9/l (750/mm³)
≤ 3 days (preterm)	Up to 1.0×10^9/l (1000/mm³)
> 3 days (term and preterm)	Occasional only
Eosinophils	
Term babies	0.7×10^9/l (700/mm³)
Preterm babies	0.6×10^9/l (600/mm³) by 1st week, increasing to 1.0×10^9/l (1000/mm³) by 1 month
Basophils	
All neonates	rare
Monocytes	
All neonates	1.0×10^9/l (1000/mm³)

*from Xanthou (1970)

first few days when the reticulocyte count is $150–200 \times 10^9$/l (about 4–5%), it stays below 50×10^9/l (about 1–2%) for most of the first 1–2 months in all babies (Table G.1).

The white blood count varies considerably during the first month of life in term and premature babies. The normal values for neutrophils and lymphocytes are given in Table G.2, and for other white cells in Table G.3.

The platelet count in the neonate averages $150–450 \times 10^9$/l (250 000–300 000/mm³), but it may be up to 600×10^9/l

$(600\ 000/\text{mm}^3)$ by 2–4 months. Platelet function is virtually normal in the neonatal period; although abnormalities of function can be demonstrated in a test tube the bleeding time is normal.

Table G.4 Reference values for coagulation tests in healthy term infants and in the adult (Andrew *et al.* 1987)
Means and 1 standard deviation

Test	Day 1	Day 5	Day 30	Adult
PT (s)	13 ± 1.43	12.4 ± 1.46	11.8 ± 1.25	12.4 ± 0.78
APPT (s)	42.9 ± 5.8	42.6 ± 8.62	40.4 ± 7.42	33.5 ± 3.44
TCT (s)	23.5 ± 2.38	23.1 ± 3.07	24.3 ± 2.44	25 ± 2.66
Fibrinogen (g/l)	2.83 ± 0.58	3.12 ± 0.75	2.7 ± 0.54	2.78 ± 0.61
II (U/ml)	0.48 ± 0.11	0.63 ± 0.15	0.68 ± 0.17	1.08 ± 0.19
V (U/ml)	0.72 ± 0.18	0.95 ± 0.25	0.98 ± 0.18	1.06 ± 0.22
VII (U/ml)	0.66 ± 0.19	0.89 ± 0.27	0.9 ± 0.24	1.05 ± 0.19
VIII (U/ml)	1.00 ± 0.39	0.88 ± 0.33	0.91 ± 0.33	0.99 ± 0.25
vWF (U/ml)	1.53 ± 0.67	1.40 ± 0.57	1.28 ± 0.59	0.92 ± 0.33
IX (U/ml)	0.53 ± 0.19	0.53 ± 0.19	0.51 ± 0.15	1.09 ± 0.27
X (U/ml)	0.40 ± 0.14	0.49 ± 0.15	0.59 ± 0.14	1.06 ± 0.23
XI (U/ml)	0.38 ± 0.14	0.55 ± 0.16	0.53 ± 0.13	0.97 ± 0.15
XII (U/ml)	0.53 ± 0.20	0.47 ± 0.18	0.49 ± 0.16	1.08 ± 0.28
Plasminogen (U/ml)	1.95 ± 0.35	2.17 ± 0.38	1.98 ± 0.36	3.36 ± 0.44

All factors except fibrinogen and plasminogen are expressed as units/ml where pooled plasma contains 1.0 U/ml. Plasminogen units are those recommended by the Committee on Thrombolytic Agents.

Table G.5 Reference values for coagulation tests in preterm infants (Andrew *et al.* 1988)

Means and confidence intervals given

Test	Day 1	Day 5	Day 30	Adult
PT (s)	13 (10.6–16.2)	12.5 (10.0–15.3)	11.8 (10.0–13.6)	12.4 (10.8–13.9)
APTT (s)	53.6 (27.5–79.4)	50.5 (26.9–74.1)	44.7 (26.9–62.5)	33.5 (26.6–40.3)
TCT (s)	24.8 (19.2–30.4)	24.1 (18.8–29.4)	24.4 (18.8–29.9)	25 (19.7–30.3)
Fibrinogen (g/l)	2.43 (1.5–3.73)	2.8 (1.6–4.2)	2.54 (1.5–4.14)	2.78 (1.56–4.0)
II (U/ml)	0.45 (0.41–1.44)	0.57 (0.29–0.85)	0.57 (0.36–0.95)	1.08 (0.7–1.46)
V (U/ml)	0.88 (0.41–1.44)	1.0 (0.46–1.54)	1.02 (0.48–1.56)	1.06 (0.62–1.50)
VII (U/ml)	0.67 (0.21–1.13)	0.84 (0.3–1.38)	0.83 (0.21–1.45)	1.05 (0.67–1.43)
VIII (U/ml)	1.11 (0.50–2.13)	1.15 (0.53–2.05)	1.11 (0.5–1.99)	0.99 (0.5–1.49)
vWF (U/ml)	1.36 (0.78–2.1)	1.33 (0.72–2.19)	1.36 (0.66–2.16)	0.92 (0.5–1.58)
IX (U/ml)	0.35 (0.19–0.65)	0.42 (0.14–0.74)	0.44 (0.13–0.8)	1.09 (0.55–1.63)
X (U/ml)	0.41 (0.11–0.71)	0.51 (0.19–0.83)	0.56 (0.20–0.92)	1.06 (0.7–1.52)
XI (U/ml)	0.30 (0.08–0.52)	0.41 (0.13–0.69)	0.43 (0.15–0.71)	0.97 (0.67–1.27)
XII (U/ml)	0.38 (0.10–0.66)	0.39 (0.09–0.69)	0.43 (0.11–0.75)	1.08 (0.52–1.64)
Plasminogen (U/ml)	1.70 (1.12–2.48)	1.91 (1.21–2.61)	1.81 (1.09–2.53)	3.36 (2.48–4.24)

Table G.6 Reference values for the inhibitors of coagulation in healthy full-term infants (Andrew *et al.* 1987)

Means ± standard deviation

Coag inhibitor	Day 1	Day 5	Day 30	Adult
AT III (U/ml)	0.63 ± 0.12	0.67 ± 0.13	0.78 ± 0.15	1.05 ± 0.13
α_2 M (U/ml)	1.39 ± 0.22	1.48 ± 0.25	1.50 ± 0.22	0.86 ± 0.17
α_2 AP (U/ml)	0.85 ± 0.15	1.0 ± 0.15	1.0 ± 0.12	1.02 ± 0.17
C_1-INH (U/ml)	0.72 ± 0.18	0.9 ± 0.15	0.89 ± 0.21	1.01 ± 0.15
αAT (U/ml)	0.83 ± 0.22	0.89 ± 0.20	0.62 ± 0.13	0.93 ± 0.19
Protein C (U/ml)	0.35 ± 0.09	0.42 ± 0.11	0.43 ± 0.11	0.96 ± 0.16
Protein S (U/ml)	0.36 ± 0.12	0.50 ± 0.14	0.63 ± 0.15	0.92 ± 0.16

Table G.7 Reference values for the inhibitors of coagulation in preterm infants (Andrew *et al.* 1988, Andrew *et al.* 1990)
Means and 95% confidence intervals given

Coag inhibitor	Day 1	Day 5	Day 30	Adult
AT III (U/ml)	0.38 (0.14–0.62)	0.56 (0.30–0.82)	0.59 (0.37–0.81)	1.05 (0.79–1.31)
α_2M (U/ml)	1.10 (0.56–1.82)	1.25 (0.71–0.77)	1.38 (0.72–2.04)	0.86 (0.52–1.2)
α_2AP (U/ml)	0.78 (0.40–1.16)	0.81 (0.49–1.13)	0.89 (0.55–1.23)	1.02 (0.68–1.36)
C_1-INH (U/ml)	0.65 (0.31–0.99)	0.83 (0.45–1.21)	0.74 (0.40–1.24)	1.01 (0.71–1.31)
αAT (U/ml)	0.90 (0.36–1.44)	0.94 (0.42–1.46)	0.76 (0.38–1.12)	0.93 (0.55–1.31)
Protein C (U/ml)	0.28 (0.12–0.44)	0.31 (0.11–0.51)	0.37 (0.15–0.59)	0.96 (0.64–1.28)
Protein S (U/ml)	0.26 (0.14–0.38)	0.37 (0.13–0.61)	0.56 (0.22–0.90)	0.92 (0.60–1.24)

α_2AP	α_2 antiplasmin
α_2AT	α_2 antitrypsin
α_2M	α_2 macroglobulin
AT III	antithrombin III
C_1INH	C_1 esterase inhibitor.

REFERENCES

Andrew, M., Paes, B., Milner, R., Johnston, M., Mitchell, L., Tollefsen, D.M. and Powers, P. (1987) Development of the human coagulation system in the full term infant. *Blood* **7**: 165–172.

Andrew, M., Paes, B., Milner, R., Johnston, M., Mitchell, L., Tollefsen, D.M., Castle, V. and Powers, P. (1988) Development of the human coagulation system in the healthy premature infant. *Blood* **72**: 1651–1657.

Andrew, M., Paes, B. and Johnson, M. (1990) Development of the hemostatic system in the neonate and young infant. *The American Journal of Pediatric Hematology/Oncology* **12**: 95–104.

Brugnara, C. and Platt, O.S. (1998) The neonatal erythrocyte and its disorders. In: *Nathan and Oski's Haematology of Infancy and Childhood*, 5th edn. Nathan, D.G. and Orkin, S.H. (eds), W.B. Saunders, Philadelphia, pp. 19–52.

Xanthou, M. (1970) Leucocyte blood picture in healthy full term and premature babies during the neonatal period. *Archives of Disease in Childhood* **45**: 242–249.

APPENDIX H

PHARMACOPOEIA

UNITS
1 kilogram (kg) = 1000 grams
1 gram (g) = 1000 milligrams
1 milligram (mg) = 1000 micrograms
1 microgram (μg) = 1000 nanograms
1 nanogram (ng) = 1000 picograms

A 1% (1:100) weight for volume (w/v) solution contains 1 g of substance in 100 ml of solution
A 1% (1:100) weight for volume (w/v) solution contains 10 milligrams in 1 ml
A 1:1000 solution contains 1 milligram in 1 ml
A 1:10 000 solution contains 100 micrograms in 1 ml

We have avoided using μ throughout this book (including this Pharmacopeia) because it can be confusing when written by hand. We strongly recommend writing prescriptions using "micrograms" in full.

Drug	Route	Dose	Chronological age	Frequency (times/24 hours)
Acyclovir	IV	10 mg/kg per dose (give over one hour)	0–1 week 1 week or more	2 3
Adenosine	IV by *rapid bolus*	100 microg/kg per dose *(Max 300 microg/kg per dose)*		repeatable
Adrenaline	IV IV infusion	10–100 microg/kg per dose 0.1–0.3 microg/kg/min *(Max 1.5 microg/kg/min)* 10 microg is contained in 0.1 ml of 1:10 000 solution 100 microg is contained in 0.1 ml of 1:1000 solution or 1 ml of 1:10 000 solution		repeatable

Drug	Route	Dose	Chronological age	Frequency (times/24 hours)
Amoxycillin	oral	50 mg/kg per dose	0—1 week	2
	IV, IM	(100 mg/kg in	1—3 weeks	3
		meningitis)	4 weeks or more	4
Amphotericin	IV	0.5 mg/kg per dose (give over 4—6 hours) *max 1 mg/kg/day*		1
Ampicillin	IV, IM, oral	as amoxycillin	as amoxycillin	as amoxycillin
Atracurium	IV bolus	500 microg/kg		single dose
Atropine	IV subcut, IM	15 microg/kg		single dose
Aztreonam	IV	30 mg/kg per dose	0—1 weeks	2
			1—3 weeks	3
			4 weeks or more	4
Caffeine citrate	IV, oral	Loading dose 20 mg/kg		once
		Maintenance 5 mg/kg per dose		1
Calcium gluconate	IV	0.3—2 ml of 10% sol/kg in arrhythmias or hypotensive emergencies		once
	oral	1.5 ml of 10% soln/kg per dose		4 hourly in feeds
Captopril	oral	10—50 microg/kg/dose *(max 100 microg/kg/dose)*		3
Carbenicillin	IV	100 mg/kg per dose	0—1 week	2
			1—3 weeks	3
			>4 weeks	4
Carbimazole	oral	250 microg/kg		3
Cefotaxime	IV, IM	50 mg/kg per dose	0—1 week	2
			1—3 weeks	3
			4 weeks or more	4
Ceftazidime	IV	25 mg/kg per dose (50 mg/kg in meningitis)	up to 4 weeks	2
			4 weeks and over	3
Cefuroxime		as ceftazidime		
Chloral hydrate	oral	45 mg/kg single dose		once
		30 mg/kg per dose		max 4 in 24 hours
Chlorothiazide	oral	10 or 20 mg/kg per dose		2
Chlorpromazine	oral	1 mg/kg per dose *(Max. 6 mg/kg per day)*		3
Cimetidine	oral	5 mg/kg per dose if active problem, half this if used prophylactically		4

Ciprofloxacin	IV	5 mg/kg per dose (lactate)	2
	oral	7.5 mg/kg per dose (hydrochloride)	2
Clonazepam	IV (oral)	25–100 microg/kg per dose	0–1 week	1
Desmopressin (ADH)	intranasal	5 microg/dose	1–2
Dexamethasone	IV, oral	0.1 mg/kg per dose for 7 days for CLD (p. 209)	1
	IV	0.2 mg/kg per dose starting 4 hours before extubation	3 doses at 8 hourly intervals
Diamorphine	IV	Loading dose 180 microg/kg	once
	IV infusion	Maintenance 15 microg/kg/h	
Diazepam	IV	Start with 0.2 mg/kg	single dose
Diazoxide	oral	1.7 mg/kg	3
	IV	1–3 mg/kg for hypertension	
Digoxin	loading dose oral (very rarely IV)	10 microg/kg (over 15 min) then 5 microg/kg after 6 hours then 5 microg/kg after a further 6 hours	loading regimen only
	oral	2–4 microg/kg per dose	2
Dobutamine	IV infusion	5–15 microg/kg/min	
Dopamine	IV infusion	Low dose 2–5 microg/kg/min High dose 6–10 microg/kg/min	
Doxapram	IV	Loading dose 2.5 mg/kg	once only
	IV infusion	Maintenance 0.3 mg/kg/h (Max. 1.5 mg/kg/h)	
	oral	6 mg/kg per dose (best after IV loading dose)	4
Edrophonium	IV	40–150 microg/kg give the first 20% very slowly and have atropine available to control hypersalivation	once only
Epoprostenol (PGI₂ prostacyclin)	IV infusion	10 nanog/kg/min	
Erythromycin	IV, oral	15 mg/kg per dose (give over one hour if IV) 2 mg/kg for gut dysmotility	3 3
Erythropoietin	subcut. injection	250 units/kg per dose	three times *per week*
Fentanyl	IV	10 microg/kg	repeatable

Drug	Route	Dose	Chronological age	Frequency (times/24 hours)
Flucloxacillin	IV, oral, IM	50 mg/kg per dose (for meningitis or osteitis use 100 mg/kg per dose)	0—1 week 1—3 weeks 4 weeks or more	2 3 4
Fluconazole	IV, oral	6 mg/kg per dose	0—2 weeks 2—4 weeks 4 weeks or more	once every 3 days once every 2 days 1
Flucytosine	IV, oral	50 mg/kg per dose		2
Frusemide	IV, IM, oral	1—2 mg/kg per dose		1 or 2
Fucidin (sodium fusidate, fusidic acid)	IV	10 mg/kg per dose sodium fusidate *over 6 hours*		2
	oral	15 mg/kg fusidic acid		3
Ganciclovir	IV	5 mg/kg/dose		2
Gentamicin	IV, IM	5 mg/kg		1
Glucagon	IM, IV	200 microg/kg		once only
	IV infusion	0.3 microg/kg/min		
Heparin	IV loading	50—75 units/kg	use lower loading dose under 36 weeks	once only
	IV infusion	25 units/kg/h and monitor APTT		
Hydralazine	IV	300—500 microg/kg/dose maximum 3 mg/kg/24 h		once (repeatable)
Hydrocortisone	IV	25 mg (with IV dextrose) in Addisonian crisis		once
	oral	2.5 mg		3
Immunoglobin	IV	400 mg/kg over several hours		once (repeatable)
Indomethacin	IV, (oral)	loading dose 0.2 mg/kg then 0.1 mg/kg for 5 days		once 1
Insulin	IV	0.5—1.0 units/kg/h with TPN		
	IV	0.3—0.6 units/kg/h with glucose for hyperkalaemia		
Isoniazid	oral	5 mg/kg 10 mg/kg	0—2 weeks more than 2 weeks	1 1
Isoprenaline	IV infusion	0.02 microg/kg/min *(Max 0.3 microg/kg/min)*		
Labetalol	IV infusion	Start with 0.5 mg/kg/h Double the dose every 3 hours until a satisfactory BP level is reached. *(Max 4 mg/kg/h)*		
Lignocaine	IV IV infusion	Loading dose 2 mg/kg Maintenance 2 mg/kg/h *(Max 6 mg/kg/hour)*		once

Magnesium sulphate	IM (deep) IV IV infusion	100 mg/kg per dose Loading dose 250 mg/kg Maintenance 25–75 mg/kg/h		2 once
Mannitol	IV	1 g/kg over 10–20 minutes		repeat once after 6 hours if needed
Meropenem	IV	20 mg/kg/dose double in meningitis		2
Metronidazole	IV, oral	Loading dose 15 mg/kg Maintenance 7.5 mg/kg per dose	0–3 weeks 4 weeks or more	once 2 probably 3
Miconazole	oral topical IV	apply 2.5% gel apply 2% cream 6 mg/kg per dose (give over one hour)		2 after feeds 2 3
Midazolam	IV infusion	10–60 microg/kg/h		
Morphine	IV boluses IV IV infusion	100 microg/kg per dose (can be doubled if ventilated) Loading dose 120 microg/kg Maintenance 10 microg/kg/h		2 or 3 once
Naloxone	IM IV	100 microg/kg 40 microg/kg		repeatable
Neostigmine	IV IM IV	for diagnosis 50 microg/kg for treatment 0.15–0.3 mg/kg per dose 80 microg/kg for reversal of pancuronium (after 20 microg/kg of atropine)		once 3–6 once
Netilmicin	IV, IM	6 mg/kg		1
Noradrenaline	via central vein	0.1 microg/kg/min of noradrenaline *base* *(Max 1.5 microg/kg base/min)*		
Nystatin	oral, topical	100 000 units (1 ml) per dose		4 (after feeds)
Pancuronium	IV, (IM)	initial dose 100 microg/kg repeat doses 50 microg/kg		once as needed, usually 4–6
Paracetamol	oral (rectal)	10–15 (max 60 mg/kg in 24 h)		3
Paraldehyde	deep IM rectal	0.2 ml/kg 0.3 ml/kg of paraldehyde mixed with olive oil 1:1		repeatable once once
Penicillin G (Benzylpenicillin)	IV, IM	30 mg/kg per dose (60 mg/kg in meningitis)	0–1 week 1–3 weeks 4 weeks or more	2 3 4
Pethidine	IV, IM	1mg/kg		max 2
Phenobarbitone	IV, IM IV, oral	Loading dose 20 mg/kg Maintenance 4 mg/kg (increase to 5 mg/kg after 2 weeks)		once 1

Phenytoin	IV *only*	Loading dose 20 mg/kg (give over 20 minutes with ECG)		once
	oral	Maintenance usually 2.5 mg/kg per dose		2
Propranolol	oral	0.25–0.75 mg/kg per dose		3
Propranolol	IV	25–50 microg/kg once		
Prostaglandin E$_2$ (Dinoprostone)	IV infusion	0.6 microg/kg per hour (= 10 nanog/kg/min)		
Prostaglandin I$_2$	See Epoprostenol			
Pyridoxine	IV	50–100 mg bolus (with EEG monitoring)		once
	oral	start with 10 mg/kg		1
Ranitidine	IV	0.5 mg/kg per dose slowly to avoid arryhthmias		4
Rifampicin	IV	6 mg/kg per dose over 60 minutes		2
	oral	12 mg/kg		1
Salbutamol	nebulised	2.5 mg nebulised		repeatable
	IV	4 microg/kg over 20 minutes		once
Spironolactone	oral	1 or 2 mg/kg per dose		2
Streptokinase	IV infusion	3000 units/kg loading dose then 500–1000 units/kg/h maintenance		once only
Suxamethonium	IV	2–3 mg/kg		single dose
Teicoplanin	IV	16 mg/kg/load		once
		then 8 mg/kg/dose		1
Theophylline	IV	Loading dose 6 mg/kg aminophylline		once
		Maintenance 2.5 mg/kg per dose		2
	oral	Loading dose 9 mg/kg choline theophyllinate		once
		Maintenance 4 mg/kg per dose		2
Thyroxine	oral	10 microg/kg		1
Tobramycin	IV, IM	4 mg/kg		1
		5 mg/kg		1
Tolazoline	IV	1 mg/kg bolus		once only
	IV infusion	0.2 mg/kg/h		
Trimethroprim	oral (IV)	3–4 mg/kg per dose		2
		2 mg/kg for prophylaxis		1
Vancomycin	IV	15 mg/kg per dose (give over one hour)	*less than 28 weeks*	1
			28–35 weeks	2
			36 weeks or more	3

REFERENCE

Northern Neonatal Network (1998) *Neonatal Formulary*. BMJ Books, London.

INDEX

Note: Page references in *italics* refer to Tables; those in **bold** refer to Figures

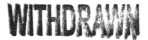